Health Policy

Reform

Driving the wrong way?

Health Policy

Reform

Driving the wrong way?

A Critical Guide to the Global 'Health Reform' Industry

JOHN LISTER

Middlesex
University
PRESS

First published in 2005 by Middlesex University Press

ISBN 1 904750 45 1

A CIP catalogue record for this book is available from The British Library

Book design by Helen Taylor

Printed in the UK by Hobbs the Printers, Hampshire.

Middlesex University Press, Queensway, Enfield, Middlesex EN4 3SF

Tel: +44 (0)20 8411 5734: +44 (0)20 8880 4262 Fax: +44 (0)20 8411 5736
www.mupress.co.uk

John Lister can be contacted at www.healthemergency.org.uk
email: info@healthemergency.org.uk

Acknowledgements

This book could not have been completed without the help, inspiration and encouragement of a number of individuals who have played a vital supporting role.

I would like to thank my PhD supervisory team, Dr Edwin Griggs, Dr Alistair Hewison, and Professor Colin Francome, whose constructive criticism helped me structure and focus my studies. For taking on the publication project and guiding the revamping of the thesis into a book, I have to thank the team at Middlesex University Press: Paul Jervis, Celia Cozens, Matt Skipper and others behind the scenes. As ever, I thank them for helping with what has gone right, while absolving them from responsibility for any errors that may have slipped through the net, and which are down to me.

I have also been lucky enough to get support and encouragement from family and friends, including Nobs and his benevolent Foundation, Doreen, and my Mum and Dad. I learnt a great deal from visiting friends working in health care in Kenya (Andrew and Shelley) and in Canada (Ian and Joanna), from work with affiliates and supporters of London Health Emergency, which has effectively sponsored this work, and from colleagues at Coventry University.

I must reserve special thanks to those other friends and family members who have with so little complaint allowed me to devote a seemingly endless number of weekends, bank holidays, weeknights and odd moments to solitary writing, rather than spending time with them. In particular I want to thank Kevin, Elaine, and grand-daughter Kaitlin.

Perhaps above all I owe a tremendous debt of gratitude to my wife Sue, not least for her practical assistance on the references and other issues, especially in the final stages. Thank you, Sue – I couldn't have done it without you. Thanks for just being there: now at last there should be some spare time for me to be there too!

Contents

Chapter 7 – Country summaries: Africa and Asia

Introduction

The research for this book was prompted by the decision of Tony Blair's New Labour government to abandon its pre-1997 promise to scrap the controversial 'internal market' reforms imposed on the National Health Service in the early 1990s by Margaret Thatcher's government.

Already by 1997 the costly and bureaucratic split of a previously integrated and relatively low-cost system into counterpoised 'purchasers and providers' had brought a sorry combination of lengthened waiting lists, 'self-governing'Trusts saddled with rising deficits, and mounting unspent surpluses in the practice accounts of 'fundholding' GPs.

As a long-time researcher and campaigner against cutbacks, closures and all forms of privatisation in the NHS, I had for 13 years been among the many trade unionists, pensioners and others actively pressing for an alternative approach.

The Tory governments had consistently refused to conduct any evaluation which might demonstrate whether or not their market-style reforms achieved their stated objectives of improving the cost-efficiency and quality of NHS services. Until 1997, the Labour Party, as the founder of the NHS, had always been seen as offering an alternative, and the need to 'save the NHS' had remained a key component of Blair's successful campaign.

What new model of health system was Blair's government now aiming to establish in place of the centralised, publicly-owned and funded 'Beveridge' system established in 1948? Was there any prospect of a 'Third Way', or was the New Labour rhetoric of 'modernisation' and 'partnership' merely a mask, partly concealing a further round of market-style measures?

Related questions immediately arose. How closely were the British reforms linked politically and ideologically to apparently similar reforms and suggested reforms in New Zealand, the Netherlands, Sweden and elsewhere? Had the long-standing separation of purchasers and providers in insurance-based systems such as France and Germany brought additional efficiency, or simply increased costs?

And what of the developing and least developed countries, where a host of problems and the rampant HIV/AIDS epidemic confront relatively undeveloped health care systems: to what extent did the existing models of health care systems in wealthier countries offer any guide to positive and achievable change?

My early investigations revealed a continuing international debate over 'health sector reforms'. The debate involved academics and consultancies in many countries, but was largely ignored by the mainstream press and mass media. It also became clear that – encouraged by the World Bank and USAID – a set of pro-market assumptions and a similar concept of 'reform' had already been extended to the much less developed health care systems in the developing countries – including the poorest countries of sub-Saharan Africa.

This combination of factors makes it appear that there has been a drive to export a general, global blueprint for a 'one size fits all', market-style reform of health care systems. I wanted to investigate the extent to which this could be shown to have happened, but also to answer the more important question: were the resulting policies either appropriate or viable? And was there any evidence that they could, in fact, deliver the improvements they promised?

That investigation is the essence of this book. Unlike most other volumes offering 'comparative' studies, which are generally written by a variety of specialists in particular countries, this is an attempt at an integrated, global overview. It seeks to identify and to analyse consistently the main 'menu' of health system reforms, and the driving forces behind them.

After a prolonged exposure to the literature of health care reform in the UK and around the world, in which the language and jargon used appears both to create and exploit ambiguities, I was also keen to offer some more general guidance for readers seeking to grasp the essence of this type of material in varying contexts. This has resulted in the inclusion in this study of a 'toolkit' which can highlight ambiguities in language and jargon, and assist in the assessment of the motivation, and likely trajectory and impact, of policies and proposals for health care reform.

The concluding chapters test out the early analysis by looking more closely at a large number of countries across five continents. They explore the extent to which the stock reform menu has been taken up and the impact such reforms have had on health services.

My objective throughout is to widen out the discussion, and develop a consistent critique of market-style reforms which – despite the inflated costs of implementation – have yet to be shown to deliver the promised benefits. I believe a first step to the adoption of a more progressive and socially responsible policy has to be the critique of the prevailing 'wisdom' of market mechanisms and individual 'patient choice' as the basis for health care systems. Such approaches discard any pretence of social solidarity as they siphon an ever-growing share of the resources for social insurance into the pockets of private providers and suppliers.

Implicit throughout this critique is my conviction that there is an alternative that offers more evidence and prospect of success, one that is more popular than the cold theories of neo-liberalism and the empty rhetoric of 'public-private partnership'.

This begins with the necessity of rejecting bureaucratic and wasteful market-based policies. Instead it embraces inclusive systems based on the collective sharing of risk, on the socialist principle 'from each according to his/her ability: to each according to their needs'.

Part I

Chapter one

The desperate need for reform: inequalities and pressures on health care systems

Introduction

The aim of this chapter is to explore the pressures on health care systems that are tending to increase costs, and which in some cases require reforms. This sets the context in which later chapters will look in more detail at specific changes or 'reforms', and ask how appropriate the reforms appear to be as a response to the issues that have been identified.

Inequality: the context of reforms

Fundamental changes are required in health care systems around the world if they are to be enabled and equipped to meet the challenges of the 21st century. The most obvious need for reform is to redress large and growing inequalities in health and in access to health services around the world, which mirror growing inequalities in wealth and power.

Health care spending is almost completely inversely proportional to the global burden of disease. The World Health Organisation's *World Health Report 2000* pointed out that 84% of the world's population shared just 11% of global health spending, but suffered 93% of the world's burden of disease (WHO 2000).[1] By the mid 1990s the top 29 countries, grouped in the Organisation for Economic Cooperation and Development (OECD), accounted for 90% of total world expenditure on health, leaving the vast majority of the world's population to share the remaining 10% (WTO 1998).

Statistics showing the widespread disparity between global population and health spending underline the scale of the inequality that has been generated by the current mix of systems and policies.

- The United States, with around 5% of the world's population, spends over 40% of the world's total health budget, in a system that is so inefficient and expensive to administer that as little as 50-60% of each dollar paid in insurance premiums finds its way to front-line health providers, and which costs an estimated $399 billion per year in administration costs alone[2] (Woolhandler et al 2003)

---

1 For more comparisons between population, economic strength and health spending see Appendix A.

2 $399 billion is almost four times the combined national health spending of the 62 lowest spending countries, including India and China (World Bank 2003b: Appendix A).

- Japan, with almost the same size population as Nigeria, spends 270 times more than Nigeria on health care

- Medical and pharmaceutical research is strongly biased towards the health priorities of high-income countries. The Global Forum for Health Research[3] was established in 1998 in an attempt to shift the priorities of the pharmaceutical industry, which, driven by the quest to generate profits, devoted just 10% of research resources to diseases that affect 90% of humanity (GFHR 2002)[4]. Although there are many other social and environmental factors over and above health spending that determine levels of health morbidity and mortality, the unequal levels of premature mortality also mirror broadly the same pattern

- While in Europe the median age at death is 75, the median for Africa is just five: meaning that half of all African deaths occur in children who have not reached their fifth birthday (Turshen 1999)[5]

- In developing countries in 1995 over nine million children under five died avoidable deaths – more than the entire population of Sweden (Filmer et al 1997). 98% of deaths among children under five occur in developing countries (Sachs 1999). The most recent figures show 530,000 women a year dying in childbirth in the world's poorest countries (Costello et al 2004)

- A government study in Nicaragua in 1998 found that extremely poor children were ill 50 times more often than children who were not poor (PAHO 2002)

- And while poor countries are pressed to restrict spending to minimal 'sustainable' levels, global multinationals are using offshore companies and tax havens to evade payment of taxes totalling billions of pounds a year on their operations (Campbell 2004).

These are just a few of the more glaring inequalities and contradictions from health care systems operating within a capitalist system that prioritises profit rather than human health, perpetuates extremes of inequality between and within countries, and that gives preference to the operation of market forces rather than planning and redistribution of wealth. With inequalities on this level, and evidence that there are also gross inequalities in health spending and access to care for those most needing it *within* particular countries, there is clearly a need for reforms in the organisation and delivery of health care.

Gender, race and other specific forms of inequality

The global pattern of inequality between rich and poor countries is also replicated within individual countries, and often also at an even more local level between different areas of the

---

3 Backed by the WHO, the World Bank, various national governments, academic institutions, international charities and NGOs.

4 Seven years later the Mexico Summit on Health Research noted that despite a rapid growth in global spending on research, the same inequalities prevail, urging governments in poor and donor countries alike to take action to redress the balance (GFHR 2004, Abbasi 2004).

5 The situation is getting worse: in ten African countries under-five mortality rates increased in the decade 1990-2000. Twenty-three of the 49 African countries with data had a lower life expectancy in 1999 than 1990 (Labonte et al 2004).

same city or region. Studies have shown substantial inequalities between the level of health and the availability of affordable health care services in rural and urban areas, with rural populations customarily losing out in terms of provision (Xing 2002).

However within each section of the population there are further levels of inequality, varying according to local culture, creed and political context, between men and women, and between ethnic groups. There is also a widespread issue of discrimination on grounds of sexuality, which often makes it harder for gay men, lesbians, transgender and bisexual individuals to access appropriate health care, but is also reflected in a relative lack of research on relevant public health issues (Boehmer 2002).

Schuftan (2003) argues that poverty – one of the main drivers of ill-health – 'is becoming increasingly feminised [70% of all the poor are women]'. Clearly a more detailed analysis of the health care systems in any of the countries touched upon in this study would need to address these issues of equity and access, and to weigh the success or failure of health care reforms in the context of their ability to improve the health and meet the needs of the most deprived and oppressed sections of society.

Doyal (1998, 2004) has argued for 'creative methods' of research to 'put women into the research process', and Standing (2000) has raised a number of important issues on the impact of health reforms on women. PAHO (2001) has developed a guide for this type of evaluation, although there is still little in the way of published results. However, while welcoming all of these proposals, this book is restricted in length, and is focused on general issues of policy. In many cases the specific data required to show the impact of health care reforms on particular oppressed groups – such as women, or ethnic minorities – are still lacking.

Policies are therefore analysed here from the standpoint of their likely general impact on the poorest and the most vulnerable: the assumption is that this will often result in added disadvantage for those already suffering discrimination or exclusion. The fact that we cannot here explore each of these important areas of discrimination and disadvantage should not be seen as in any way detracting from their significance.

However there are two specific groups which in almost every country suffer special levels of discrimination from health care systems – the elderly, and people with mental illness. With the possible exception in some countries of the growing burden of HIV/AIDS – on which there is at least a substantial and growing literature and active campaigns fighting for adequate resources at local, national and international levels – the sheer scale of the problems posed in meeting the current and future needs of these two groups is far larger than any other factor shaping health care and health policy in the next two decades. A case study examining the scale and varying impact of the pressures presented by the growing prevalence of mental illness in developed and developing countries can be found in Appendix B.

The failure of the health reform agenda adequately to incorporate the needs of these very substantial, but disadvantaged and socially vulnerable sections of society can be seen as further evidence that the global menu of health reform flows from economic and ideological considerations, and not from health needs.

Unequal power and influence

Many proposals for health care reforms in developing countries refer to the scale of social inequalities, inequalities in health, and inequalities in access to health care services for the poorest. However the content of most reform proposals indicate that inequalities represent the context, rather than the starting point for the reform agenda.

As Ollila and colleagues[6] argue, far from resolving these major issues, current reform policies run the risk of increasing inequality, failing to address crucial health concerns, and 'misallocation' of public health care spending. They point out that traditional analysis of health policies has primarily focused on national contextual issues, with little emphasis on the influence of international forces. Yet today it is precisely such international forces outside the health sector which are proving the key element, driving governments to:

> ...redefine the framework for health policies that countries can put into practice, influencing the capacities to allocate resources to the health sector, the structures and modes of functioning of the health care system, as well as the extent to which countries can practice healthy public policies outside the health sphere (Ollila et al 2002:243).

It is significant that in few instances, if any, have major reform programmes in developing countries been proposed, initiated or in any way led from within those countries themselves: instead the initiatives flow from outside, from global bodies such as the World Bank, or other organisations working to their own political priorities and assumptions (Lee and Goodman 2002). Instead a 'menu' of reforms that will be shown to be unrelated to the biggest problems facing health systems, and ineffective at delivering their promised benefits, has dominated the international health agenda for the last two decades.

Health and health care policies have to be understood as the product not just of the efforts and interventions of health care professionals and developments in medical science, but of wider processes of social, economic and political change. Within these complex social processes, not all of the actors are of equal power and influence.

Capitalism remains a system that preserves – and on a global scale even *increases* – the inequality between the (minority) propertied ruling 'corporate' class on the one hand, and the large majority of working classes who live by their labour, on the other. Except in the most exceptional circumstances, or in issues of relatively minor and parochial concern, the needs, concerns, and ideas of the ruling classes predominate over those of the majority (Hofrichter 2003).

Identifying pressures on health care systems

While reforms, developments and expansion are vitally needed at national and international level to meet the health challenges of the 21st century, the development of medical technology under capitalism is a far from even process. Research does not go forward on all possible fronts equally and simultaneously – it is concentrated on areas of greatest potential financial return. Nor do innovations and research relate primarily to social or health need (though *some* need must be present, or the new technique, tool or drug developed will lack use value, and thus be unable to realise its exchange value, and prove a costly failure[7]) but first and foremost to the possibilities of realising profit.

All health care systems must over time change in size, in scope, and in organisational structure to adapt to objective demographic patterns and pressures, which increasingly impact

---

6 Summing up a literary 'forum' on 'Globalisation and national health policies'.

7 There are occasional exceptions, such as instances where marketing can create a demand among the wealthier classes for what many professionals regard as an unnecessary or cosmetic treatment or product.

on all countries. But this does not pre-determine the character of these reforms, or their overall direction.

The pressures and challenges faced by health care systems are somewhat different in developed and developing countries, reflecting factors such as average incomes, the degree of income inequality, living conditions of the poorest, and the degree of investment that has already been made in health care resources.

In the wealthier, developed economies the predominant problems can be summarised as:

- Escalating provider-driven costs of health care and technical innovation
- High and rising popular expectations that the most recent advances will be made generally available to the insured population
- The 'epidemiological transition', in which the scourges of communicable disease and diseases of poverty have been largely eclipsed as health problems by cancers, cardiovascular disease, arthritis, and dementia, which tend to take an increased toll in the later years of life
- Continued entrenched professional power in the hands of a medical elite, which may obstruct reforms and drive up costs
- Increasing problems in recruiting sufficient qualified nursing and professional staff to sustain expanding health care services.

In developing countries, however there is a combined and more complex series of challenges, reflecting the partial advances which have begun to increase average life expectancy in the last 50 years, but also the prevailing lack of economic development, resulting in mass poverty, extreme inequalities, poor living conditions, and a chronic lack of investment in health care personnel and facilities:

- High levels of communicable disease, diseases of poverty, and preventable mortality
- Poor infrastructure of primary and secondary health care, worsened by shortages of skilled nursing, medical and professional staff
- Inequalities in access to health services between rich and poor and rural and urban populations, often compounded by user fees for treatment, which deter the poor despite their level of need
- The beginnings of an 'epidemiological transition', in which diseases and problems of an ageing population come on top of unresolved problems of communicable disease
- Economic weakness alongside the high cost of modern medicines and medical equipment techniques, most of which have to be imported at world market prices
- In many cases the inequalities and inadequacies of the health care system combine with the absence of local control and democratic or accountable local or national governments, and the continuation of arrangements which ensure preferential access to private or publicly-funded care for the wealthy, and the elite of the armed forces and civil service.

It might be expected that if reforms were driven solely by the type of objective pressures outlined above, there would be much greater diversity in the pattern of change, in which plans at national and local level would represent a varying combination of national specificities, influenced by local needs as much as by wider global patterns, and in which evidence of effectiveness would be much more of a prerequisite in convincing governments and health care planners of the need for new policies. Instead it appears that a very similar 'menu' of reform policies is being urged upon all countries, including the poorer countries, whose choices are being shaped by global agencies such as the World Bank, and by academics and consultancies sponsored by them.

As can be seen from the diagrammatic view below, the pressure for reform and development of health care systems is by no means purely the result of changes in governments, or in the prevailing ideological or political climate. Material forces and factors are compelling governments and health care providers to examine closely the ways in which services and treatments are provided and financed. Figure 1 summarises the different combinations of pressures encountered by health systems in the wealthier and poor countries. The pressures are further divided into two overlapping but separable categories: one defined as 'social and historical factors', the other as ' " epidemiological transition" and pressures from demographic change'.

Social and historical factors

1a Burden of communicable disease

It is immediately clear from Figure 1, which compares the pressures on advanced and developing countries, that while many of the problems of coping with the epidemiological transition affect both the wealthy countries and those in the developing world, the poorest nations face an *additional* burden, which both increases the pressures and costs on health care systems and debilitates their economies – the continued high levels of communicable disease, and much higher levels of maternal and child mortality[8].

Only part of the improvement that has been made in average life expectancy in recent decades can be attributed to medicines and medical care: living standards and social conditions play a major role, and the UN singles out the importance of better diet for special mention (UN 1997). Improvements in housing and physical environment are also widely recognised as factors in improving overall health and raising life expectancy – which helps explain why within the general averages, many countries, especially in sub-Saharan Africa, have lagged behind this pattern of improvement. In the poorest countries the spread of disease has a doubly destructive impact on the affected population: the treatment costs escalate, as the potential to generate income is reduced. According to the WHO, Africa's GDP would have been up to £100 billion higher in 2001 if not for malaria, while the impact is also felt at the level of the individual and their family:

> A malaria-stricken family can spend over one quarter of its income on treatment. A person with tuberculosis loses on average 20% to 30% of annual household income because of illness (WHO 2001e).

---

8 In 1990, over half of all children in the global poorest 20% died before the age of 15, compared with less than 4% among the richest 20% (Murray and Lopez 1996). But there is also a big difference in the causes of death in the poorest countries: in 1996 infectious and parasitic diseases were responsible for 43% of deaths in developing countries, but just 1.2% in developed nations, including transition economies (Labonte et al 2004:39).

Figure 1: Pressures on health care systems

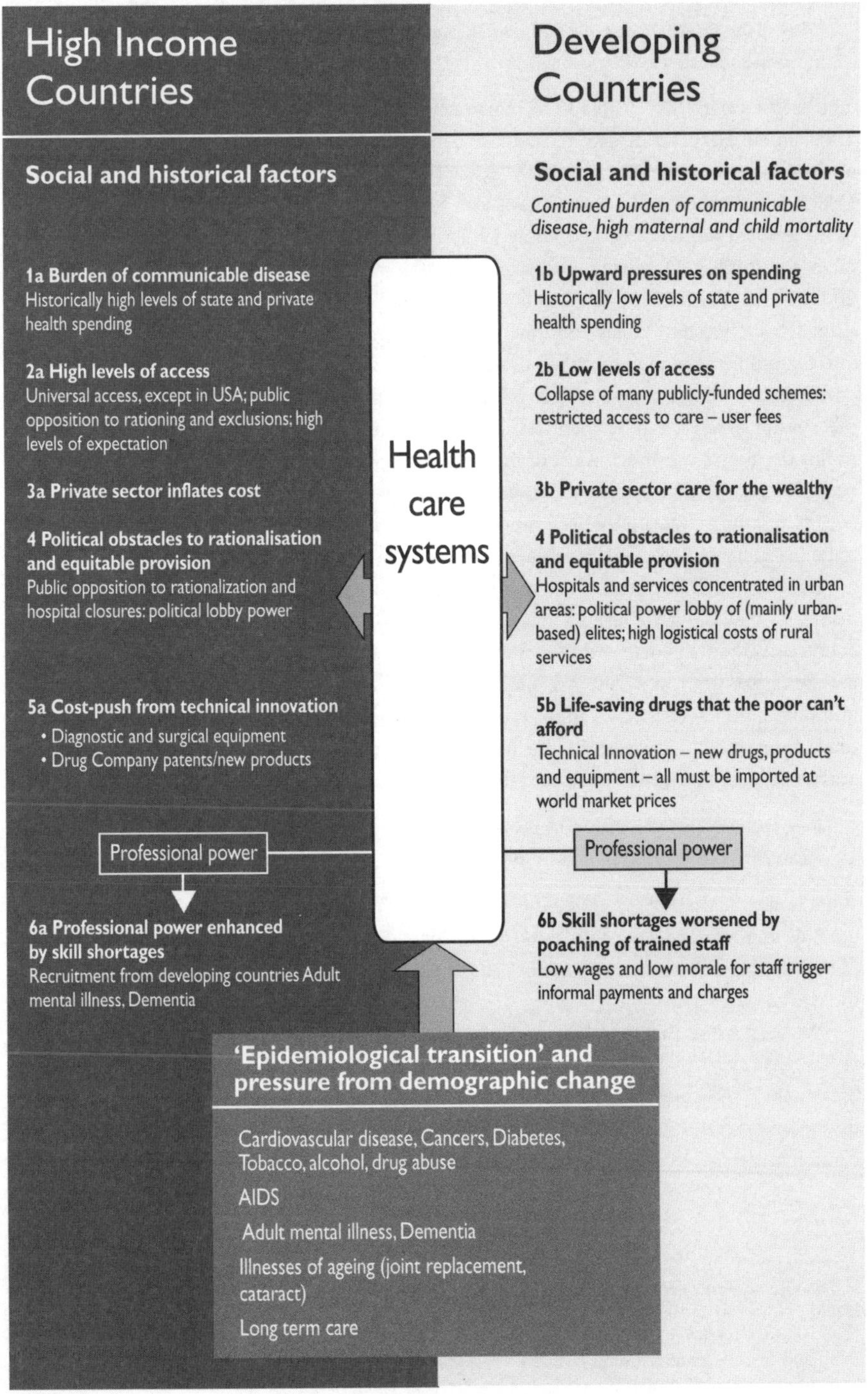

High Income Countries	Developing Countries
Social and historical factors	**Social and historical factors** *Continued burden of communicable disease, high maternal and child mortality*

Health care systems

High Income Countries

1a Burden of communicable disease
Historically high levels of state and private health spending

2a High levels of access
Universal access, except in USA; public opposition to rationing and exclusions; high levels of expectation

3a Private sector inflates cost

4 Political obstacles to rationalisation and equitable provision
Public opposition to rationalization and hospital closures: political lobby power

5a Cost-push from technical innovation
• Diagnostic and surgical equipment
• Drug Company patents/new products

Professional power

6a Professional power enhanced by skill shortages
Recruitment from developing countries Adult mental illness, Dementia

Developing Countries

1b Upward pressures on spending
Historically low levels of state and private health spending

2b Low levels of access
Collapse of many publicly-funded schemes: restricted access to care – user fees

3b Private sector care for the wealthy

4 Political obstacles to rationalisation and equitable provision
Hospitals and services concentrated in urban areas: political power lobby of (mainly urban-based) elites; high logistical costs of rural services

5b Life-saving drugs that the poor can't afford
Technical Innovation – new drugs, products and equipment – all must be imported at world market prices

Professional power

6b Skill shortages worsened by poaching of trained staff
Low wages and low morale for staff trigger informal payments and charges

'Epidemiological transition' and pressure from demographic change

Cardiovascular disease, Cancers, Diabetes, Tobacco, alcohol, drug abuse

AIDS

Adult mental illness, Dementia

Illnesses of ageing (joint replacement, cataract)

Long term care

The central issue in these developing countries is the lack of adequate resources targeted at the main destructive diseases:

> Most of the 13 million deaths a year from infectious diseases can be prevented with existing tools,
> medicines and strategies… (op. cit.)

The WHO argues that deaths from malaria could be cut by as much as 97% by the correct intervention. However despite the extensive lobbying that had preceded the decision process at the Genoa summit of the world's eight richest countries, the establishment of a Global Health Fund against Aids, Tuberculosis and Malaria has so far failed to deliver anything close to the amount required. By 2003 only $2.3 billion had so far been offered towards the WHO target for 2002-2004, leaving a projected shortfall of $1.4 billion in 2003 and $3.3 billion in 2004 (Global Fund 2003). With additional economic problems facing the poorest countries as their debts to western banks continue to mount, this is unlikely to make any serious inroads into the problems of disease and ill-health (Rowson 2001)[9].

Even limited allocations of new money almost inevitably come with some restrictions on the ways in which it can be spent. Much of the money was to be used by the poor countries to buy drugs and vaccines – most of them from suppliers in the 'donor' countries. There have been complaints that the global bodies overseeing the 'partnership' between governments, NGOs and the private sector are unrepresentative, unaccountable to those they are supposed to be assisting, and selected by arbitrary means (Brugha and Walt 2001).

Brugha and Walt question the methods and priorities of these global bodies, notably the insistence that funds for the strengthening of health care systems and services in recipient countries will only be released *after* they have achieved higher levels of immunisation, despite the fact that improved systems may well be needed to reach the people in need of immunisation. There are pressures to re-shape services – to ensure that they use more modern (and more costly) drugs from the major pharmaceutical giants. But with no long-term guarantee of further cash to flow into the Global Fund, there are fears things could get worse:

> Poor countries that alter their drug policies to incorporate expensive new drugs could be left with
> unsustainable costs at a future date (Brugha and Walt 2001).

What is clear is that this type of aid is not a way of 'reforming' health care systems: instead it upholds and reinforces the status quo – the dependency of the poorer countries, the poverty of the very poorest in each population, and the monopoly control over medical technology in the wealthy countries.

Worse, it seems that the focus on developing services based on high value drugs – not least in the treatment of HIV/AIDS victims – is diverting from the need for much cheaper preventative measures, which can cut off the route by which the disease is spreading throughout much of Africa. Shelton and Johnston, analysing UN data, found that provision of condoms, the most cost-effective means of prevention, had barely increased during the

---

9 The Global Fund's executive director, Richard Feachem, (a former director of the World Bank's Health, Nutrition and Population division) has called for a scaling up of capital investment, but has been less than forthright in challenging the miserable $200 million allocation proposed by George W Bush and the US administration in 2003 – less than a tenth of their 'fair share' calculated on the basis of the US share of the UN budget (Labonte et al 2004:43-45).

previous five years, and was only around a quarter of the level required to match the highest provisions in African countries, giving a 'condom gap' of 1.9 billion. The additional condoms required could be produced for only an extra $48m (Shelton and Johnston 2001).

1b Upward pressures on spending

The impact of the combined demographic, social and historical pressures on health systems is to force the costs of health care upwards. This is true in wealthier countries – where spending is already higher; but it also affects the poorer countries, where historically low levels of spending have left such a poor infrastructure of health care that substantial investment is required to create sufficient capacity to tackle new and additional tasks – especially if they involve delivering care outside of the urban areas.

2a High levels of access: high expectations in wealthy countries

In most of the wealthier countries[10] collectively funded tax or insurance-based systems have been established which provide health care services to virtually 100% of the resident population (OECD 2003). While this offers possibilities to share the costs and risks across far wider sections, or even (in Beveridge-style systems) the whole population, it also helps to build expectations and create obstacles to any subsequent policies that might cut back on services or benefits. In particular there is a public expectation (and thus a political pressure to ensure) that every latest new drug and technique will swiftly be made generally available.

This type of pressure has ensured that explicit rationing of health care, for example, though discussed by academics for some years, has not been introduced in any industrialised country (Saltman 2002). Health care systems have become significant political issues, and any potential reforms and restructuring are scrutinised by a critical public. Governments nationally and locally have suffered the consequences of antagonising public opinion by imposing unpopular policies[11].

2b Low levels of access: user fees as obstacles to care

By contrast many of the developing countries which established publicly-funded, often free health care immediately after independence have been forced by economic pressures including Structural Adjustment Programmes to reverse these progressive measures. Many have cut back public provision; many more have imposed user fees for treatment, including treatment in publicly-owned hospitals. In many middle income countries health care insurance schemes cover only a relatively small section of workers employed in the formal sector of the economy,

---

10 With the notable exceptions of the USA (24%), the Netherlands (74%) and Germany (91%).

11 Examples include New Zealand, and the UK. In New Zealand the National Party which had brought in market oriented reforms in the teeth of professional and popular opposition in 1993 lost its majority in the next general election and was forced to conclude a coalition deal with New Zealand First, a party that had campaigned against the reforms – and effectively reverse direction on some of the key market-style proposals (Hornblow 1997). In the UK, the warning to electors that they had 'ten days to save the NHS' helped ensure Tony Blair's defeat of the Conservative government in 1997: but in the subsequent general election one of Blair's junior ministers, David Locke, lost his parliamentary seat to an independent after endorsing the closure of his local hospital in Kidderminster as part of a rationalisation designed to fund a privately-financed NHS hospital 30 miles away in Worcester (Gulland 2001).

leaving very large numbers of the poorest with no cover. Any moves to reform health care on a more equitable basis in these countries will inevitably require increases in state spending.

3a Private sector inflates costs

Many of the wealthier countries have also encouraged the development of private sector hospitals, including a 'for-profit' sector, which depends for its market upon the failure of public sector providers to deliver sufficient volume or speed of response, and the existence of a wealthy minority and a private health insurance sector. With few exceptions it is admitted that this private provision runs at higher costs than public provision, and that it serves to 'cherry pick' more lucrative operations and treatments, leaving the more expensive caseload to the public sector (Carlisle 2003, Devers 2003, Woolhandler and Himmelstein 2004). Private providers also tend to compete directly with the public sector for professional and medical staff, pushing pay levels higher and intensifying the pressure on emergency services.

3b Private sector cares for wealthy

World Bank advice to poorer countries centres on restricting publicly-funded health care to a basic minimum package of largely primary care services, leaving more advanced hospital care to the private sector – and thus largely restricting its accessibility to exclude the poor (World Bank 1987, 1993). And as in the wealthier countries, doctors and other qualified staff, trained through the public health care system, are frequently drawn to work for higher salaries and in better conditions in the private sector[12] (Nandraj 1997).

However, the availability of modern medical treatment for the richest sections of society – which also tend to be concentrated in the urban centres – removes the political pressure that might have persuaded governments to invest in publicly-funded hospital care, which could in turn benefit the poor and the rural population.

4 Political obstacles to rationalisation and equitable provision

In wealthier and poorer countries alike, any attempt to rationalise health care resources is likely to fall foul of intense political lobbying, in which a range of interest groups can unite: local populations facing the loss of local hospital facilities as specialist services are centralised may combine with sections of health workers, professionals, and local politicians. In some cases, protests can force retreats, and the retention of services at the expense of anticipated financial savings.

In developing countries, in line with the inverse care law, the more advanced facilities tend to be centred in urban areas, closest to the more affluent – and influential – sections of the population. The most senior professionals are often reluctant to extend services into rural areas – especially if it results in any diminution of their 'power base' in the major hospitals. The most dominant health care professionals, often with links to government, also tend to be drawn from the secondary care sector, making it more difficult to reallocate resources to improve primary care services.

---

12 In Brazil, there are 120,000 private doctors covering a quarter of the population, but just 70,000 to cover the other 75% (Sexton 2003).

5a Cost-push from technical innovation

Technical innovation continues to be a key motor for change in health care, especially in the more advanced economies in which health care systems are already relatively well-developed. New drugs, new diagnostic equipment and methods, new anaesthetics, new surgical techniques, new methods for rehabilitation all offer to prolong and improve the lives of patients as they have done over the last 100 years – but bring with them various new requirements, such as investment of new money in equipment, drugs or in the training and recruitment of new specialists or community teams. However they have subsequently served to reduce unit costs, by avoiding prolonged hospitalisation. Average lengths of stay for each hospital admission have been progressively reducing (OECD 2000).

Established examples of technical advance have included the use of anti-ulcer drugs to avoid the necessity for hospital treatment and even surgery (Rivett 1998)[13]; increased options for chemotherapy delivered on an outpatient basis to cancer patients; new anaesthetics which expanded the scope for day surgery; and assertive outreach teams, which can dramatically reduce dependence on hospital services for mental health patients (Ayonrinde et al 2000, Chisholm and Ford 2004).

5b Life-saving drugs that the poor can't afford

The priorities of the R&D departments of the big pharmaceutical companies do not necessarily coincide with the most pressing health needs, either in the wealthier countries, or across the world. Though some drugs can save lives and massively reduce the spread of illness, their development remains in the hands of giant transnational companies, which defend both their profits and their right to decide which areas they will pursue in research and development.

New and expensive drugs have been brought to market promising to tackle what might be seen as social rather than medical issues, and life-style rather than life-threatening problems, with the drug corporations invoking consumer power to bring pressure to bear on political leaders to ensure they are made widely available.

In poorer countries, where per capita health care spending is so much lower, access to these and other new drugs and treatments is often seen as financially out of reach. An exception to this has been the pressure for the provision of modern cocktails of drugs to contain the effects of the AIDS virus, which has taken its heaviest toll in sub-Saharan Africa. The battle between the major drug companies and the South African government over the supply of cheaper drugs to treat HIV/AIDS patients has underlined the lack of any accountability by the pharmaceutical firms to the people in need of treatment.

But there are other conflicts: Oxfam has launched a campaign naming Pfizer, the world's largest pharmaceutical supplier, criticising its refusal to lower prices of the life-saving drugs it exports to developing countries, and its relentless efforts to enforce its patent rights, preventing any development of cheaper, generic, locally produced equivalents (Oxfam 2001).

---

13 Drug therapy for ulcers in the US cost just $900 a year in the early 1990s, compared with $25,000 for surgery: and the use of beta blockers to prevent second heart attacks was by 1993 claimed to be saving between $1.6 and $3 billion a year from health bills in the USA ten years earlier (Goldberg 1993).

6a Professional power enhanced by skill shortages

In the wealthier countries, despite the very generous pay and benefits available to senior medical professionals, the further expansion of health care systems has been hampered by a lack of sufficient numbers of the right types of trained doctors, nurses and other therapeutic staff. The logic of such shortages would be a sharp increase in the prevailing rates of pay in order to attract and retain recruits with the right type of educational background: to some extent this is taking place, and costs are being driven up [14].

Managers attempting to break though these barriers have in recent years undertaken a programme of recruitment of staff from a range of developing countries where levels of training are regarded as generally comparable: Britain and the USA in particular have centred on the English-speaking countries, notably the Philippines, where nursing staff are trained to degree standard, but also sub-Saharan African countries such as South Africa, Zimbabwe, Zambia, Kenya and Nigeria. This has been challenged by a growing body of professional and trade union opinion and by leading NGOs, who have underlined the high costs and negative consequences for health care in the developing countries which suffer the outflow and in effect 'prop up' the NHS and other health care systems (Buchan 2005, Martineau et al 2002).

However tightened restrictions on immigration and residence have meant that the USA and EU countries may be worsening the levels of staff shortages they face in key areas for health care [15] (Paral 2004).

6b Skill shortages worsened by poaching of trained staff

The result of such recruitment campaigns on developing countries, themselves often seeking to build a more comprehensive health care system, is the persistent loss not so much of new recruits but of a skilled 'middle layer' of nursing and other qualified staff who have begun to show their value in hospitals and other sections of health services.

In Kenya, a large proportion of the small numbers of specialised hospital nurses trained each year are enticed out of the country to work in British hospitals (Stenton 2002). Such policies often bring only temporary solutions for the wealthier countries, while causing long-term damage and expense in the poorest countries (Laporte 2005, Save the Children 2005).

---

14 South Africa's public sector has resorted to a system of paying hefty bonuses for doctors with 'scarce skills', and a further 20% of salary to those who agree to work in rural areas, which otherwise would have no medical cover. Labonte et al (2004) point out the drain of talented nurses and medical professionals from developing countries to the developed health care systems is a combination of the 'pull' of higher salaries, status, resources and career progression abroad, and the 'push' arising from the lack of all of these at home, especially in rural areas.

15 Paral's (2004) detailed report for the US Immigration Policy Center found that 1.1 million immigrants made up 13% of the US health care workforce. Foreign-born staff accounted for 25% of all physicians in the US, 17% of all nursing assistants, 16% of clinical laboratory technicians , 15% of pharmacists and 12% of registered nurses.

'Epidemiological transition' and pressures from demographic change: the rising cost of age and disease[16]

In the wealthier countries the main focus of health care services long ago shifted from communicable disease to the diseases and conditions which more commonly occur in later life and also affect the more affluent – notably cardiovascular disease, diabetes and cancers. There are of course also substantial problems in terms of a still virulent AIDS epidemic, high levels of adult mental illness, and the range of diseases and health problems relating especially to old age – the debilitating effects of arthritis, requiring a rising number of joint replacements; cataract; and dementia. See Appendix B for a case study of mental health.

Statistical research by Gwatkin and Guillot shows that communicable diseases are by far the biggest factor in the health gap between the world's richest and poorest quintiles of population. While non-communicable disease, notably ischaemic heart disease, is the main single cause of death among the global rich, accounting for 23.4% of deaths in 1990, it comes well down the list of fatal diseases among the global poor. Conversely, respiratory infections, which accounted for 13.4% of deaths among the world's poorest 20% in 1990, brought about the deaths of only 4.8% of the richest 20%. The authors argue that it is cheaper to reduce deaths and disability from communicable diseases than to reduce the death toll from non-communicable conditions – and that such a policy would overwhelmingly benefit the world's poor (Gwatkin & Guillot 2000).

The WHO, in seeking to address global inequalities in health, also wants to see extra spending on tackling communicable diseases (and other preventive measures, including a reduction in tobacco consumption) adding up to $10-$20 billion in the developing countries, some of which could come from debt relief. The reluctance of the wealthier countries to commit this level of extra resources can perhaps be explained by the fact that it would offer little obvious benefit to their own population, among whom communicable disease accounts for fewer than one death in every ten.

However there is no doubt that as the transition begins to take effect there will be an ever growing section of population in the poorest countries suffering from long-term illnesses. The WHO estimates that by 2020 70% of health needs in developing countries will involve chronic diseases and mental disorders, meaning that older people now and in the future are likely to be among the main client group requiring care (HAI 2002a:8, UN 2002:84). In some cases health promotion measures or early intervention now can reduce the prospect of more expensive treatment being required later on.

As people get older, they become more vulnerable to non-communicable diseases, including diabetes, cancers and circulatory disorders, which in turn can require relatively

16 'Epidemiological transition', a phrase coined by Abdel R Omran (Omran 1971), and popularised from the late 1980s (Frenk et al 1989) is a term often used to describe the changing profile of disease and health problems in countries where rising life expectancy and living standards take effect, reducing the proportionate burden of communicable disease and increasing the incidence of cancers, coronary vascular disease and chronic conditions associated with old age (Gribble and Preston 1993). It has also been criticised as a means of diverting from social and political factors determining poverty and ill health, as an approach embodying the 'ethnocentrism' of 'a coloniser's model of the world', and carrying assumptions and ideology which implicitly endorse and sustain the status quo (Aviles 2001).

expensive forms of treatment. Diabetes is estimated to affect 143 million people around the world, and accounts for 8% of health budgets in the advanced economies (WHO 1998).

The risk of mental illness also increases with age. Numbers of older people suffering from senile dementia, estimated at around 22 million throughout the world in 1996, could top 80 million in the developing economies of Africa, Asia, and Latin America alone by 2025 (WHO 1996).

Responding to this challenge, one NGO, Help Age International spells out on its website a very clear and simple agenda for the improvement of health care for older people, especially in developing countries. It calls on all governments to implement the resolution passed in 1982 by the World Assembly on Ageing in Vienna, which urged them to formulate and implement policies on the basis of specific national needs and objectives. It calls for action to change the prevailing negative attitudes, which deter older people from accessing health services in primary care and other health facilities, and for services to be brought closer to the rural areas where many older people live.

Despite this reasonable plea, so far there is little evidence that HAI's appeal has in any way influenced the reform agenda of governments and global bodies. As the next chapter will discuss, the source of these reforms is in general not the needs of particular groups of service users or those requiring health care, but political, ideological and economic pressures.

Chapter two

Mixing up the wrong prescription:
analysing the 'reforms' and the reformers

Introduction

'Reforms' to health care systems are commonly presented in terms which strip them from their context and effectively deny their ideological and political content. This chapter briefly explains the analytical method that will be adopted to confront this problem, and questions the appropriateness and evidence base of the most common menu of reforms. The historical evolution of today's health care industry, and the emergence of social, political and economic pressures to reform are discussed.

Positive changes?

The changes under examination in this study are commonly termed 'reforms'. The implication is that a flawed system is being made better, and that 'reform means positive change' (Berman and Bossert 2000). Berman (1995:15) defines health sector reform as 'sustained, purposeful change to improve the efficiency, equity and effectiveness of the health sector'. However, critics of the process take a different view: Schuftan and Dahlgren (1999) argue that in the context of current reforms, the term means little more than 'market-led interventions in the health and nutrition sector', and Marmor (2001:22) expresses reluctance to use the word because of 'discomfort with the marketing connotations of reform'. By contrast, the World Bank's Preker and Harding (2003:2) happily draw analogies with the 'new public management' policies introduced into other privatised utilities and services, and approvingly sum up many of the changes as 'marketising reforms'.

It is not reform as such that is being questioned here, but the specific reform *measures* which have dominated the political agenda for the past two decades. The question is whether they can meet the demands of the new situation. Structural, managerial and policy changes have been taking place within virtually all of the world's health care systems since the early 1990s (Mills et al 2001, ICHSRI 1997, EHMA 2000, PAHO 2000, Whitehead et al 2001). But are these 'health care reforms' driven primarily by the health needs of the wider population in the countries concerned, or do they flow from non-health considerations – the financial, political and ideological concerns of governments and global institutions?

Since the fall of the Berlin Wall in 1989, and the collapse of the Soviet Union, capitalism has been the overwhelmingly dominant economic framework in almost every country. All of the reforms that have been brought forward since the late 1980s – whether in wealthier countries or the poorest countries of Africa, Asia and Latin America – have been shaped within this broad framework.

Under capitalism most goods and services are exchanged – bought and sold – on the basis of a market system, in which a variety of manufacturers, retailers and service providers compete with each other for market share on the basis of price, quality, and availability. It is argued by advocates of capitalism that in most, if not every case this market mechanism offers the best way to maximise the efficient and cost-effective delivery to meet the needs and wishes of the consumer.

One finding from this study is that health reform packages premised on the role of markets, competition and a growing role for the private sector have not been restricted to the advanced economies. While governments in the wealthiest OECD countries have been developing their own repertoire of reforms, developing countries have also been urged in the direction of similar reform measures by global bodies, notably the World Bank and the IMF, and by donor organisations such as USAID and the various consultancies and academic research they have sponsored in the last 20 years (as will be discussed in more detail in Chapter three below).

The reform agenda depicted in Figure 2 (see the Introduction to Chapter four) summarises a variety of remarkably similar proposals that have been advanced both for developed and developing countries[17].

Reforms that cut costs – and those that don't

As in Figure 2, this study draws a distinction between two very different types of 'reform' which can be seen being implemented in many different parts of the world. One school of reforms openly professes the aim of *restructuring* previously planned, centralised or regulated health care systems in order to create, extend or 'manage' market-style mechanisms: these (listed above) will be referred to in this study as 'market-style' reforms. Others, which this study categorises as 'market-driven' measures, seek only to cut or contain costs. The impact of these two types of reform can be quite different, and they tend to arise from different political and economic pressures.

Market-driven reforms are not new: as 'the blunt instruments of budget constraint and cost shifting' (Tuohy 1999:4), such policies have a history reaching back at least to the 1970s. There is little doubt about the pressures driving measures to constrain or reduce health care spending. Whether or not they are presented as 'reforms', these changes are essentially a response to wider economic pressures, external to health needs: indeed the cash limits that are set and the resultant restrictions on services can increase any gaps between capacity and demand for service, generating waiting lists or other symptoms of service shortfall. Their effect on health services varies according to two main factors: the scale of the cutback imposed, and whether this represents a real terms reduction in spending, or simply a restriction on the rate of increase.

---

17 A variant version of a similar combination of reforms (though without the subdivision into market-driven and market-style reforms) is set out in Labonte et al (2004:185), citing similar work by Cassels (1995,1997) and Breman and Shelton (2001). There has been an extensive debate over the most appropriate way to characterise the poorer countries, as Labonte and colleagues (2004:ix) note in their introduction. This study will follow their approach, and adopt the usage most often employed in the main literature, referring to 'developed', 'developing' and 'least developed' countries.

Spending restraints obviously have a greater impact where they are enforced on health systems that are already inadequately resourced to meet prevailing health needs. Some methods of attempting to cut expenditure result in a more substantial transfer of costs from public budgets to individual service users and their families. These measures represent a response to the pressures of the competitive world market on national economies – and are not strictly speaking *reforms*, since they leave existing organisational structures largely unchanged. In a few cases similar policies (such as user fees or the reform of provider payment systems) may appear on either the 'market-driven' or 'market-style' agendas – or on both.

However while cost-saving measures aim precisely to cut costs and if possible improve efficiency, no such simple explanation applies to the distinctive new market-style reforms ('an epidemic of reforms based on various forms of market principles' (Leppo 1997:3);'market type mechanisms' (Pollitt 2003)) that have increasingly been introduced to health care systems around the world over the last 15-20 years. There is very little evidence to show that these type of policies – such as the separation of purchaser and provider, decentralisation, competition, contracting out of support services, corporatisation of hospitals, user fees, public sector use of private finance, and private health insurance – can either reduce costs or deliver on their claims to improve the efficiency and effectiveness of services.

This doubt is compounded by the fact that some of the pioneers in market-style reform of health services have been the most resistant to any evaluation of its effects[18]. While some improvements have been noted in some areas of health care delivery after such reforms have been introduced, this has generally been in the context of substantial increases in overall spending and resources, and other developments in technique and technology. The few evaluations that have been made are often marred by lack of solid baseline information to isolate the impact of reform measures, and inform a genuine comparison of 'before' and 'after' the introduction of market type mechanisms (Gilson 1999, Pollitt 2003).

Their impact on efficiency may be open to doubt[19], but there is significant information suggesting that these reforms serve to *increase* administrative costs[20]. To make matters even worse, market-style reforms are often highly controversial and politically unpopular with the wider electorate as well as health care professionals and support staff (Ranade 1998). The

---

18 Analysts have commented on the refusal of the British Conservative government to support any evaluation of its controversial market reforms of the early 1990s (Smith 2000:4, Robinson & LeGrand 1994). Scott and colleagues (1999) asked how the 1993 health system reforms in New Zealand affected technical efficiency, allocative efficiency, clinical outcomes, consumer satisfaction and equity of access: but they were forced to conclude that 'No comprehensive examination has been done in these terms' (Scott et al 2003:324). Maynard (2002) notes in the case of Britain, where the resistance to evaluation is undiminished, that 'The failure to learn by systematic evaluation and use of evidence is impressive'.

19 Boyle et al (2004) describe efficiency as a 'slippery concept', and against the conventional notions of economies of scale, they counterpose 'diseconomies of scale' which can result from the 'sheer wastage' in establishing ever larger institutions 'where staff feel they have no stake' and where costly mistakes and levels of cross-infection are maximised.

20 A World Bank study has found that health care systems which incorporate insurance-style separations between purchaser and provider incur much heavier administration costs than those which do not (Dunlop & Martins 1996). Paton (2000) argues that there is no evidence that the purchaser/provider split is a worthwhile market-style reform, and that it may be the case that the separation of planning from implementation 'makes policy less coherent' (Paton 2000:16).

reforms also signally fail to address many if not all of the major objective challenges confronting health care services in the 21st century – in particular the health needs of a rapidly expanding elderly population, and the worldwide increase in demand for mental health services.

So why – given that they do not appear related to health needs, to popular demand, or to the generalised pressure for economic savings – should such reforms have become so widely accepted, discussed and implemented on a world scale? And since – despite varying conditions and systems into which they are being introduced – the underlying 'menu' of reforms is so similar (Mills et al 2001), the explanation must be more than just a succession of national peculiarities, or the dominance at a certain conjuncture of a particular political party. What global pressures have led to the adoption of these policies by governments of various political allegiances, in high- and middle-income countries and in the poorest developing countries?

Are these the 'right' reforms – and do they work?

It is an underlying premise of this study that far-reaching reforms are needed to enable health care systems around the world to grow and change in order to meet health needs and develop an equitable system ensuring full access for the poorest and most socially excluded. However this by no means suggests that any and all forms of reform are equally effective – or ineffective.

While this study largely focuses on the inadequacy of many of the stock reforms, other measures can offer progress. Don Berwick, for example, in a recent *BMJ* overview article has outlined innovative ways of working that can be shown to deliver improved quality of care in some of the poorest developing countries – while incorporating no market-style methods, rejecting competition, and focusing instead upon the development of teamwork, cooperation and commitment among health workers (Berwick 2004). Molyneux and Nantulya (2004) have shown ways in which parallel disease control programmes in Africa can be linked to improve effectiveness and efficiency.

In Brazil, a new publicly-funded health care system, making extensive use of private sector providers, but delivering a statutory right to health care free of charge for all, funded through a fixed levy on tax income at national, state and municipal level, has been introduced by governments far removed from socialism, offering an alternative model for other middle income countries (Fleury 2001).

In Britain the New Labour government since 2001 has injected dramatically increased resources to health care, and succeeded in reducing the maximum waiting time for treatment: but while this has been carried through in the context of a continual process of 'modernisation' and structural reform, there is little evidence that the reforms, rather than the additional billions in spending (which also represents a form of 'reform' and a sharp change of policy) have been responsible for the improvement.

The World Bank has conceded the spectacular health gains achieved by the Cuban health care system: but this has been achieved largely on the basis of ignoring the World Bank's menu of reform, and combining the public health measures of the World Health Organisation with the development of modern, hi-tech hospitals and pharmaceutical production (World Bank 2003b).

The question must be asked: regardless of their origin and underlying motivation, do the various reform packages promoted by neoliberal and 'third way' politicians and by the World Bank and its co-thinkers ask the right questions, and do they offer the right answers from the point of view of service users and their health needs?

The judgement of success or failure of health care systems depends upon what aspects are judged. A private hospital corporation will assess its success by the profits in its end of year balance sheet, while a publicly funded health care system will tend to be more focused on the delivery of care, and will compare 'outputs' (patients successfully treated) against 'inputs'[21]. The criteria by which this study has sought to judge the success or failure of proposed reforms are:

- Whether or not they enable a health care system to deliver more health care on an affordable basis to those in greatest need;

- Whether there is evidence they can deliver the results they appear to promise in terms of efficiency, quality and effectiveness in delivering care;

- Whether they enable a health care system more adequately to deal with the type of rising pressures identified in Chapter one above.

The 'baseline' for the evaluation has to be the level of accessibility and availability of health care to the poorest sections of society prior to the reform process: if the reforms themselves, rather than any accompanying increased allocation of resources, can be seen to widen access and increase the volume of care available to those who need it, then they can be judged to have succeeded from the point of view of service provision.

If on the other hand reforms can be seen to exclude those who might previously have used services, to restrict the level of services, or increase overhead costs without generating improvements in the quality of care, then they must be regarded as a backward step for health care, and the motivation for such 'reforms' needs to be examined.

There is of course another way of appraising a reform package: establishing whether the reforms themselves are based on any genuine evidence of effectiveness. The key question with reforms is whether or not they can be seen to 'work': yet here is one of the strangest gaps in the available literature. Some efforts have been made at comparative and evaluative analysis of the reform process. Berman and Bossert (2000) begin to raise useful questions when they ask what has been learned from a decade of health sector reforms in developing countries. But there are few clear answers on offer.

It is clear that market-style policies have been introduced in a wide variety of countries – with very little attempt either to support them with evidence of success, or to monitor the impact of the reforms to show they achieved the intended results. The World Bank's 2004 *World Development Report* notes the lack of evaluation of new interventions as one of the problems in poorer countries, but also warns that such evaluation must be specific, taking account of the concrete circumstances: 'relying on research from other countries, while useful, is not enough' (World Bank 2003b:26). It is important not to exaggerate apparent similarities and lose sight of national specifics: the pattern of reform, and the political background to it, varies in each country. But recognising diversity in both the underlying models and the specific examples can be a major obstacle for a 'comparative' study, potentially leaving the researcher not with a genuine comparison but with a rather shapeless collection of studies of diverse single countries (Cochrane et al 2001).

---

21 A recent report for the Organisation for Economic Cooperation and Development notes that 'The value of health care is, generally, measured by inputs and fails to take into account the value of improved quality of care arising from advances in medicine' (Docteur and Oxley 2003).

Another limitation has been that the underlying pro-market assumptions behind the few evaluative studies that have taken place can limit their effectiveness and result in further reinforcing a defective model.

Comparing changes, not systems

The potential problems of seeking a worldwide comparison between health care systems were underlined by the World Health Organisation's highly controversial *World Health Report 2000* (WHR2000). After many years of publishing its own *Health for All Statistical Database* (launched in 1987, and comprising over 500 different indicators (WHO 1999a)), the decision to synthesise some of the information into a direct comparison between different national systems led to a major dispute over the validity of the comparative data. WHR2000 attempted (albeit in an appendix rather than in the main body of the report) to rank 191 health services from all over the world in a single league table – based on contentious calculations of 'healthy life expectancy' for the country's population, 'responsiveness' of the service to patients, and the 'fairness' of the financing system. It triggered a wave of angry responses, as will be discussed in below.

However the intention of this study is not to compare or rank systems *per se*, but to focus on the extent to which a bewildering variety of different symptoms – chronic problems facing health care systems in wide variety of different contexts – have been confronted by a resort to a single, essentially similar, ideologically-based prescription – a dose of market-style policies and New Public Management.

A methodology for analysing changes

Marxism

Unlike many existing comparative studies of the reform process[22], this study employs a Marxist framework, seeking to develop an approach which is able to offer a coherent explanation of events, economic forces, policies and ideologies, while also embracing complexities, contradictions and tensions. A Marxist approach offers the possibility of a consistent and critical analysis of the context, the content, the motivation, and the material (class) interests served by particular policies and 'reforms'.

By contrast, the contending analytical methodologies offer a choice between a variety of relatively static, apolitical and ahistorical approaches. This study is primarily one of health care policy reforms rather than philosophy and methodology, so unfortunately there is no space for an in-depth explanation and critique of the multiplicity of possible alternative approaches[23].

The strength of the Marxist method, as exemplified in Doyal's landmark study *The Politics of Health* (1979), is that it recognises that history is made by a complex interaction of

---

22 These include Flood (2000), Freeman (2000), Moran (1999), Preker and Harding (2003), Ranade (1998), Saltman and Figueras (1997), Saltman et al (1998), Saltman et al (2002), Schieber (1997), Scott (2001),and Tuohy (1999).

23 It is not the purpose of this study to engage in a detailed examination of, or polemic with, the various academic Marxists, neo-Marxists, post Marxists and critical theorists, in the hands of many of whom, in the period since the rise of Stalin, and especially since the post-war period, 'Marxism' has evolved in a very different direction, back towards the levels of abstraction and contemplative disengagement which Marx himself rejected in 1845 (Pierson 1998, Therborn 1996).

individuals, interest groups and social classes – 'all the many wills' that combine to make history, though not in a manner of their own making or choosing (Marx 1852). The underlying roots of ideology, politics and culture are seen to lie in the material conditions of societies divided along class lines.

Moreover, as one of the component parts of a modern 'political economy' approach, Marxism's inherent strength is understanding the integral relationship between politics and economics, recognising that the health sector has to be understood as an issue of both political and economic significance (Armstrong et al 2001). As a tool for analysing the development of the health reform agenda, Marxism also sets the development of social and political phenomena in a historical context, and recognises that ideas and policies change and evolve over time, rather than emerging ready-made in the minds of individuals.

Marxism does not reject the need for progressive reforms, or dismiss the possibility of achieving significant improvements for working people even within the framework of capitalism: but Marxists do not automatically conclude that all reforms are socially progressive, and neither do they see reforms as an end in themselves[24].

Rather than assuming that in every case 'Reform means positive change' (Berman and Bossert 2000), a Marxist analysis of 'reforms' to the health care system within a capitalist framework will explore the inevitable limitations, contradictions and unresolved political aspirations that will arise from even ostensibly progressive measures implemented by capitalist governments.

A number of the global bodies whose policies have helped drive reforms in health care, and which are central to this study – notably the World Bank, the International Monetary Fund (IMF), the Organisation for Economic Cooperation and Development (OECD), and USAID – are themselves 'the financial agencies of international capital' (Alcock 2001:4), institutions founded with the specific and declared objective of sustaining and developing capitalism (and, in the case of USAID, supporting US foreign policy). This makes it especially relevant to subject their proposals and their involvement in health care policy to a Marxist critique.

The predominant line of criticism and opposition to market-style reforms and neoliberal-influenced policy reflects not a Marxist but a reformist perspective, which sees it as possible to resolve or at least ameliorate the gross inequalities which persist within global capitalism through a series of policy reforms that leave the underlying system (and its class divisions) intact. Many of the policies of the World Health Organisation derive from precisely this reformist approach, and a Marxist standpoint offers the possibility to distinguish the socially progressive aspirations of such policies, while also demonstrating the recurring contrast

---

24 *The Communist Manifesto* notes the success of British workers in forcing the legislation of the Ten Hours Bill, and stresses (Section IV) that 'The Communists fight for the attainment of the immediate aims for the enforcement of the momentary interests of the working class, but in the movement of the present they also represent and take care of the future of that movement' (Marx and Engels 1970). The Communist International in the *Theses* of its Third and Fourth Congresses developed tactics and a programme, which required the new Communist Parties to be involved in every 'individual and partial' demand of the workers (Adler 1980). Trotsky's 1938 *Transitional Programme* also insisted that 'The Fourth International does not discard the programme of the old "minimal" demands to the degree to which these have preserved at least part of their vital forcefulness. Indefatigably it defends the democratic rights and social conquests of the workers' (Breitman and Stanton 1977:113-4).

22   CHAPTER TWO

between progressive rhetoric and less progressive reality – the ideal and the material.

Most of the literature and documents on which this study must be based assume that the capitalist market – especially if regulated in some way – offers a suitable model for the development and reform of health care services. Many studies and policy proposals reflect the prevailing 'health care reform agenda' which as Drache and Sullivan (1998:1-2) point out:

> ...has been dominated by economists and policy-makers narrowly focused on deficit reduction and spending controls. [...] All advanced economies now admit some role for markets in their financing and delivery systems.

The underlying contradiction of health care under capitalism

Health is by no means simply a product of health care and medical intervention: it is socially constructed, inevitably reflecting class differences in living standards and conditions. However the focus of this study is specifically on health services, and on the content and objectives of reforms to health services, which can have an impact on the poorest members of society, whose health care needs are likely to be the greatest.

Analysis of the health system reforms has to begin from a grasp of what is a fundamental underlying contradiction: each of the structural and managerial reforms that will be examined is an attempt to remedy the continuing – possibly inevitable – failure of the profit-driven capitalist system to deliver a suitable and affordable supply of health care goods and services to a global market which is driven by 'need' rather than 'want', and which is dominated numerically by people too poor to pay a profitable rate for them (Drache & Sullivan 1999).

Another way of looking at this same contradiction is that while most health care is required by poor people, whose average levels of chronic ill-health are far higher than the wealthy, most political and economic power lies in the hands of the rich[25].

Perhaps the simplest current embodiment of this contradiction is the dilemma facing the pharmaceutical companies over the development of a vaccine to prevent further infection in people already suffering from the AIDS virus. Dyer (a *Financial Times* correspondent) aptly sums up:

> The economics of such a vaccine would be difficult. Dr Berkley points out that the target market would be in poor countries. There would be little demand in the wealthy markets where vaccine developers might hope to recoup investment (Dyer 2003b).

---

25 This in turn may be seen as an updated variation on the 'inverse care law' identified by Tudor Hart more than 40 years ago, according to which the provision of accessible health care is inversely proportional to the level of need (Hart 1971).

Economic overview

1 A major global industry

Health care is one of the world's biggest industries, accounting for global spending just short of $3 trillion in 1997, or almost 8% of the world gross domestic product. It is also a major employer: the health care workforce, numbering upwards of 35 million worldwide[26] is the biggest of any industry (WHO 2000). Policy decisions affecting health care systems therefore affect not only service users, but also potentially the jobs, pay and conditions of the staff employed as professionals, and the large numbers – often on very low comparative rates of pay – providing support services.

Health-related industries, notably those manufacturing pharmaceuticals and modern diagnostic equipment, along with US private health insurers and health maintenance organisations, are among the world's biggest companies, with turnover in tens of billions of dollars. They also generate huge returns for shareholders: for over 30 years from 1960-1991 the US pharmaceutical industry was first or second in the *Fortune 500* league table of post-tax profitability (Mossialos and Mrazek 2002).

This level of commercial investment places additional pressures on health care systems: for example, one of the hardest factors to control in health services anywhere in the world has been the upward pressure in pharmaceutical spending – and the profit margins jealously guarded by the multinational corporations which dominate this market.

2 Health care as a special type of commodity

Capitalism is a system driven by the accumulation of capital, through the production and exchange of commodities. Commodities, as Marx analysed in *Capital*, embody two contradictory values: their use value, without which they would not be saleable in the marketplace; and their exchange value – defined by the hours of necessary labour time for their production. It is from the labour of the working class, itself sold to the capitalist enterprise in the form of a unique commodity, *labour power* – the ability to work – that the capitalist enterprise derives and appropriates surplus value, a portion of which can be retained as capital (Marx 1970, Vol 1 43-161).

Marx begins his critique of the whole system with the analysis of the commodity, seeing in it a microcosm of the social and economic relations within society. An analysis of the health care episode can in similar fashion offer a basis on which to appraise the predominant values and social relations in a given society.

Health care shares with other commodities the combination of 'use value' (in this case additional healthy life, which for the patient remains the key factor). But also, since it is the product of human labour, embodying necessary hours of work (and in many cases access to modern, capital-intensive 'means of production') it embodies potential 'exchange value'. Like other industries under capitalism, health care has moved from small-scale and often primitive 'petty' production (the early predominance of the individual practitioner) to larger-scale

---

26 There is also a very large workforce indirectly linked with health care. Moran (1999:9) calculates that while 2.2 million workers in Germany were directly employed in health care, a further 2 million jobs were dependent upon the health care system.

socialised production (the development of large and complex modern hospitals and health care systems, which rely on the combined efforts of a wide variety of professionals, technicians and support staff).

As a system, capitalism has consistently demonstrated its tendency to develop and revolutionise the productive forces, and with them science and technology (Hoggett 1994): but has not done so evenly. The underlying quest to accumulate surplus value dictates which techniques and which areas of production receive the greatest level of investment.

In health care, since the emergence of scientific medicine, the most profitable areas have been hospital-based and pharmaceutical-based treatments: and on a global scale the greatest investment has focused on the health issues affecting the wealthiest countries – with the greatest ability to pay.

3 The limits of markets

Markets as a means for the exchange of commodities and the realisation of surplus value are the natural state of capitalism. Goods and services are primarily produced *not* for their use value (to match social need), but for their *exchange value*, to generate profit. In a classical market, producers compete to maximise profits while minimising the costs of production: the logical conclusion of successful competition is to win maximum market share, and to force competitors out of business (Malin et al 2002).

Perversely, therefore, the outcome of the ultimate in competition can be its very opposite – *monopoly* control of a market by a few large-scale producers. While competition can be seen as a means to force producers to hold down costs and prices, monopoly gives producers the opportunity to maintain *high* prices, and to exclude new entrants to the market. As Lenin argued in 1916 in his keynote analysis *Imperialism, the Highest Stage of Capitalism*, the extension of the capitalist market and major corporations onto the global level opened up the possibility of *worldwide* monopolies, delivering 'super-profits' to the ruling rich minority at the expense of poverty and exploitation in developing (many of them then colonial) countries (Lenin 1973).

The inherent drive to monopoly within the competitive dynamic appears to be little discussed by advocates of the market system. Instead neoliberals, and the classical economists harking back to Adam Smith, emphasise the role of each individual being free to maximise their own income and happiness, guided only by the 'invisible hand' of the market:

> ...a competitive system is an elaborate mechanism for unconscious coordination through a system of prices and markets (Samuelson 1967, cited in Malin et al 2002:67).

Preferring this 'unconscious' mechanism to conscious attempts at planning provision to meet need, neoliberals seek a minimal role for the state, which they see as distorting the market through attempts to intervene, regulate and control. They take strongest exception to measures such as public funding and provision of health care, which effectively 'decommodifies' and removes a large section of this industry from the market.

Market-style systems have been seen one-sidedly by their proponents as a means of increasing efficiency in health care, and reducing the costs of treatment by stimulating competition – whether this is between financing bodies (insurance funds or HMOs which purchase care on the behalf of the patient/consumer) or between health care providers (hospitals and other facilities) working under contract for the purchaser. Competition between rival funds is commonly termed 'managed competition', while competition between providers can form part of a system of 'managed care' (Flood 2000).

The European Health Care Management Association investigated the proposition that market mechanisms increase productivity – and found little evidence to support it. But they also investigated other propositions: that market mechanisms increase costs, that they separate public health policy from other reforms, and that they reduce the autonomy of professionals. They found evidence from various countries in Europe to support each of these views, while noting that market systems are general incompatible with greater equity in access to health care (EHMA 2000).

The EHMA study demonstrates that it is not necessary to embrace a Marxist analysis to conclude that unbridled market mechanisms are incompatible with the equitable provision of health care. That represents the overwhelming consensus view of academics, economists and governments, and is disputed only by the most fundamentalist of neoliberal theorists (Glennerster and Midgley 1991)[27]. Even the much-constrained 'managed' competition and 'planned markets' that have been proposed as a means to utilise what is seen as a progressive dynamic of competition to improve publicly-funded services have proved controversial, and offered little evidence of success.

4 Market failure in health care

The various sources of 'market failure' have been frequently rehearsed and debated by a wide range of authors from very different standpoints, so this study will examine the argument only briefly. World Bank studies summed up by Dunlop and Martins (1996:196) concur that market mechanisms for the financing of health care:

> …will not ensure either equity or economic efficiency, because of the characteristics of the health care market on both the supply and demand side, which suggest the presence of market failure conditions.

What then are these characteristics? According to Dunlop and Martins (1996:190) the supply side (health care providers) is characterised by imperfect competition and monopolistic practices, among other reasons because:

- Too many economic units are large enough to exert an influence on the prices of goods and services
- There are too few providers to allow competitive pressures to drive down prices, creating effective monopoly positions
- It is prohibitively expensive for new providers to enter the market, and difficult for existing providers to pull out
- There is insufficient standardisation of quality
- There is unequal knowledge on the part of both consumer (patient) and supplier (provider).

---

27 Among the many varied authors embracing the consensus view that a free market mechanism is inappropriate for health care systems, while not necessarily sharing a common analysis of what systems are appropriate, are Saltman and von Otter (1992), Walt (1994), Mohan (1995), Dunlop and Martins (1996), Laurell and Arellano (1996), Enthoven (1997), Appleby (1998), Figueras et al (1998), Drache and Sullivan (1999), Buse and Walt (2000b), Deber (2000), Freeman (2000), Ferge (2001), Leys (2001), Scott (2001), Malin et al (2002), Koivusalo (2003).

On the demand side, the characteristics which undermine the workings of a free market are seen as including:

- Unequal knowledge (dependence on the professional expertise of doctors and nursing staff), which opens up the possibility of supplier-induced demand – or of patients failing to receive adequate care

- The prevalence in advanced economies of 'third party' payment systems (public or private insurance or tax-funded systems) meaning that neither the doctor nor the patient has any incentive to minimise the cost of care

- Demand for health care is often uneven and uncertain: previously healthy individuals may suddenly suffer catastrophic and costly accidents or illness, raising the need for risk-pooling

- A patient suffering pain or life-threatening illness is less likely to 'choose' not to have treatment than a customer for other, more optional, goods and services

- Patients – especially those with chronic conditions or from low income groups – may be excluded from insurance cover through 'adverse selection', while conversely young and fit, prosperous adults of working age and low risk of illness may be 'cherry-picked' by insurance companies, reducing the risk pooling, and increasing the cost to individuals

- Insurance systems are also seen as vulnerable to 'moral hazard' (excessive use of services once the cost for the individual patient is covered by insurance)[28].

An additional problem arising from a market mechanism for the financing and delivery of health care is that it may well not provide for 'externalities' – the provision of immunisation or other public health measures which necessarily extend even to those lacking insurance cover: such a service will benefit the population as a whole by reducing the risk of communicable disease, but financing and delivering such a service effectively require state intervention.

5 Free markets, politics and social forces

Whether or not there is an attempt to realise the exchange value, by trading health care as a conventional commodity (or service, like hair-dressing) for sale in the market-place, is determined by a combination of social, political and economic factors – all of which are *external* to the health care episode itself. Drache and Sullivan offer three possible approaches, variously regarding health care as:

- A service like any other, to be bought and sold in the market

- A 'public good that only states can effectively provide'

---

28 'Moral hazard', although referred to as an established fact by some health economists (Dunlop and Martins 1996) might more realistically be seen as a largely imaginary creation of health economists, under which patients may in theory be tempted to avail themselves of additional unnecessary treatment if it were available to them free of charge. However as Deber (2000) points out, even where health care is available free, demand for it is far from infinite: people demanding it are restricted to those suffering the appropriate condition: 'I doubt if many readers ... would gladly accept free chemotherapy or free open-heart surgery, unless they "needed" it.'

- Something 'closer to what Adam Smith described as a non-market "necessary" for the support of life, that no society can afford to be without'.
(Drache and Sullivan 1999:5)

Clearly the answer to this will depend in each case upon a complex balance of forces, including the politics and electoral or other social base of the government in the country concerned, and the extent to which key decision makers face political or social pressure from different social classes.

The post-war development of welfare state provision in many European countries brought an extension of publicly-funded services or universal social insurance which effectively 'decommodified' health care and other benefits[29]. The extent to which welfare services have been decommodified is one measure used by Esping-Andersen to categorise and compare different types of welfare state (Esping-Andersen 1990), while critics of latter-day social democracy in Britain warn of the 'recommodification of the residual public sector, to promote the role of market forces' (Leys 2001, also Jessop 2003).

The commercial trading of health care as a commodity serves above all the interests of those who are in a position to profit personally from such trade, and who feel themselves sufficiently wealthy and/or powerful to be able to withstand the costs of any treatment they or their families may themselves require. By contrast it may be argued – not least because the 'exchange value' of health care treatment, drawing as it does on the skills and training of specialist and professional staff, means that it can command a price higher than most working people could afford to pay – that the commodification of health care is against the interests of the working class and the rural poor.

Hart argues that the limitations to the expanded production of health care arise not from the boundaries of knowledge, which continue to widen, but the 'ruling assumptions about the nature of the medical care economy':

> The minds of politicians with their hands on state power recognise only one possible kind of economy and one possible mode of production, capitalist production for the market, expanding not to meet human needs but to maximise profit (Hart 2003).

6 When is a market not a market?

Many of the new generation of health system reforms that have emerged in the 1990s claim to make use of the dynamics of market forces such as competition, 'quasi-markets' and market-style measures, not, it is said, primarily to maximise profit, but to improve the efficiency of public health care services. Various contradictory phrases have been coined to sum up this new, supposedly benign application of a system which is inherently unplanned and ill-equipped to secure equity in access to services.

Saltman and Von Otter (1992) responding to market-style reforms in Sweden, Finland and

---

29 After years in which it was largely unchallenged, many health care professionals and consumers have come to see the post-war 'social democratic' consensus of socially funded health care provision as a moral principle, and would tend to agree with Vienonen et al (1999) that 'Markets are amoral'. Yet the failure of health care in the free market is not a moral problem: as has been discussed above, economic factors and the social relations of production under capitalism make health care an exceptional commodity.

the UK, argue the case for 'a hybrid territory between politics and markets'. However the notion of 'planned markets' (in which patient choice between providers becomes the driving force of 'public competition') is as inherently oxymoronic as the fashionable notion of 'managed competition' promoted by Flood (2000) but derided by Marmor (2001, 2002).

Saltman and Von Otter seek to distinguish between 'planned markets' and 'regulated markets', and propose a system of 'public competition' which:

> ...partially uncouples health sector management from political control on matters of economic productivity, but retains public responsibility for normative outcomes... (1992:152)

However the notion of exploiting market-style incentives to remodel publicly-funded services, while not embracing the classical operating objectives of genuine markets (personal gain, corporate profit) is even more problematic in the context of other government objectives – such as reining in state spending, and reducing taxation. Saltman and Von Otter[30] argue that under the new paradigm:

> ...the patient's decision about where to obtain care becomes the decisive factor for steering system-wide resource flows (1992:153).

The contradiction is that – partly because it is NOT a genuine free market, in which the providers would have free access to additional borrowing for capital investment – this new regime cannot ensure the availability of sufficient resources to enable the public sector providers to meet the wishes of patients, even though it appears to prioritise the patient's choice. Full and unfettered availability of services to allow any patient to choose any provider would require a surplus of capacity among public sector health care providers – thus diminishing efficient use of resources, increasing unit costs, and creating new pressure to increase global budgets to facilitate expansion. Meanwhile there is always the underlying threat that if the public sector cannot deliver the capacity and resources to meet levels of expressed demand, the private sector can be expected to take advantage of the opportunity to pick up additional work, and drain precious resources from public sector budgets.

Elsewhere Saltman, apparently oblivious to the contradictions inherent in the concept, has upheld the view that 'the idea of a planned market is a straightforward one' (Saltman 1996). Differentiating between three variants of 'planned markets', to be based on price, on quality or on market share, he argues that:

> A central element of these planned market models is that only system-level expenditures are capped. In both the price-based and the quality-based approach a particular provider doesn't have a fixed prospective global budget... (1996:9)

The tension between a globally fixed budget and competition between providers, in which 'each provider competes for a bigger share of a fixed pie' (1996:10) is that if any providers make gains, others will lose out in revenue terms, while the system overall cannot expand to offer the additional capacity required to offer genuine free choice, or to remedy problems of quality or inadequate capacity in individual providers. With no overall increase in resources, providers seeking to increase their 'efficiency', to reduce prices, or cope with reduced budgets

---

30 Foreshadowing the 'Patient Choice' and 'financial flow' policies ushered in by Britain's New Labour government in 2003.

will have no choice but to cut jobs or squeeze increased effort from their workforce.

Perhaps an even bigger problem is ignored by the Saltman formula: the *cost* of implementing market-style reforms, in terms of increased complexity in administration and accountancy. The British market-style reforms, which introduced a new system of pricing, billing and annual contract negotiations between a large number of purchasers and providers, dramatically increased the previously very low administrative costs of the National Health Service, requiring thousands of additional managerial and clerical staff (Paton 2000). The decision of the New Labour government to retain the purchaser/provider split has meant a further substantial (59%) increase in numbers of senior managers since 1997 (DoH 2004)[31].

Behind this ostensibly 'straightforward' suggestion of applying competition to publicly funded health services, therefore, is a fundamental shift from planning, solidarity and cooperation to division, conflict, competition and fragmentation. Any efficiency savings achieved in the delivery of front-line health services can be undermined by increased costs of more complex bureaucracy, and by the alienation of staff and less coherent treatment of patients in larger, impersonal units (Boyle at al 2004).

And the maintenance of global cash limits may appear to squeeze better value out of public services, but can result in the longer term in a shortfall in investment which leads to a growing reliance on private sector provision. In other words, 'planned' markets carry with them all of the contradictions of 'unplanned' markets.

As noted above[32] the study explores the extent to which changes stem from, lead to, or tacitly reinforce and legitimise defective market-based models, and ask how far it is reasonable to conclude that the new policies can be expected to result in a less egalitarian, less efficient and eventually more expensive system, that will hold back rather than assist improvements in the health and health care of millions.

7 The limits of 'globalisation' as an explanation for reforms

Despite the use of the word 'global' in its title, this study is not primarily focused on exploring the concept of 'globalisation' and its alleged impact on the politics of health care and welfare states. Globalisation alone has generated a substantial literature, but little agreement from the various authors, either on the definition of 'globalisation', or on the extent to which it can be seen to influence health sector reform[33] – and whether that influence can be seen as for better or for worse, or a combination of the two (Labonte et al 2004:1-12). Palier and Sykes (2001:2) argue that globalisation is a 'buzz-word' used to suggest 'a whole range of phenomena'. Yeates (2001:4) also argues that:

> Globalisation is a highly contested term, the frequent use of which has tended to obscure a lack
> of consensus with regard to what it entails, explanations of how it operates and the directions in

---

31 Management numbers in proportion to front-line nursing and administrative staff have also increased, with almost 25% fewer admin and clerical staff, and 50% fewer qualified nurses per manager in 2003 than in 1995 (DoH 2004).

32 Chapter one, page 5

33 As Palier and Sykes (2001) point out, so many accounts have been developed since the mid 1990s that it is not feasible here to cite all of the available references on globalisation, let alone to explore them in this study. Palier and Sykes recommend textbooks by Held et al (1999) and Baylis and Smith (1999), although much more has been published since then.

which it is heading.

Yeates, citing Petrella (1996), elaborates seven types of globalisation, relating to:

- Finances and ownership
- Markets and strategies
- Technology and knowledge
- Modes of life, consumption patterns and culture
- Regulator capabilities
- Globalisation as the political unification of the world
- Globalisation of perception and consciousness.

(Yeates 2001:5)

However while some or all of these variants of globalisation as analysed by Yeates can be seen to play a role in the developing pressure on health care systems, none relates specifically to the reform process within health care systems that is the main focus of this study. As Yeates argues, reference to 'globalisation' has been used to help explain changes in very different areas of enquiry: political science, economics, geography, sociology and social policy among them (2001:15). Yeates is also careful to distinguish between the concepts of 'strong' globalisation as an irresistible economic force compelling governments into action, which she criticises as economistic, deterministic and reductionist: and a more nuanced version which incorporates issues of political agency and social conflict.

Palier and Sykes draw a similar distinction between 'apocalyptic' versions (attributed to Mishra 1999), and versions in which globalisation is 'as much a political and ideological phenomenon as an economic one' (2001:5). These authors argue that there is a two-way process of pressure and legitimisation, in which the ideological globalisation perspective of bodies such as the World Bank, OECD and European Commission 'provides welfare reformers with a certain repertoire of reforms' (often neoliberal), while:

...the threat of globalisation provides governments with ideological justification for their welfare state changes (2001:11).

The 'globalisation of the social policy process' is described (Yeates 2001:28) as centred on 'general agreements reached by participants in international fora such as the UN or G7 summits': yet while these bodies (though very different) can be seen as gatherings of equals, health system reforms appear in the main to have been transmitted from the wealthier countries to the poorest not through voluntary engagement and agreement, but through the pressure and even through the intervention of less egalitarian global organisations. In this context Deacon (2001) draws attention to the 'hidden politics' of the World Bank, IMF, WTO and OECD, and their role in encouraging neoliberal forms of globalisation.

Accounts often suggest that globalisation is not so much one uniform process, but a collective label for a variety of pressures on governments. Yeates, echoing Deacon et al (1997) points to the preoccupation of governments and 'international bureaucracies' with the regulation of global capitalism. Yet she also notes the strength of neoliberalism, which favours minimal – if any – regulation of the capitalist market, and concludes that there is little sign of the emergence of a unitary view or ideology on welfare policy 'either within or between international institutions'.

Historical and political overview

a) The material and political roots of reform

The reforms examined here are relatively recent, and represent a new stage in the evolution of health care policy. In many cases they appear to have been inspired by what George and Wilding (2002:64) sum up as a 'globalised faith in market mechanisms'. However, it is useful to recall that today's reforms are in many cases re-shaping systems which were themselves the product of substantial earlier reforms, and which were also a response to material and political circumstances and ideological pressures.

From his earliest writings developing a materialist view of history, Marx (in *The German Ideology*) argued that:

> The ideas of the ruling class are in every epoch the ruling ideas, i.e. the class which is the ruling material force of society, is at the same time its ruling intellectual force (Marx 1970:64).

If this general statement – which is intended to locate the material and class origin of 'ruling ideas' which otherwise might simply be seen as abstractions – were taken too literally, one might assume that market-style policies would have enjoyed continued dominance for as long as the capitalist system remains in place. But no political process is that simple. Marx also makes clear that there is always scope for differences of opinion and a degree of disunity within the camp of the ruling rich, just as there is within other social classes.

This is because thought and ideas inevitably reflect the material world, within which constant and complex changes take place, requiring adjustment to both theory and practice. As Kelsey (1995) argues, analysing New Zealand's reforms in the 1980s, governments may be confronted by objective pressures and situations – but these do not lead automatically to any one inevitable conclusion: governments always have choices.

b) The post-war welfarist consensus

One of the key historic periods of choice came in 1945, when Europe's weakened and bankrupt ruling classes faced a new post-war political reality. They had to devise a new approach that could safeguard stability and rebuild a system that had been shattered and destabilised by war. The emergence of Keynesian economics and a 'welfarist' consensus in much of Europe reflected a new balance of class forces, in which capitalist classes found themselves having to deal with the expectations and demands of a more militant working class (reflected also in the strengthening of social democratic and Communist parties) which they were poorly placed to confront.

Only the USA, where the economy had been relatively untroubled by the war, and where the absence of even a social-democratic party of the working class helped ensure that the post-war wave of trade union militancy remained largely confined to economic rather than political objectives, remained largely unaffected by the new situation (Armstrong et al 1984).

The new economics and welfarism were no threat to capitalism, but a means of ensuring its survival. Even the 'socialists' and 'Communists'[34] within post-war reformist and coalition governments in Western Europe lacked either the courage or the political commitment to press for socialist solutions, but instead joined with the capitalists – who in turn embraced the Bismarck technique of cooption, and purchased a degree of social peace by offering concessions to the working class and the middle classes. The policy was shared by most major political parties: in Britain, for example, where some of the most sweeping changes took place[35], the post-war Labour government's development of a welfare state as part of a reconstructed capitalist state followed social policies drawn up by a Liberal, and reflected a broad (if not precise and detailed) consensus with the Conservative Party (Doyal 1979, Timmins 1995).

The political consensus around this type of 'post-war settlement' dominated much of Western Europe through the boom years of the 1950s and 1960s, during which time health care and other welfare spending grew substantially (Alcock 2001): but a generalised recession in 1974-5 ended what had been a prolonged period of economic growth and expansion of welfare state provision, and most OECD governments have since then been seeking policies to contain what had been an inexorable rise in health care spending from the early 1960s (Abel-Smith et al 1995, OECD 1995a).

As Saltman and von Otter sum up, by the 1980s:

> The logic of neo-classical economics had begun to replace that of classical democratic politics as the core theoretical basis upon which to evaluate all types of social activity. Markets were increasingly seen to embody the virtues that politics, and with it public sector organisation, appeared to lack... (1992:6)

c) Constrained consensus: market-driven reforms

Although statistics of health care spending show that these efforts at containment were generally less than completely successful – and in most of the wealthiest countries health care has continued to consume an ever-growing share of national wealth and of government spending (Moran 1999:2-3) – most observers agree that in this early period policies for restructuring and rationalising health services were often drawn up more for financial than health reasons. An OECD study, analysing changes in the 30 years to 1990 argues that:

> ...the combined weight of medical technology *and of financial pressures* contributed to a rationalisation in the supply of [acute] beds (OECD 1992:166).

The same OECD report also noted the extent to which cost-cutting measures in the wealthier countries were driven by the wider pressures of a competitive world market. The signs of an 'overall convergence' in the health care policies of OECD countries were seen as:

> ...the result of market forces which lessen each country's discretion to go its own way (OECD 1992:16).

These measures are therefore examined in this study under the general heading of 'market-driven' reforms. However it is also necessary to explain why they need to be addressed as 'reforms' at all, rather than as economy measures: the issue is one of political presentation.

---

34 Despite the abolition of the Communist International during the war, Communist Parties in Western Europe were at this stage still firmly controlled by the Kremlin, and followed Stalin's general strategy of 'peaceful coexistence' with capitalism, including the 'Parliamentary Road to Socialism' (Black 1970, Wohlforth & Westoby 1978).

35 Not least with the nationalisation of the hospital network and establishment of a new National Health Service offering universal access free at point of use, based on need rather than ability to pay (Armstrong et al 1984).

Most cost-saving measures, involving cutbacks in popular publicly funded services, are inherently politically unpopular, especially when they declare their intentions openly: most Western European-style health care systems offer near-total coverage of the entire population[36], and are so dependent upon public (government) spending that any attempt to cut or even hold down health spending becomes a highly-charged political issue (Chinitz et al 1998, Armstrong et al 2001:2). One consequence of this is that cost-cutting changes are often presented not as straightforward economies, but as 'reforms' – 'centralising', 'rationalising' or 'modernising' services.

Although such thin disguises are seldom sufficient to conceal the underlying purpose[37], these market-driven measures are therefore analysed in this study as one part of the 'menu' of reform.

d) Breaking the consensus: market-style reforms

However the other main strand of reform has very different political and ideological roots. Many market-style reforms have actually brought a commitment to *increased* state and private spending – not least the sharply increased costs of administering the new 'market-style' NHS in Britain after 1991 and New Zealand after 1993, and the higher costs of private health insurance which had been encouraged by government tax incentives in Australia (Ham 1999, Drache & Sullivan 1999, Birrell et al 2003).

The key driving factor in these changes has *not* been financial pressure (Moran 1999, Mossialos and Dixon 2002). Rather, they flow from the ideological New Right, a political current championed by Hayek and Milton Friedman, which had never disappeared in the US, or relented in its opposition to welfare state provision and Keynesian economics (Harrison et al 1990). In a context of growing economic crisis from the mid 1970s, this strand of ideology began to influence a new section of right wing political leaders seeking a break from welfarism, who now felt strong enough to opt for confrontation with the working class, rather than consensus. It led to a new approach based on 'rolling back' the 'nanny state', privatisation, competitive tendering, deregulation, reduced taxation and an emphasis on 'possessive individualism' as an alternative to collectivism and social solidarity (Jones 1994, Malin et al 2002).

As Jones (1994) argues, such ideas were also able to find a purchase in genuine problems and shortfalls in health and welfare provision: some of the arguments developed by the New Right as weapons to attack the welfare state as 'bureaucratic', 'inefficient', 'remote', and 'ineffective' were shamelessly taken from criticisms originating on the left, among campaigners pressing for more responsive, local and democratic services, protesting at the perverse incentives of the 'poverty trap' effect, and complaining of continued inequalities in health.

Margaret Thatcher's rise to the leadership of the Conservative Party coincided with, and reinforced, the gathering ideological challenge to welfarism. In parallel, Thatcher in Britain and

---

36 As such European systems have more in common with each other than any has in common with the US model (Freeman 2000, Kokko et al 1998).

37 Examples in Britain include the Worcestershire Health Authority's boldly-titled *Investing in Excellence* (1997) which involved the loss of more than a quarter of the county's acute beds including all in Kidderminster Hospital, and West Hertfordshire's Choosing the Right Direction (1998) which again centred on substantial cost-saving rationalisation.

Ronald Reagan from the Republican right in the US bid for office arguing that 'big government' was strangling enterprise (Clarke et al 2001). Thatcher's election victory in 1979 brought in a Conservative government which could experiment with some of the policies devised by the New Right[38]. For health care, this began with a combination of market-driven constraints on health spending, coupled in the mid 1980s with two policies which anticipated elements of what was later to be branded as the 'New Public Management':

- Managerialist changes designed to break from the old ethos of NHS administration and consensus, and strengthen the hand of management in dealing with senior medical professionals; and...

- The imposition of competitive tendering for most non-clinical hospital support services ('steering, not rowing').

e) The neoliberal agenda: a 'Washington consensus'

These were the opening shots in a 'new right' offensive on welfarism, the underlying ideology and assumptions of which combine the neoliberal[39] assertion that the private sector is

---

38 However, the health service remained so hugely popular with the electorate that even Thatcher repeatedly insisted it would be 'safe in our hands'. Her government also resisted continual efforts from the right wing of the Conservative Party to promote more radical, right wing reforms such as wholesale privatisation, voucher schemes, opt-out schemes – and other devices that would expand private provision at the expense of declining services for the poor and elderly (Caldwell et al 1998).

39 'Neoliberal' is the general description of a set of economic policies related to economic liberalism, the notion of allowing the fullest freedom of the market, originally associated with the writings of Adam Smith. His study The Wealth of Nations, published in 1776 has inspired a new generation of 'free market' fundamentalists since the late 1960s, amid the decline of the post-war Keynesian/Social Democratic consensus. Among the more prominent and influential neoliberals have been University of Chicago economist Milton Friedman (whose 'Chicago Boys' advised the Pinochet dictatorship in Chile from 1973), and philosopher-economist Friederich von Hayek. Backed by important sections of the US super-rich, their ideas have been promoted by a powerful network of right wing foundations, institutes and research centres. Neoliberals and neoliberal policies have also been prominent in the work of the IMF, the World Bank and USAID. Von Hayek was a direct influence on British Prime Minister Margaret Thatcher, while neoliberal institutes have long been linked with the US Republican Party: the Heritage Foundation, the principal think-tank for Ronald Reagan's administration, has remained an influential force in US politics. The main elements of neoliberalism can be summed up as:

- The rule of the market, liberating 'free' private enterprise from any restrictions or regulations and de-unionising workers
- Cutting public expenditure for social services, health and education
- Deregulation
- Privatisaton of state-owned enterprises, including utilities supplying power and water as well as health care, schools, railways and roads
- Eliminating the concept of 'community' and the 'public good', replacing them with individual responsibility.
  (Martinez & Garcia 1997, George 1999, Coburn 2000)

The influence of neoliberal ideology in the formulation of health system reforms has been noted by many critics, including Collins and colleagues who point specifically to the links with so-called 'user choice', promotion of the private sector, the introduction of competition, markets, decentralisation and new incentives, limits on the public sector, and changes in the finance of health care including user fees and private health insurance (Collins et al 1999:76).

inevitably more efficient and more responsive as a provider of services, and the neo-Conservative emphasis on the traditional role of the family and the individual (Clarke et al 2001).

On health and other areas of policy the neoliberals aimed to:

- Reduce the role of the state
- Change the role of the state from provider to purchaser and regulator
- Break up the state monopoly of welfare provision
- Encourage 'consumers' to make choices about the services and service providers they used.

Such structural reforms can run alongside cost-cutting: soaring spending on both public and privately-funded sectors of health care in the USA in the 1970s had brought a succession of measures aimed at curbing costs[40]. The new Reagan administration from January 1981 lost no time in pressing home cuts in spending and a deregulation of medical care, but followed this with more elaborate measures to hold down spending, introducing the concept of Diagnosis Related Groups of treatments which would receive fixed payments (Patel and Rushefsky 1999).

The monetarist, free-market, policies of the British and US governments of Margaret Thatcher and Ronald Reagan brought wider acceptance of what became the dominant 'neoliberal' model for politics and economics, the basic package of which was summed up by Williamson (1990) as the 'Washington consensus'. Among the ten basic broad propositions for policy reform at the centre of this 'consensus' were five which relate directly to the subject of this study:

- Fiscal discipline
- A redirection of public expenditure priorities toward fields offering both high economic returns and the potential to improve income distribution, such as primary health care, primary education, and infrastructure
- Liberalisation of inflows of foreign direct investment
- Privatisation
- Deregulation (to abolish barriers to entry and exit to and from the market). (Williamson 2000:252-3)

Williamson now argues that his list stopped short of some of the more extreme neoliberal propositions. Writing for the World Bank's own journal, he insists that the 'consensus' he described should have been seen not as a policy prescription based on the most hard-line free market principles, but as a 'lowest common denominator' of the reforms 'Washington' could agree on for Latin America in 1989. He argues that the term 'consensus' was merely intended to sum up the dominant approach of both the US government and the Washington-based institutions shaping the world economy – the World Bank and the IMF, and that by 1990 some

---

40 Including support from the Nixon administration for the launch of the first Health Maintenance Organisations in 1973, and failed attempts by Jimmy Carter's administration to impose limits on hospital costs, thrown out by Congress in 1980 after three years of debate (Patel and Rushefsky 1999).

of the most radical free-market policies had been toned down or dropped:

> ...the market fundamentalism of Reagan's first term had already been superseded by the return
> of rational policymaking (2000:255).

However Williamson also concedes that the various Washington policy makers *were* looking to develop global models that would be applied to a very wide range of diverse countries. Interestingly, he admits that in this sense there *was* at that time a form of underlying 'blueprint' for all developing countries, so that:

> ...there probably would not have been a lot of difference if I had undertaken a similar exercise
> for Africa or Asia (Williamson 2000:254-5).

The 1990s saw the 'Washington consensus' widely applied as the basis of policy advice and prescriptions from global bodies to developing countries. And while the primary targets were lower state spending, privatisation and the maximum deregulation of the market, the accompanying neoliberal rejection of notions of social solidarity was summed up by Margaret Thatcher's insistence – echoing von Hayek and a long tradition of laissez-faire advocates of individualism going back to Adam Smith and de Tocqueville – that:

> There is no such thing as society. There are individual men and women, and there are families
> (Timmins 1995:433).

f) The limitations of neoliberalism

Although the term 'neoliberal' is widely (and often loosely) used by critics to describe the ideology and reforms proposed or inspired by sections of the New Right, the most radical section of neoliberals embrace policies which very few politicians or publicly accountable health care planners could be seen to endorse.

One example of this extreme view is Aubrey, a doctor writing in the *Medical Sentinel*, who explicitly defends the idea that medicine should properly be seen as 'a commodity produced by profit-seeking entrepreneurial physicians, working in a free market, and purchased by their patients' (Aubrey 2001). Pauly (2000), approvingly introducing a volume of neoliberal essays, states:

> Is health care so different from other goods and services that a dominant role for government is
> inevitable or desirable? American Health Care addresses that important question and answers it
> with a qualified 'no' (Pauly 2000:ix).

Any policy designed to ensure equity in health care, especially if it involves government intervention to regulate private sector providers in the health care marketplace, or the raising of progressive taxation to subsidise care for the poor, is likely to incur the wrath of the hard-line defenders of the free market.[41] In American neoliberal publications, and US websites such as the Heartland Institute and Independence Institute, doctors, right wing theorists and academics decry as 'socialism' or even 'fascism' any attempt by government to intervene in the

---

41 'Any limit on technology, any restraint on drug firm profits, any fee schedule for doctors – all will apparently ruin the quality of US health care. Those willing to challenge that assumption are hard pressed to gain access to the media' (Marmor 1999:262).

market or to 'manage' competition (Aubrey 2001, Dorman 1999). For such ideologically driven proponents of the free market, even such elementary public health precautions such as gun control and discouragement of smoking tobacco are unreasonable intrusions into the lives of individuals.

Neoliberalism has been well described by Bourdieu (1998) as a 'utopia of endless exploitation'. However health care systems, like other aspects of the economy in democratic countries, are shaped and driven not only by economics, and ideology, but also by *political* considerations and interests. In democracies, governments have to be elected, and policies have to win the backing of an appropriate alliance of forces in order to be implemented: key players include the pharmaceutical industry, other major suppliers of health care equipment, medical professionals, and of course the main political parties, each with an eye to the practical and electoral consequences of the policies they adopt.

For neoliberals, therefore, there is a serious and insoluble problem: their ideas presume the workings of a free and perfect market, which clearly does not, and cannot, exist. Worse: their ideas are so inherently unpopular among the majority of the population that it is almost impossible for any democratically-elected government to implement and test them out (Mills et al 2001, Collins et al 1999). Decades of experience in the USA, the most heavily private health care system in the OECD, with the world's most powerful lobby of neoliberal pressure groups and academics, have left American neoliberals frustrated and bitterly critical of successive governments' failure to carry through their favoured model[42] (Health Policy Consensus Group 2001, Armey 2001, Scandlen 2003).

Indeed even when democracy has been swept away, and political obstacles crushed, the inherent contradictions of a completely liberalised, privatised, free market health care system have restricted the options of the most brutal dictatorships. General Pinochet's regime, which privatised so much of the economy during its period of military rule in Chile, left a health care system in which private hospital capacity and private insurance had been expanded for the wealthy, but the public sector had also been retained as a safety net service for the most serious and costly health problems of those too poor to pay private premiums or hospital bills (De La Jara and Bossert 1995, Fiedler 1996, Reichard 1996, Trumper and Phillips 1997, Bertranou 1999, Bitran et al 2000, Taylor 2003).

Because of this inherent problem, the pressure from neoliberalism has been channelled into other, more pragmatic 'market-style' policies, centred not so much on establishing the full freedoms of the market, but on attempting to devise or copy (especially from the USA) methods of maximising the role of the private sector while restraining and 'managing' the market, competition and entrepreneurialism, to avoid their worst, most wasteful, excesses (Enthoven 1985, 1997, 2003, Hunter 1998, Laurell and Arellano 1996, Saltman and von Otter 1992, Saltman et al 2002).

Laurell and Arellano (1996) and Deacon (2001) are among those who have detected the confusion and contradiction running through many of the policy documents of the World

---

42 Their anger is paralleled by the disappointment of those seeking a more socially progressive reform, which also foundered under the Clinton Presidency, having also failed to construct a suitably broad coalition of political support (Marmor 1998). The influence of neoliberalism in the USA is underlined by the fact that even socialist campaigners have in recent years focused on socialising the finance rather than the provision of health care (PNHP 2003a, 2003b).

Bank, which is instinctively aligned with neoliberalism, but which feels obliged in its policies to make reference to 'equity'. Indeed the Bank's more astute analysts appeared by the end of the 1990s to have begun to concede pragmatically that the neoliberal model cannot be fully implemented in the area of health care, and that public provision must play a key role if key areas of health care are to be delivered to those in greatest need:

> ...it is evident that government intervention is essential to ensure equitable and efficient delivery and financing of health care (IFC 2002:16).

Significantly, the Bank (here represented by its sub-division the International Finance Corporation[43]) intends this public sector intervention to restrict itself to those low-cost peripheral areas of public health, health education, immunisation and preventive services which the private sector is least interested in providing.

g) Neoliberalism meets Social democracy: the 'Third Way'

Doyal (1979) argues that even among those most wedded to the capitalist mode of production there have been different approaches to the question of whether health care should be bought and sold in the same way as any other commodity. Many political parties are committed not to abolishing, but to reforming capitalism. The most influential of these have been 'social democratic' (sometimes calling themselves 'socialist') parties, which – having decades ago renounced their Marxist origins in the Second International – have become wedded to the notion of purely parliamentary action to secure progressive legislation for reforms benefiting their largely working class electoral base.

The post-war 'social democratic consensus' led governments of various political parties in most of the industrialised countries to develop 'welfare state' provision, including health care[44]: other European governments followed suit developing public health care systems at a later stage[45] – as did Canada, which broke from a US-style private insurance system to establish Medicare in 1971. These developments took place in the context of generalised economic expansion, partly on the basis of post-war reconstruction, and partly driven by an expansion in mass production of consumer goods.

Even the most expensive of the publicly-funded schemes have also proved to be relatively cost-effective systems for capitalism, incurring only a fraction of the massive overheads in administration costs which help inflate the costs of US health care. Indeed, while proposals for publicly-funded health care have been largely unsuccessful in the US, there has nevertheless been a degree of socialisation of financing of services for the elderly, children and the very poor through Medicare, Medicaid and state-level funding of public hospitals. These, plus extensive

---

43 The IFC's main concern is expanding the role of the private sector (Lethbridge 2002).

44 Welfare state systems can be seen as concessions to the strength of the working class, or as a means to ensure the active or passive acquiescence of a strong working class in the continued operation of capitalism (Saltman and von Otter 1992, Navarro 1992a). However, social concessions to coopt workers are by no means the prerogative of left wing or social democratic governments: the authoritarian Bismarck government in Germany was the first to identify an advantage in binding the otherwise alienated and increasingly organised working class to the capitalist state with a social insurance system in the late 19th century (Freeman 2000).

45 Italy (1978), Portugal (1979), Greece (1983), Spain (1986)

provision of tax breaks for privately-financed insurance schemes[46], have meant that the result has been a situation in which the US population is 'Paying for National Health Insurance, but not getting it' (Woolhandler & Himmelstein 2002).

However the end of the period of capitalist 'boom' opened a new period of intensified global competition, bringing a rise of neoliberalism and the simultaneous erosion of old-style social democratic parties and politics. According to Saltman and Von Otter (1992), the reason why the health policy debate in Northern Europe increasingly began to focus on the question of the introduction of competition into publicly operated health services was linked with the demise of 'classical democratic politics' as a result of various factors, including:

- A decline in the strength and organisation of the working class, leaving governments freer to mould services to the more individualistic, consumerist needs and wishes of the middle class

- Younger people increasingly reluctant to accept standardised services

- The service sector was larger than manufacturing in most Western economies, looking to improve efficiency; health care as the biggest service industry became a focus for attention.

While all of these factors are empirically verifiable, this analysis of the forces driving change appears to focus more on the conditions in which a political offensive *could* be waged than on explaining why governments would feel obliged to run the political risks involved in forcing through controversial changes in highly popular public services. The fact that some governments have advanced far further and more rapidly than others on market-style reforms suggests that more overtly political and ideological factors are driving the process of change, rather than general and objective trends.

The new conditions have helped create a new dominant element within social democracy, that has been described as the 'Third Way' – a political approach supported by such leading politicians as former US President Bill Clinton, British Prime Minister Blair, Brazil's President Lula, and German Chancellor Schroeder. Its events have been sponsored by sections of big business, and have incorporated elements of the neoliberal agenda while discarding some of the concepts which previously defined social democracy[47] (Elliott 2003, Madarasz 2003).

The Third Way seeks to distance itself from class politics and collective 'socialist' objectives, and to focus instead on the individual consumer, and on 'partnerships' between public and private sectors. It also embraces the main precepts of the New Public Management, and seeks to smooth away inequalities through reforms designed to appear 'radical', but remain amenable to the wealthy capitalist elite (Blair 2001, 2003).

While traditional social democracy favoured reforms involving planning and active

---

46 According to neoliberal critics, the tax-break subsidy for employment-based health insurance in the US is worth an estimated $125 billion a year (Health Policy Consensus Group 2001).

47 Elliott (2003) sums up by arguing that 'third wayers are free marketers who have learned how to play the chords to Stairway to Heaven'. The conference in the UK was attended by 400 think tank analysts: it was followed by a summit meeting of leaders from 14 nations, including Germany, Canada, Poland, Hungary, Romania, Czech Republic, Chile, Argentina, Brazil, New Zealand, South Africa and Ethiopia.

management of capitalism, Third Way politicians have moved substantially towards the neoliberal approach, favouring the free working of the capitalist market system, with a minimum of regulation[48] – summed up in Britain as 'Thatcherism with a Christian Socialist face' (Jessop 2003). The Third Way also differs sharply from traditional social democracy in drawing no distinction between the purchase of services from the private or public sector.

In Britain this has led to the use of private capital to finance 94% of new hospitals since 1997 through the Private Finance Initiative[49], a new 'Concordat' with the private sector to treat more NHS-funded patients (Leys 2001), the establishment of a new network of private, for-profit Diagnostic and Treatment Centres delivering care to NHS patients, and the establishment of a new 'patient's choice' system that is already beginning to divert more NHS patients to private hospitals, financed from the public sector budget[50] (Plumridge and Kemp 2004). This is a more subtle approach than simply 'privatising' care: it enables the private sector to select its chosen areas and services, and to benefit from popular public sector budgets. As Tudor Hart points out:

> There is no question of total privatisation in the sense that medical care for the mass of people will ever be returned to the market. The new global capitalism is a true and devoted partnership between governments and multinational corporations (Hart 2003).

h) Pressures to conform

By the 1980s many governments were already embracing the ideology of the free market in many areas of economic activity: many were seeking to privatise public services and utilities, and step away from direct ownership and control. This helps explain why, even as European governments struggled to hold down the costs of largely state-funded health services, they became more receptive to ideas drawn from the very different, hugely expensive, but technically very advanced health care system in the USA. Moran argues that even though the UK had developed a health care system that was very good at cost containment, the new model for health system reform became the 'stunningly expensive' US, where health care was a 'complete policy fiasco':

> More generally the diffusion of institutional innovation seemed to be from the system that was conspicuously failing at cost containment: it was the United States, not the United Kingdom or Scandinavia, that was state of the art as far as health care reform was concerned. In the international diffusion of health care reforms, apparently nothing succeeded like failure (Moran 1999:xi).

---

48 Clearly minimal regulation is not the same as no regulation at all – which despite the enthusiasm of today's neoliberals and their predecessors has not prevailed as a policy with any government since the brief heyday of 'laissez faire' economics in Britain in the early 19th century.

49 PFI was aptly described by Conservative Chancellor Kenneth Clarke in 1993 as 'Privatising the process of capital investment in our key public services, from design to construction to operation' (Lister 2002:1).

50 Tony Blair in an article on 'Where the Third Way goes from here' goes even further, suggesting 'We should be far more radical about the role of the state as regulator rather than provider, opening up healthcare for example to a mixed economy under the NHS umbrella, and adopting radical approaches to self-health. We should also ... be willing to experiment with new forms of co-payment in the public sector' (Blair 2003).

In this context one of the influential figures who won an audience among western governments was American economist Alain Enthoven. He was one of the many economists, politicians and academics seeking ways of 'managing' the chaotic and ruinously expensive private market in health care in the USA. His proposals for restricting the costs of private medical insurance through the introduction of 'managed care', offering a restricted range of funded treatments from a restricted range of 'preferred providers' (Enthoven 1978), led to an influential paper on the British NHS (Enthoven 1985). This pamphlet, with its proposal for a competitive 'internal market' within the NHS, was acknowledged to be the kernel of the Conservative government's market-style reforms,[51] once the more outlandish New Right notions from back bench Conservatives had been discarded.

The British health care reforms, in turn, served to encourage other governments to contemplate their own market-style reforms, notably New Zealand, which also looked to Enthoven for inspiration as it implemented its own variant of a 'managed market' system in 1991 (Enthoven 1988).

In most cases, such as in Sweden during a brief three-year period of conservative-liberal government in 1991-4, the changes which resulted have been slower and much more partial than those in the UK (Freeman 2000). However these pioneering health care reforms triggered a new worldwide interest both in the corporatisation of hospitals (established as NHS Trusts in the UK, Crown Health Enterprises in New Zealand) and in the introduction of competition and quasi-markets into publicly-funded health services (Preker and Harding 2003). The early 1990s saw further moves towards private sector involvement in public services, with the development in the UK of the Private Finance Initiative (PFI) as a means to privatise the capital investment programme in publicly-funded health care (Sussex 2001, Lister 2001, IFC 2002).

i) Ideological bias of reforms

The overall political thrust of the reforms in the last 20 years has been politically rightwards, away from notions of social solidarity. The range of alternative policies for welfare backed by global (World Bank and IMF) and supranational (OECD) organisations is limited, and 'currently confined to variants of liberalism', while:

> ...there is a marked absence of any international institution advancing a social democratic or
> redistributive agenda (Yeates 2001:29).

Deacon (2001) draws a similar conclusion – that no international organisation, with the possible exception of UNICEF, embraces a Scandinavian-type redistributive approach to social policy. Sections of the political left have found it too easy to refer to 'globalisation' as the root cause of social problems such as unemployment, poverty, austerity and 'structural adjustment programmes', without recognising the extent of complicity and corruption of national governments and political leaders. Such political factors can be decisive: Ferge, examining developments in Central and Eastern Europe, raises the issue of the ideological driving force behind the reform process:

---

51 Embodied in the White Paper *Working for Patients*, and the subsequent NHS & Community Care Act (DoH 1989, DoH 1990, Ham 1999).

In the short term, cutbacks in state spending are an economic necessity. This does not fully explain, however, why the welfare system had become the main target of cutbacks, and why the cuts are implemented in a way that affects long-term commitment in all areas of public well-being (Ferge 2001:150).

Arguing that 'politics matter', Yeates (2001:127) criticises the excessive weight given to economic forces and the downplaying of political factors by all those who argue a 'strong' role for globalisation as a force 'bulldozing' reluctant governments into policies. She stresses the importance of political counter-pressures which can limit the scope for implementation of market-style reforms, notably social conflict, political opposition and class struggle at a national level, and notes that this has increasingly led to international pressures and campaigns explicitly challenging capitalist globalisation. Pierson, too, argues that:

> Few serious commentators on social policy accept the globalisation story in its simplest and most draconian form (Pierson 1998:64).

But of course globalisation has its supporters: the political right and 'third way' social democrats have welcomed 'globalisation' as offering new opportunities and advances, while ignoring the negative side-effects of growing inequality and social exclusion on a global level.

This study recognises a global dimension to health system reforms, and is focused on the role of global bodies as well as pressures for reform which cannot be reduced to the specifics in single countries or even groups of countries. But because the focus is on variation and diversity in the application of a common 'menu' of reforms, there will be little focus on 'globalisation' as such.

Nevertheless, the very existence of a common global 'menu' of reforms, and the prevalence of market-style reforms despite the lack of evidence to show them to be effective or efficient, strongly suggests the existence of some form of global pressure towards reform. The next chapter outlines some of the organisations which can be seen to play an active or passive role in the proliferation of a limited range of reforms, and their relationship to the political and ideological forces discussed above.

Chapter three

In the driving seat:
International agencies and the transmission of policy ideas

This chapter will look at some of the organisations whose policies and influence have shaped the international reform agenda, exploring the economic, historical, and political context and content of the policies they promote. It begins with perhaps the most influential of them all, the closely linked 'Bretton Woods' institutions, the World Bank and International Monetary Fund, before examining other organisations and policy circles promoting neoliberal and market-style reforms. These include the European Central Bank, the OECD, the WTO and regional free trade areas, as well as academics, institutions and NGOs sponsored by the Bank and USAID. The chapter concludes by analysing the historical and political evolution and the political influence of the World Health Organisation.

World Bank

Historical origins

The World Bank, like the IMF, was established in 1946 as one of the institutions charged with stabilising and assisting the development of world capitalism after World War 2, and as Williams (1994:111) notes:

> The World Bank has never pretended to be anything other than a capitalist enterprise with a commitment to free trade, the optimisation of investment flows and the support of free enterprise.

While the IMF's task has been to extend loans to relieve balance of payments deficits and ensure stable currencies and economies, the Bank's role was originally to lend for long-term development, beginning with the reconstruction of war-torn Europe, and then focusing on industrialisation. Only since the 1980s has the Bank's focus (and influence) concentrated on the poorest developing countries, though it was denounced as early as 1982 as:

> ...perhaps the most important instrument of the developed capitalist countries for prying state control of its Third World member countries out of the hands of nationalists and socialists who would regulate international capital's inroads, and turning that power to the service of international capita (Payer 1982:20, cited in Williams 1994).

More recently the Bank has claimed to have embraced poverty reduction as its overarching goal, emerging as 'the world's foremost development agency' (Williams 1994:101).

The Bank[52] now covers 184 member countries, but although it purports to be in favour of democracy, openness and accountability, its internal structure has left it vulnerable to veto by the US or ideological capture by the most powerful of the wealthy countries, as the recent appointment of George Bush's neo-conservative nominee Paul Wolfowitz – the eager architect and proponent of the war in Iraq, and advocate of further use of military force to export the US notion of 'democracy' – to take over the presidency so vividly underlines. Its governance arrangements reflected the initial reality when the Bank was first established, when it depended upon the industrialised countries for funding. But funds from these 'donor' countries now represent only a small share of the Bank's lending[53], much of which is raised through loans on the financial markets and from interest payments on the billions already extended in long-term loans (Christian Aid 2003)[54].

Nevertheless the balance of voting strength reflects the post-war situation in which, in addition to the US, seven countries (the UK, France, Germany, Japan, Saudi Arabia, Russia and China) have a full vote in their own right – leaving the remaining 176 member countries to share 16 seats on the Board. The US alone has 16% of the votes, while just 15% is required to block a decision by either the World Bank or IMF Board. Five of the world's richest G7 countries, none of which borrows from the Bank any more, share over 20% of the votes, while the world's 80 poorest countries have a combined voting strength of just 10% on the Bank's Board, and the combined voting strength of 50 African countries is less than half that of the US[55]. Only European members and the US can nominate candidates for the two top jobs in both Bank and the IMF. In 2002 92% of the Bank's Board and 100% of the IMF Board were men (Christian Aid 2003).

To some extent even this summary gives an exaggerated view of the level of accountability and democracy in the Bank: in practice the influence of even executive directors in the operational running of the Bank has been marginalised since 1947, while all of the Bank's presidents have been US citizens (Williams 1994). It is small wonder that many of the poorest countries complain that their interests and concerns are not properly prioritised by these agencies.

Those defending the nomination of Wolfowitz point to his experience of living three years in a developing country, while he was US ambassador to Indonesia. But far from displaying any commitment by Wolfowitz himself, or the US State Department, to 'democracy', that period 1986-89 represented a high point of the repressive regime of General Suharto, whose CIA-backed dictatorship rose to power through a coup in 1965, slaughtered upwards of 500,000 communists and other opponents, and remained in control until 1998, amassing a corrupt personal empire for Suharto and his family valued anywhere from $16 billion to $35

---

52 In fact the Bank consists of a Group of five linked institutions: the International Bank for Reconstruction and Development (IBRD), the International Development Association, the International Finance Corporation (IFC), the Multilateral Investment Guarantee Agency, and the International Centre for the Settlement of Investment Disputes. The first three of these are the most relevant to the development and implementation of health care reforms.

53 The Bank loaned $18.5 billion to more than 100 developing countries in 2003 (WDR 2004).

54 This dependency on the private sector, requiring it to maintain its 'triple A' credit rating, has preserved its essential character as a bank, rather than a donor agency.

55 In the IMF, which describes its 184 member states as 'shareholders', just five countries – the US, Japan, Germany, France and the UK - hold 29% of the votes (IMF 2003).

billion in industries ranging from hotels and transportation, to banks and automobiles (Washington Post 1999). Human rights activists and anti-corruption campaigners recall receiving no support from Mr Wolfowitz during his time in Jakarta, and note that he continued to support the regime throughout the 1990s, praising Suharto's 'strong and remarkable leadership' in testimony on Indonesia before the US House Appropriations Subcommittee on Foreign Operations in 1997 (Donnan 2005). The nomination of such a controversial political figure with such a poor track record[56] underlines the extent to which the World Bank is seen by Bush as little more than a front for US policy, while his subsequent unanimous endorsement by the Bank's Executive Board – in the absence of any other candidate – spells out the lack of serious democracy or accountability at the top level of the Bank.

There are unlikely to be any big political changes as a result of Wolfowitz's appointment: based in Washington, and strongly influenced – though not directly controlled – by successive US governments, the Bank and the IMF have been identified since the early 1980s with the political and economic policies of neoliberalism (Bayliss and Hall 2002, Williams 1994)[57].

While such policies initially centred on the IMF's imposition in developing countries of 'structural adjustment programmes', this evolved in the direction of more specific Bank involvement in health policy. Though its first lending for health services was not until 1980, the expansion of the Bank's role in this area was rapid: by the end of that decade it was the largest funder of health sector activities, having overtaken the WHO, lending an average of $1.5 billion per annum in the early 1990s (Walt 1994)[58].

The Bank adopts a health policy

In 1985 a major document *Paying for health services in developing countries: an overview*, arguing the case for user fees for health care (de Ferranti 1985), was followed by a more developed neoliberal policy for health care in developing countries in an official Bank document

---

56 Wolfowitz is also a prominent member, alongside other Bush confidants, of the far-right think tank Project for a New American Century, which set out its basic principles very clearly:

- 'American leadership is good both for America and for the world'
- 'Such leadership requires military strength, diplomatic energy and commitment to moral principle'
- 'Too few political leaders today are making the case for global leadership'.
  (http://www.newamericancentury.org)

57 Washington-based campaigners The Development GAP (Group for Alternative Policies) sum up the impact of the IMF 'imposing its will' on developing countries:

'Its new role as judge and financier of anti-poverty programs is a frightening prospect given that the institution remains wedded to an orthodox adjustment paradigm and has demonstrated that it knows considerably less about poverty than the Third World poor know about classical economics...

'For decades, the Fund has imposed its will on the countries of the South, reshaping their economies with virtually no input from the millions of people affected by their policies. Farmers, workers, consumers, small entrepreneurs, indigenous people and many others have taken to the streets to express their anger and frustration, but to little avail.

'Not only has the Fund failed to respond, but it has ensured that governments are unresponsive as well by threatening a cut-off of all international financing if its adjustment policies are not implemented' (Development GAP 1999).

58 The Bank's cumulative lending portfolio had reached $13.5 billion by 1996 (World Bank Group 1997). It lent over $9 billion between 1990 and 1999 (Stott 1999).

Financing health care: an agenda for reform. This restated the case for user fees in the context of a concerted argument for a reduced role for the state and increased reliance on market mechanisms and the private sector (World Bank 1987).

To develop its policy, influence and input into the reorganisation of health care systems around the world, the Bank has consciously fostered an image of itself as a 'knowledge-based institution'. It employs some 10,000 'development professionals' in its Washington HQ and 109 country offices – and spends around $100 million each year on research, commissioning work from hundreds of academics and professionals, and publishing hundreds of reports each year on a wide range of social policy issues, including health care (Caufield 1997). Much of the research has tended to reflect what Williams (1994:119) describes as the Bank's 'consistent policy of support for neoliberal principles and market solutions'.

The Bank also runs a 'Flagship Program', a project for training the top managers and civil servants running health services in developing countries and Eastern Europe in the assumptions and values the Bank wishes to promote. They receive an 'intensive, four week course' in Washington, at the end of which participants are expected to be able to:

> ...speak a common language about dimensions of health care reform and sustainable financing options (World Bank 2004)[59].

Perhaps the most influential policy document shaping health policy for developing countries in the 1990s was the Bank's 1993 *World Development Report*[60]. This effectively proposed the consolidation of a two-tier global health care system, in which the wealthy countries would remain free to spend as much as they wish, but publicly funded hospital care in developing countries would be reduced to a rudimentary minimum, or privatised. The same report itemises and estimates the costs of an 'essential public health package' designed for the poorest developing countries, which, the Bank concedes, should be subsidised, partly or completely, from public funds (Musgrove 1994).

The 'essential package' includes:

- The Expanded Programme on Immunisation (EPI), including micronutrient supplementation
- School health programmes, to treat worm infections and provide health education
- Programmes to increase public knowledge about family planning and nutrition, self cure and indications for seeking care
- Programmes to reduce the consumption of tobacco, alcohol and other drugs
- AIDS prevention programmes with a strong STD component.

  (World Bank 1993:106)

---

59 This type of training lends weight to Williams' 1994 warning that the responsiveness and sympathy of the Bank to the needs of Third World peasants or workers is unlikely to be guaranteed by the incorporation of more citizens of Third World countries into the Bank's staff and apparatus: 'These officials are just as likely, through their education in the West and socialisation into the organisational ideology, to be divorced and alienated from the rural sector and urban poverty as their Western counterparts.' (1994:117)

60 Still promoted on the Bank's website as of June 2004.

The estimated cost of this minimal – largely educational rather than health care – package was put at $6.80 per head of population per annum in 1990 prices. However the same World Bank document was concerned to restrict the range of health care services provided, again stipulating a 'minimum package of clinical services'. It warned that:

> ...government-run health systems in many developing countries are overextended and need to be scaled back (1993:108).

Bank guidance is very explicit:

> Only by *reducing or eliminating* spending on clinical services that are outside the nationally defined essential package can governments concentrate on ensuring essential clinical care for the poor. Two key ways to reallocate government spending are to increase cost recovery, especially by charging the wealthy for services in government hospitals, and to promote unsubsidised insurance for middle and upper-income groups (1993:108).

The Bank also conceded that an essential package would have to include treatment of minor infection and trauma, as well as 'advice and alleviation of pain for health problems that cannot be fully resolved with existing resources.' Hospital capacity should aim at providing about one bed per 1,000 population – but would be subject to very strict limits:

> ...the hospital would have to perform only basic surgery. No higher-level hospital is required for the delivery of the basic package (1993:113).

A minimum package of care

The Bank's document estimated that delivery of a 'minimum clinical package' along these lines would cost an average of about $8 per person each year in low income countries, and $15 in middle income countries such as Latin America.

> When the cost of selected public health interventions is added, total costs rise to $12 per capita in low-income countries and $22 in middle income countries (World Bank 1993:116).

But there was another warning:

> The case for government financing of discretionary clinical health care – services outside the essential package – is far less compelling. In fact, governments can promote both efficiency and equity by reducing – or when possible eliminating – public funding for these services (1993:119).

Of course the decision that such services should not be publicly funded means that any such services could only develop in the private sector, levying charges which will not be affordable by the poor. The Bank makes no secret of the fact that, on a world scale, completely different rules are being applied to poorer countries than to the richest members of the OECD, most of which finance comprehensively defined essential packages for virtually all their citizens, whereas:

> In low income countries where current public spending for health is less than the cost of an essential package, some degree of targeting is inevitable.

The equity of such a system therefore is very limited, since the wealthy few will continue to gain access to services which are not available to the vast majority. Charges could also lead in the opposite direction. Gertler and Hammer argue that:

If the wealthy are willing to pay but the poor are not, then this policy could lead to a reallocation of public subsidies from the poor to the wealthy (Gertler and Hammer 1997:21).

The ability of governments to square this circle and compensate for the chronic and inevitable failure of the market is limited by their lack of resources. Even raising the level of health provision to supply the World Bank's essential 'minimum package' was estimated to require a quadrupling of poorer countries' spending on public health from $5 billion to $20 billion a year in 1993 prices: but the World Bank is reticent on exactly how this money should be raised:

> Paying for an essential package will require a combination of increased expenditures by governments, donor agencies and patients and some reorientation of current public spending for health (World Bank 1993:11).

For slightly wealthier countries – those 'with the financial resources and political will to go beyond the minimum package' – the Bank proposed more scope to offer additional interventions, such as treating diabetes, medical treatment for mental illness, screening and treatment for breast and cervical cancer and 'inexpensive management of angina and heart attacks'. Other possible additional treatments could include hernia repair, treatment of meningitis in children and cataract operations.

The World Bank conception of a 'minimum' or 'essential' package, set out in this 1993 policy statement, achieved an extremely wide currency. Indeed it could be argued that what began as a 'minimum' provision became increasingly perceived as a *target*, effectively a 'maximum' for organisations such as the WHO, in a context in which many of the poorest countries were spending substantially less than the $12 per head per year (Laurell and Arellano 1996). It helped shape WHO and other policies for the remainder of the decade, and remains a factor into the 21st century (Pearson 2000, Navarro 2000).

Politics and economics of Bank policy

User fees

The Bank (and to a lesser extent the IMF, which has little direct involvement in health policy) have perhaps above all become identified with the advocacy of user charges for health care, again especially in less developed economies where they have more political influence, and often as part of a wider austerity programme[61]. By 1998 about 40% of the Bank's Health Nutrition and Population projects – and almost 75% of those projects in sub-Saharan Africa – included the introduction or increased use of user fees (Dunne 2000).

The Bank has argued that imposing a price on certain forms of care brings a series of benefits, in that charges:

• Deter unnecessary or frivolous use of services

• Encourage appropriate use of first contact and referral services

• Encourage the use of important services by exempting them from charge

• Encourage providers to limit over-supply

---

[61] By the 1990s the Bank and IMF 'routinely' applied strict conditions to countries seeking loans or rescheduling of debts, despite the 'generally negative' effect that these policies have on people's health (Labonte et al 2004:17).

- Act as an incentive for providers to improve quality
- Contribute to resources for spending on health care.

(Shaw 1995, Wang'ombe 1997)

There is no doubt that user fees do have a deterrent effect, and therefore reduce the usage of services. Schieber (1997) suggests that cost sharing is therefore a means to combat 'moral hazard', and Wang'ombe also (optimistically) suggests that the 'right' people are deterred: 'Presumably part of that reduction is due to a reduction in frivolous demand' (Wang'ombe 1997:151). Unfortunately there is little evidence of 'frivolous demand' in developing countries and, as most of the Bank's arguments acknowledge, those most likely to be deterred are the poorest: in fact this effect is the most consistent and predictable result from any cost-recovery programme (Creese and Kutzin 1995). Cotlear shows the scale of the problem in his analysis of the minimal health care system available to the poor in Peru, where drugs and medical inputs are charged to the user at full cost plus a mark-up, meaning that for the poorest 20% these costs account for over 80% of health spending. Yet fewer than one in five of the poor is exempt from payments (Cotlear 2000).

All of the empirical evidence appears to confirm the initial assumption that the imposition of charges will reduce the utilisation of services: the scale of the reductions observed ranges from 52% in Kenya (Mwabu et al 1995) to 64% in Zambia (Kahenya and Lake 1994). Other countries where the same effect has been observed include Ghana, and Zaire (Shaw 1995). High levels of user fees 'which exclude the poor' are seen by donor groups as a problem in Mozambique (Brown 2000a) and Uganda (Brown 2000b), where outpatient numbers doubled after user fees were abolished in 2001 (Okuonzi 2004, Deininger and Mpuga 2004)[62].

The Bank recognises that user fees deter the poorest from even such basic health care as immunisation – but this has not prevented the policy being applied in some countries. A major WHO report on user fees in immunisation services in 2001 concluded that it raised little money but had many disadvantages, and offered a blunt three-point summary:

- User fees discourage people from seeking vaccination
- Public funding is the most equitable way to finance essential immunization
- Essential immunization services should be free of charge.

(England et al 2001:6)

It is self-evident that an immunisation programme whose fees deter a section of the poor is going to be less effective – and thus less efficient – than one that erects no such barriers (Segall 2003). The exclusions always hit the weakest of the poor. Among the poorest social groups, those most likely to be excluded from treatment by user fees are children and the elderly. Bennett (1989) reports a fall of 40-51% in the use of government services in Lesotho, with children suffering the greatest reduction. Oxfam argues that the main victims of a cost recovery policy are women and young girls. A study in Indonesia found that imposing charges served

----

62 The UN Research Institute for Social Development has concluded that 'Of all measures proposed for raising revenue for local people, this [user fees] is probably the most ill advised. One study of 39 developing countries found that the introduction of user fees had increased revenues only slightly, while significantly reducing the access of low-income people to basic social services' (UNRISD 2000, cited in Whitehead et al 2001).

as a deterrent to seeking treatment not only for relatively minor illnesses, but also for more serious medical problems: another effect was to persuade users to delay seeking treatment, making any later intervention less effective (Gertler and Molyneaux 1997, Oxfam 1994).

Of course in many developing countries neither the 'ability' nor the 'willingness' to pay for treatment can be taken for granted. The Bank's insistence upon a norm based on the imposition of user charges for all treatment other than immunisation, with minimal if any exemptions from payment for the very poorest of the poor (Shaw 1995), took shape in a context of a grossly unequal world economy, in which there are vast pools of extreme poverty[63].

This has given rise to debates on how to calculate the appropriate prices to be charged for health treatment to generate the maximum possible revenue, while deterring as few users as possible. This is complicated by the fact that ill-health is predominantly concentrated among the poor, so that charging for care at all risks increasing the proportional use of services by the wealthy at the expense of those with greatest health need (Gertler and Hammer 1997).

Fees and 'equity'

The World Bank's technical department director covering Africa, Kevin Cleaver, has offered a remarkable and all-embracing claim for the importance (no matter how destitute may be the population involved) of:

> …user fees and self financing health insurance not simply as a way of raising more money, but as tools to help improve efficiency, equity, sustainability and private sector participation in national health systems (Shaw 1995, Foreword).

Some may regard Cleaver's inclusion of 'equity' alongside the other (more predictable) World Bank goals of 'efficiency, sustainability and private sector participation' as an inconsistency, if not an outright contradiction. Yet for Griffin and Shaw (1995) 'equity' actually means not equality, but a two-tier system, in which the wealthy use one health service, and the poor get equal access to another, state-funded safety-net:

> A sensibly designed insurance system, even if targeted to the richest 10-20% of the population, will almost certainly improve equity if only by ushering the rich into a system that they, rather than the rural poor, support financially.

The 'inequality' to which the advocates of market reforms refer in a whole raft of Bank-sponsored 'benefit incidence studies', showing what proportion of public health spending benefits each quintile of population in different continents and countries[64] is not in practice the main concern. User fees have little or nothing to do with equity: defenders of the policy admit that of the 31 African countries that had been persuaded by World Bank and other advisors to implement user fees, almost all were simply seeking to raise money, while only four

---

63 According to World Trade Organisation Director General Mike Moore, a quarter of the globe's population, 1.2 billion people, were surviving in 2000 on an income of less than one dollar per day, and two-thirds of the world's population is obliged to survive on two dollars per day or less. So widespread is extreme poverty that the World Bank's global definition of 'middle income' begins with an average of just over two dollars per day, while the least developed countries accounted for less than a fifth of the world's poorest people (Moore 2000, Labonte et al 2004).

64 For example the Asian Development Bank (1999:10) stresses that in Indonesia the wealthiest 20% consume 41% of the public subsidies for hospitals.

claimed that either 'efficiency' or 'equity' was an objective[65] (Leighton and Wouters 1995). Schieber concedes that user fees, collected at point of service use 'may be viewed as a tax on the sick' but nevertheless defends them as a means to combat 'moral hazard', and thus achieve 'allocative efficiency' (Schieber 1997:23) despite the relatively small amounts of revenue generated, and 'some evidence of adverse effects on health outcomes'(1997:24).

There is no consensus among health policy analysts in support of user fees: the Bank itself has in recent years backed away from its more overt promotion of the policy, even claiming in a *BMJ* interview that it is not Bank policy at all (Abbasi 1999c). Saltman and Figueras (1997) and Dahlgren (2000) are among those who argue that direct user fees 'constitute the most regressive approach to health care financing'. Dahlgren argues that access to health care services must be according to need rather than purchasing power. A study by the UN Research Institute for Social Development has also concluded that:

> Of all measures proposed for raising revenue from local people this [user fees] is probably the most ill-advised (UNRISD 2000)[66].

In defence of the Bank's rationale, it might be argued that rather than *creating* inequality, a policy of seeking a minimum package of care coupled with user fees to help cover the costs is simply recognising the reality of existing inequality, and the lack of any economic basis for a more advanced and equitable health care system. This is a genuine problem. Trotsky, seeking to explain the bureaucratisation of the Soviet Union in his 1936 study *Revolution Betrayed*, repeatedly stresses the limitations on even a revolutionary government taking power in a backward, war-ravaged economy and subjected to isolation from the latest developments in technology. He cites Marx from 1875, who argued:

> Law can never be higher than the economic structure and the cultural development of society conditioned by that structure (Trotsky 1936:61).

Along similar lines it might be argued that Lenin recognised the necessity of a tactical, temporary retreat from socialist reconstruction to the New Economic Policy in order to secure food production in the war-torn Soviet Union of 1921. However, while seeing economic backwardness as part of the explanation for political setbacks and limitations, Marx, Lenin and Trotsky were not seeking a reason to accept the status quo: they were focusing on aspects of objective reality, which they believed needed to be *changed* through conscious intervention.

The problem with the Bank's approach is not so much that it acknowledges the (inescapable) chronic lack of basic resources and the poverty which leaves the poorest states with no scope to invest in health care, but that it *institutionalises* and *consolidates* that situation into a conscious policy, which threatens to leave many least developed countries permanently deprived of modern medicine, hospital care and any prospect of training their own doctors and other health professionals: worse, it would restrict public health services to the most basic services for the poorest of the poor, consolidating a situation in which any more advanced hospital-based health care, and all health care for the middle and ruling classes would be the

---

65 A finding echoed in a separate study of user fees by Russell and Gilson (1997).

66 Nonetheless it appears that user fees for primary health care and for education are included in some Poverty Reduction Strategy Papers proposed by the Bank for the poorest countries (Labonte et al 2004).

exclusive preserve of the private sector. The Bank's policy offers no dynamic for progressive change. Rather than seeking ways of bringing in extra international resources to assist the development of health care systems, it offers ways to persuade poor countries to accept that they must do without them. This exacerbates inequity rather than promoting equity.

Health insurance – and market failure

Far from promoting equal access to comprehensive health services for the poor, the Bank's policy is primarily driven by the more overtly neoliberal ideals of minimising state spending, minimising (and where possible 'rationalising' or even privatising) state provision of services, and maximising the private sector, both as health providers and as insurers:

> Health insurance is virtually the only practical instrument through which governments can get out of the expensive business of across the board subsidies for hospital care, and thus release funds for public health, preventive and primary services that benefit the poor (Griffin and Shaw 1995).

The Bank and advocates of free market policies want to encourage those who can afford to do so, even in the poorest countries, to take out private medical insurance – thus shifting a portion of the cost of health care from the state to the individual. User fees therefore play a much bigger role than might appear to be the case: they are seen not just as a means of generating income to sustain a basic health care system, but as a way to introduce more complex insurance systems. Indeed the ideal combination of policies from the neoliberal point of view would be to offer relatively affordable private insurance premium payments, coupled with high fees for hospital treatment, that would persuade the maximum number of wealthier (and less wealthy) people to subscribe[67] (Shaw 1995).

However by 1997 there was sufficient evidence of the failure of policies along these lines for the Bank's Health Nutrition and Population Sector Strategy to conclude that:

> Because of cost and the pronounced market failure that occurs in private health insurance, this is not a viable option for risk-pooling at the national level in low and middle income countries (World Bank Group 1997:8).

The persistent evidence of another surge in medical cost inflation in the already costly US health care system (Docteur et al 2002, Hewitt Associates 2003), coupled with the negative recent experience of privatisation of health services in Australia, where private sector costs are significantly higher than those in publicly funded hospitals (Richardson et al 1999), should serve as a warning that the effect of World Bank and other pro-market reforms will be neither to cut costs, nor to boost 'efficiency', but to promote private sector involvement regardless[68].

---

67 The Bank's Kevin Cleaver argues explicitly that the imposition of charges plays a key role prodding the middle classes in the direction of health insurance:

> Countries cannot jump into self-financing health insurance schemes without first passing the hurdle of imposing user fees in government facilities, especially hospitals. The reason is simply that when people have the option of obtaining health services at zero or low cost, they are unlikely to have much incentive to pay insurance premiums to cover unexpected health hazards (Introduction to Shaw et al 1995).

Ignoring the evidence of failure

Experience has indeed shown the Bank's policy to be inappropriate: one example is Zimbabwe, where Hecht and colleagues (1995) in their proposals for reforms argued that a possible doubling in fees collected would raise over Z$20 million (or 11.4% of recurrent hospital spending in 1990). However they did not mention that all of this extra money would have been taken from patients, without any contribution from the government, and therefore a minimal contribution by the wealthy. Their paper was silent on the impact the increased fees would have upon the use of services by Zimbabwe's poorest people. In practice, as a subsequent World Bank analysis of the Bank's own role in health reforms in Zimbabwe concluded, few of the hypotheses turned out to be sound[69]. The Bank's own advice and project work was later criticised in an internal evaluation, because:

> The study asserted that clients would be willing to pay more for improved quality, without analysis of how quality improvements would be achieved, and with only anecdotal evidence regarding willingness to pay (World Bank 1998:29).

The Bank has also recognised that the element of competition, which it sees as key to efficiency, is fragile in countries where incomes are chronically low. Indeed pro-market reformers fear that competition could be eliminated if services were on offer free of charge to all, including the wealthiest service users: this would deter them from either paying into private insurance schemes, or paying to use private hospitals. Shaw (1995) argues that free services at government health facilities 'undermine the efficiency of the health sector as a whole...'

The availability of free care means that potential service users cannot easily be persuaded to pay for private care instead. The question then arises:

> ...How can the private sector expand and compete under such circumstances? (Shaw 1995, p21)

The unargued assumption is that 'efficiency' is the exclusive prerogative of the private sector, and flows only from competition. Of course this is highly controversial, not least with public sector trade unions, which have stressed the limited power of individual consumers of private care, and the extent of corruption and inefficiency in parts of the private sector. Public Service International (PSI)[70], echoing the ILO, also rejects approaches which regard health care as a commodity, or as 'a tradeable good', and questions the extent to which any 'public-private partnership' can viably exist, because, as the PSI report bluntly puts it:

> ...private providers will not supply inherently unprofitable care to those who are in no position to pay (PSI 1999).

---

68 Hay (2001) also stresses that privatisation is no solution to problems of affordability in health care, since 'market provision invariably proves more expensive per capita for a given level of care than public provision' (Hay 2001:46).

69 By June 2004, Zimbabwe's largest state hospital, faced with non-payment of bills that had left it unable to provide services and drugs, was resorting to the desperate measure of refusing to allow new mothers to take their babies home until their bills had been paid. The period of imposing user fees had coincided with a three-fold increase in numbers of Zimbabwean women dying from pregnancy-related complications (Sapa-AFP 2004).

70 PSI is the international coordination of public service trade unions.

Politics of World Bank Policies

Three waves... of privatisation

Bank policies still focus on driving through three 'waves' of reform in developing countries, each wave centred on privatisation. The first focuses on privatising commercial enterprises and divesting of state assets. The second wave involves the privatisation of public sector infrastructure and utilities: and the third wave continues the privatisation process, while seeking to draw the private sector and NGOs into investment in health, education and pensions systems (World Bank Group 1997:8, Abbasi 1999b)[71].

In fact there is no evidence that the Bank's policy of increasing the role of the private sector in the provision of hospital services can make hospital services any more accessible to the poorest sections of the population – who are most likely to suffer serious illness – though it may benefit those wealthy enough to pay for their own care.

Bank and IMF economic policies, coupled with their already dependent position in the world market, have offered developing countries little scope to improve their allocation of resources to health care. By the mid 1990s, Uganda for example was spending almost six times more per head of population on debt servicing than on health care – as a rampant AIDS epidemic took hold. In Zimbabwe, World Bank-proposed policies brought not the promised improvements, but diminishing health standards year by year (Caufield 1997)[72].

Nor have the Bank's policies delivered much in the way of positive results. The Bank's own 1997 HNP Strategy noted that out of 120 ongoing projects from 1970-1995:

- Only 17% of completed HNP projects were classified as contributing substantially to institutional development

- Only 44% of completed HNP projects are rated as likely to be sustainable

- Only 59% of 68 recently completed HNP projects were rated as satisfactory, compared with 81% in education and 58% Bank-wide.

(World Bank Group 1997:15)

Interestingly, the Bank found that it had not even consistently backed its own policy advice with genuine resources:

> Although an increasing number of ongoing projects examine non-governmental roles, none of the 68 completed HNP projects included financing for privately owned facilities or activities. Furthermore health systems performance issues were dealt with mainly through public sector interventions, with little attention to the substitution effect and crowding out of private providers (1997:15).

---

71 Similar 'strings' and conditions attached to British government 'aid' to developing countries have been highlighted by organisations such as War on Want (2005), which revealed the multi-million payments to the right wing Adam Smith Institute, PricewaterhouseCoopers and KPMG to advise developing countries on the privatisation of their public services. Under pressure, British ministers have recently announced a change of policy, to drop requirements to privatise from bilateral aid (Seager 2005).

72 African countries are now paying more than $15 billion each year in debt service to rich countries – more than the total they receive in aid. Even the debt relief programmes such as the rescheduling of debts for Highly Indebted Poor Countries is expected to leave at least 10 of the 26 countries deemed to require extra support with unsustainable debt loads – while the measure of sustainability is set by the Bank and IMF at payments equivalent to 150% of a country's export earnings (Labonte et al 2004, Labonte et al 2005).

Old priorities presented as new

However the Bank's resolve to 'learn from experience' results in a series of 'HNP Priorities' – which (on the basis of no visible evidence) offer a wholesale reaffirmation of market-style methods, and a renewed commitment to fostering a rudimentary private sector:

> Governments will be encouraged to promote greater diversity in service delivery systems by providing funding for civil society and non-governmental providers on a competitive basis, instead of limiting public funds to public facilities. In many of these instances, rebalancing the public-private interface will be preferable to an outright privatisation of social assets. Quasi-market mechanisms, such as vouchers, competitive contracting-out, and the increased use of client feedback, can both improve public sector performance and encourage quality participation by the private sector (World Bank Group 1997:18).

The new, apparently modified, Bank approach is to rely upon governments to purchase, regulate, and even subsidise private sector services: once again publicly provided and funded services are seen as restricted to the areas of care that the private sector will not undertake for lack of sufficient profit. Despite the Bank's careful repackaging of itself[73], reforms based on this approach will differ slightly, if at all, from those prior to 1997.

The view of many critics was summarised by the response to the rising global pressure for Health Sector Reforms (HSRs) by academics working in Vietnam, who describe them as 'structural adjustment measures in disguise':

> ...if one does not look at HSRs critically, one can easily miss the point that HSRs have come to mean 'market oriented interventions in the health and nutrition sector (Schuftan and Dahlgren 1999).

The Bank and transitional economies

The preoccupation with extending the role of the private sector informs Bank policies, even where it is discussing the replacement of previously comprehensive state-funded health services, as for example in Eastern and Central Europe.

Bank analysts Staines and Lovelace (1998) stress on the one hand that the countries in this region 'vary greatly in their characteristics', and argue that 'no standard template for health sector reform will apply across the region'. Yet within a few paragraphs the same authors set out what amounts to... a standard template, which includes 'an expanding role for the private sector':

> In addition new payment mechanisms for health providers and new user charges policies for consumers will seek to provide balanced incentives...[the transition countries] must design new and more market-oriented health systems which steer a middle course that minimises the costs incurred from both government failure and market failure (Staines and Lovelace 1998).

This policy, too, appears to have brought problems that now concern the Bank. Its 2004 *World Development Report* notes that the move from publicly provided services to social insurance in transition economies of Eastern Europe and Asia had:

---

73 'The past decade has seen it change image from uncaring bully to compassionate stakeholder, focusing on health' (Abbasi 1999a).

...led to confusion about the government role in health, which led to the neglect of those services
and the subsequent re-emergence of communicable diseases (World Bank 2003b:140).

Is the Bank changing policy?

Other setbacks have repeatedly questioned the viability of the Bank's approach. During the
1980s, under the constraints of the world market, average incomes fell by 10-25% throughout
Africa and in much of Latin America, alongside a 50% per capita cut in education spending.
Health spending per head in the world's 37 poorest countries fell by 25% (UNICEF 1989).

Apologists argue that many of the negative developments following Bank and IMF
interventions were inherent in the scale and sources of the original crisis in the countries
concerned. Killick insists that social services in general have been relatively protected under
IMF/Bank schemes, and that the decline in health and education provision was not directly
related to the adoption of structural adjustment programmes (Killick 1995). Hopes have been
expressed in recent years that the IMF was breaking from neoliberalism and SAPs[74]. Some
have cautiously suggested that the World Bank may be easing the pressure for privatisation and
market-style policies, and 'learning some of the positive lessons from countries that have
primarily public health services' (Deacon 2001, Bayliss and Hall 2002).

However Deacon notes that:

> Many Bank documents on social policy are infuriatingly ambiguous, and the health sector
> strategy paper is no exception (Deacon 2001:61).

While Deacon detects a degree of compromise 'between several positions' in the Bank's 1997
HNP strategy text, the overriding direction of Bank policy appears to have remained largely
unchanged.

A Strategic Directions document drawn up in 2002 by the Bank's most overtly pro-
privatisation sub-division, the International Finance Corporation (IFC), appears to revert to
the original hard-line neoliberal stance. It notes approvingly that a majority of health
expenditures in most low-income countries is private, compared with less than a third in the
wealthiest countries (p8), and welcomes the opportunity for 'developing clear country and
regional World Bank Group strategies that successfully promote the integration of the private
health sector':

> The reliance solely on the public sector to address these major challenges appears to be no longer
> a viable or sustainable option in the long term because of fiscal constraints. [...] Many
> governments are rethinking the respective roles of private and public agents in the health sector,
> and are beginning to turn to market instruments to enhance the efficiency and quality of health
> care provision. The aim of much of recent health care reforms in several countries has been to
> increase the role of the private sector as the provider (rather than the financer) of care (IFC
> 2002:3).

---

74 *The Guardian's* Larry Elliott (1999) among them. However the continued impact of SAPs and
their lack of success in removing whole countries and their populations from the poverty trap was
noted by the UN in 2002: a detailed report concluded that the discredited IMF and World Bank
policies should be dropped in favour of 'development oriented poverty reduction strategies' (Denny
and Elliott 2002).

While admitting that there is no supporting evidence, the IFC strategy argues that the expansion of the private sector helps develop health services for the poor by 'producing extra capacity in the sector as a whole', leaving the public sector to 'redirect its scarce resources to those most in need' (2002:35).

The IFC focus will be on financially viable projects, delivering a profit close to the IFC average of about 5%, and therefore its strategy will be primarily centred in urban areas where (especially in poorer countries) the private market is 'most mature' (2002:36). Significantly, the IFC argues it wants to 'contribute to the financial protection against ill health and to the strengthening of the middle class,' and evinces little interest in the health of the poorest, advocating:

> ...increased involvement in private health insurance, to benefit the lower-middle and middle classes in countries without universal risk-pooling and to support growing supplementary insurance in many of our client countries (IFC 2002).

However a rather different and more ambiguous note is struck by the Bank's *World Development Report* 2004, which breaks completely new ground (and defies neoliberal 'political correctness') with a largely positive appraisal of the previously ignored health care system in Cuba[75], and which in contrast with the 1997 HNP Strategy and its emphasis on private sector solutions, declares that:

> There is no presumption that one type of provider – public, for-profit, or not-for-profit – is likely to be any better than any other (World Bank 2003b:151).

The chapter on health includes a number of passages highlighting market failure and the shortcomings of private sector providers as well as criticising examples of poor public provision. Another section offers a far less assertive defence of the imposition of user fees, claiming once again that these can 'reduce capture of supposedly free services by richer groups' (2003b:143), but noting that such policies also risk excluding the poor.

The chapter concludes by explicitly rejecting any 'one size fits all' system of accountability to ensure the best allocation of health care resources, and offering six possible variant models for health care systems – most of which include aspects of New Public Management-style contracting, but place relatively little emphasis on decentralisation, competition, privatisation, user fees and market-style mechanisms. As such they bear little relation to the policies advocated in the 1990s, and suggest that perhaps the Bank may now be beginning to recognise the extent to which previous reform packages have failed.

A word from their sponsors:
USAID and Bank funding of NGOs and academics

Alongside the World Bank and its subsidiaries, one of the largest sponsors of research and policy development in poorer countries has been USAID. Since its establishment in 1961 –

---

75 'Experience from Brazil, Chile, Costa Rica and Cuba, Iran, Nepal, Matlab (Bangladesh), Tanzania and various West African countries shows that health services, if delivered well, can improve outcomes even for the poorest groups' (World Bank 2003b:134). A two-page 'spotlight' feature on Cuba (157-8) shows that the foundations of its success have been the 1961 nationalisation of health services that left the government as sole provider, central control, tight monitoring and evaluation, and the motivation of doctors and medical staff.

in the midst of the Cold War – USAID has been explicitly tied to the US administration of the day, and to the foreign policy objectives of the State Department. Its most recent Strategy Document (2004-2009) proclaims as a core principle USAID's 'Loyalty: Commitment to the United States and the American people'. The organisation and the work it sponsors are not primarily concerned with health, but all its policies demonstrate a consistent bias towards private sector involvement, and towards socially conservative, as well as neoliberal policies (USAID 2003).

With the prospect of sponsorship from the lavish research budgets of the World Bank and USAID, there appears to be no shortage of consultants and institutions willing to help drive forward 'reforms' based on market-style measures, user fees and increased private sector involvement in health care systems. Some leading US academic institutions and teams of academics now play a supporting role as missionaries seeking to extend this market model to health systems around the world: USAID funding has underwritten work by such organisations as the Health Financing and Sustainability (HFS) Project, Partnerships for Health Reform (PHR), and Management Solutions for Health (MSH).

HFS is based in Bethesda, Maryland. One of its policy papers, *Strategies for Achieving Health Financing Reform in Africa*, explains that:

> Principal HFS activities have focused on: resource generation through cost recovery; risk-sharing mechanisms; public-private collaboration; resource allocation, use and management; and costing of health services (Leighton and Wouters, 1995).

In fact the researchers themselves, and the company they work for, epitomise precisely this link between private and public sectors – in the USA. Both Charlotte Leighton and Annemarie Wouters are members of a large team employed by Abt Associates Inc, which makes no bones about being:

> One of the largest for-profit government and business consulting and research firms in the country [the US]. […] In recent years our annual revenues have exceeded $160 million. Our staff now numbers more than 1,000 (www.abtassoc.com).

With a budget equal to the health budgets of several developing countries, Abt is well connected with 'virtually every US government agency', including those governing aid, as well as many foreign governments and businesses. These connections have brought a flow of research projects on the issue of health reform, and Abt is proud of its burgeoning health department, which publishes a newsletter listing many of its current and recent projects:

> *Healthwatch* is a quarterly publication of Abt Associates health research and consulting practices... [which] represent the activities of over 150 professionals working toward the improvement of health and health care delivery around the world (www.abtassoc.com).

From this rather less than impartial starting point (as employees of a profit-seeking consultancy firm in a project funded by the US State Department) Leighton and Wouters set themselves the task of dispelling 'myths' which might dissuade governments from introducing fee-for-service payments among the African poor:

> For example, in the absence of information to the contrary, people tend to believe that the poor are unwilling to pay for health services, that there is no role for the private sector in achieving the public health agenda, or that insurance or pre-payment mechanisms will not work in the poorest rural areas (Leighton and Wouters, 1995, p10).

The authors struggle to dispel these 'myths', despite a serious lack of evidence to support their view[76]. They and their colleagues in Abt Associates have become part of a health reform industry. The level of Abt's involvement is not always apparent from the innocuous names of the organisations through which it works.

In addition to the HFS, Abt Associates were the leaders of the USAID-funded 'Partnerships for Health Reform' (PHR) project (*Healthwatch*, Fall 1999); and they are now the lead consultants in the $44m USAID-funded project to reform – and privatise – health services in post-Saddam Iraq[77]. New pay scales will cut the salaries of state-employed doctors in primary care, pushing them towards private practice. Health provision will be opened up to foreign companies, which will be allowed to repatriate profits. Reporters assume their investment is likely to centre on the establishment of high-tech hospital care rather than rebuilding the wrecked infrastructure of primary care and immunisation services which previously cared for the poor, although it is already clear that infectious diseases are on the increase (Dyer 2004, Abt 2003, Hughes 2003, Kaplan 2003, Ali 2003)[78].

USAID backing – and often links with the World Bank – mean that in many cases the political and economic influence of the NGOs and consultancy firms promoting such models can substantially exceed that of the governments with which they are working. Acceptance of health system reform has become a classic 'offer you can't refuse' for dependent countries seeking loans, credit ratings or other aid and expert assistance to develop health and other services.

---

76 Leighton's intellectual and professional commitment to the expansion of the private sector can also be seen in her paper with Marty Makinen seeking to assess the prospects for establishing a 'niche' for a new network of 'franchised private clinics' in Zambia (Makinen and Leighton 1997).

77 According to the World Bank's website, pre-war Iraq 'developed a good infrastructure and well-performing education and healthcare system, widely regarded as the best in the Middle East' (www.worldbank.org/iq).

78 Any new government that tries to take charge of the economy and resources of Iraq will have its hands tied before it even starts: a deal signed between the US-appointed government of Iyad Allawi and the 'Paris Club' of rich nations has tied limited cancellation of debt to long-term adherence to policies laid down by the Washington based IMF. Just over $31 billion of debt run up by Saddam Hussein's regime is to be written off under the deal, which leaves Iraq still owing a possible total in excess of $200 billion.

The cancellation of 80% of the Paris Club debt comes with tight strings attached. Only 30% of the $39 billion debt was to be written off immediately: another 30% hinges on Iraq adopting an economic strategy endorsed by the IMF, and the final 20% would wait until the IMF had certified that the policies had been successfully implemented. IMF strategies typically include the privatisation of publicly owned utilities, and the imposition of user fees for services such as health care. The Iraqi Treasury has already been extensively looted by the US-led Coalition Provisional Authority, which has been revealed to have spent more than $20 billion – more than Iraq's annual GDP – during its 15 month period in control of the country's resources before the handover to Allawi's interim regime. The one Iraqi representative who was supposed to sit in on the CPA's meetings came to just two of the 43 board meetings in 2003. 'We just threw the money over the fence,' one US official told the *Financial Times*.

Millions were spent without evidence of a contract, a tender or services rendered in exchange. The health ministry spent hundreds of millions of dollars without keeping proper records or observing proper procedures. Perhaps this is the 'American way' George Bush is so keen to export? (Mekay 2004, Catan 2004).

PHR was another US-based organisation of academics, which provided guidance for reforming health care systems based on a fundamental assumption that the goal is a fee-for-service system, working with the private sector. This is made unmistakably clear in PHR's *Handbook of Indicators* for measuring the results of health reforms, which again rehearses the stock, unproven, arguments for the imposition of user fees:

> On efficiency grounds, fees should be charged in all government facilities for all services. Also as a general rule... fees should be equal to the marginal social costs of producing a service (which in competitive markets implies that in the long run they will also be equal to average, or unit costs). Charging consumers cost-based fees promotes efficient consumption of health services by consumers, because for example it can avoid excessive consumption of health services... (Knowles et al 1997:32)

PHR also backed research and reform projects in a number of countries – based on the same assumptions. But its researchers have proved reluctant to investigate questions which might undermine the logic of the imposition of charges for health care. A report on 'health seeking behaviour' in Zambia, for example, avoids addressing the impact on the poorest of user charges, and argues that the fundamental problem is not price but distance:

> ...regardless of the user fee charged... the use of services diminishes greatly with the distance at which the potential clientele are located (Diop et al 1998).

However in Niger Diop had come to rather different conclusions, warning in another PHR report that 'cost recovery mechanisms cannot replace government funding'. That report recommended that means-tested exemptions are required as a 'safety net' to protect the poor (Diop 1996).

Despite their increasingly obvious contradictions, and unanswered questions over their effectiveness, market-style measures are increasingly regarded as the norm – not only for the 'reform' of existing health care systems in more economically advanced countries, but also for the establishment of new systems in countries where economic and staffing resources are desperately short.

This is especially clear in the case of a PHR study of Cambodia conducted by a researcher from the Abt Associates team, which not only advocates user fees as a means to raise income for health care in rural areas, but goes on – without presenting the slightest scrap of supporting evidence – to assert that the 'for-profit' private sector should be encouraged as the basis of a potentially 'efficient' system delivering 'high quality' services:

> There is a need to work more with the for-profit sector, including health providers and pharmacists. The existence of a nascent private sector at the commune level in rural areas provides a unique opportunity to strengthen the quality of care in a potentially efficient service delivery environment. Some thought should be given to sponsoring a pilot activity in one province that would emphasize the use of incentives to for-profit providers to dispense high-quality basic health services (Knowles 1996).

There is likely to be little informed debate in the affected countries on the wisdom of pro-market health care reforms (which could well be perceived by the local population as an externally imposed fait accompli): often literacy levels are low, access to even the most basic news and mass media are limited, and there is limited democratic space for developed discussion.

Perhaps more alarming – especially from the point of view of those concerned about the democracy and accountability of health care systems – is the fact that debates on these policy issues have originated within, and been largely confined to, the rarefied topmost layers of international bodies and academic establishments, leaving little – if any – opportunity for health care professionals and managers of the day-to-day services at national level to discuss or challenge the policies, or the key assumptions on which they depend.

Few elected politicians, even at government level, will be aware of the origins of the reforms and changes that they have been persuaded by civil servants to implement. Few national governments can match the level of resources and research devoted by bodies such as the World Bank to promoting and developing its policy on health care, and using every available means of pressure to impose it upon governments around the world.

Small circles wield wide influence

Although they are not financially dependent upon the World Bank or the IMF, the governments and policy-making elites of high income countries are also subject to the influence of the ongoing debate on health system reform: most of the leading academics in the sphere of health policy and health economics are from universities and institutes in the richest G7 countries, who also play a role in shaping policy debates at home. This makes it a two-way flow: as Lee and Goodman (2002) point out, the debate on the public-private mix of financial sources and service providers spread to the developing countries from academic and political networks in the US and the UK.

Lee and Goodman go on to explore the various networks and the 'epistemic community' that have been instrumental in the development of health care financing (HCF) reforms, and, citing Cox, refer to the 'transnational managerial class' that is emerging as a new policy elite, which:

> ...encompasses public officials in the national and international agencies involved with economic management and a whole range of experts and specialists who in some way are connected with the maintenance of the world economy, in which multinationals thrive... (Lee and Goodman 2002:103)

Having conducted extensive literature searches, the same authors conclude that:

> HCF reform has been strongly characterised by a relatively small and tightly integrated network of policy-makers, technical advisors and scholars who have defined and shaped the content and process of policy reforms (p105).

In the 1980s in Britain a network collaborating with the WHO emerged around the London School of Economics and the London School of Hygiene and Tropical Medicine. In the US the lead was taken by USAID, which brought in consultants John Snow Inc, and through them Abt Associates. By the mid 1990s the World Bank had moved to centre stage, promoting the importance of health economics, and effectively eclipsing the WHO, which employed just one health economist.

Lee and Goodman specifically challenge 'liberal views of globalisation' that suggest that a wider range of individuals and groups are being drawn in to shaping policy, and point out that:

> Analysis of policy changes over time suggests that the process of policy initiation and formulation has been largely top-down, developed and supported through the Washington and London

hubs...

This suggests that HCF reform worldwide has been fostered by the emergence of a policy elite, rather than a rational convergence of health needs and solutions. [...]

What is different about this policy network that makes it a 'global' elite is its inclusion of public and private interests and sometimes a mixture of the two... The exertion of influence over policy reform has been through a combination of coercive and consensual means (2002:116).

In developing countries the IMF (though SAPs) or the World Bank have proved early and consistent advocates of neoliberal approaches to the funding and restructuring of health care services, and have acted as a transmission belt for the imposition of pro-market ideology and semi-privatised models of health care into countries with little or no developed infrastructure of health services[79].

Only rarely have the opinions or wishes of national leaders in developing countries been the principal factor in the policies that have been developed. As Walt (1994) and Lee and Goodman (2002) have noted, the World Bank 'largely as a result of its unrivalled financial resources' has played a leading role in reform debates, establishing 'a strong epistemic community,' which is based in academic institutions of the USA and the UK, and various global-level bureaucracies[80]. The Bank has networked on a global level with a variety of academics, health economists and consultancies to establish:

...a consensus across different institutions and national settings defining the 'problem' of health care financing reform and potential solutions (Lee and Goodman 2002:116).

However the 'consensus' often reaches no further than the elite community of policy-shapers. Critics of the impact of 20 years of health reforms on countries in Latin America and the Caribbean have drawn attention to the lack of connection between researchers and policy makers on the one hand, and the people affected by their decisions on the other:

Policy processes... must be opened up to a wider and more genuine public participation. It is simply unacceptable for health policy to be researched and conducted in small, closed circles of consultants and policy-makers. [...] It is in the very definition of good governance that people have a right to a meaningful say in the decisions that govern their lives (PAHO et al 2001, Foreword).

Many developing countries have therefore had to work within parameters set by external bankers and free market ideologists rather than by health care specialists or their own electorate (Went 2000). System reforms in developing countries may well reflect not local conditions and problems but 'a change in the economic model... as part of a philosophy of

---

79 Navarro (2000) makes a similar accusation against the WHO's 'American branch', the Pan American Health Organisation (PAHO) in its dealings with Latin America.

80 Stone (2001:352) also refers to 'epistemic communities', and notes the role of a transnational network of 'elite, technical and scientific cliques' which have been able to effect change in policy and policy agendas and become 'entrenched in bodies such as the IMF, WTO, OECD and World Bank'. Abbasi (1999b) notes the Bank's 'astuteness in recruiting staff from among its potential critics – such as the WHO and NGOs', which 'strengthens policies and dampens criticism', while its ability to recruit leading health professionals and policymakers 'gives it an unsurmountable advantage over other agencies'.

competitiveness' (Arias and Yepes, 1997).

However it would be a mistake to see all such problems as simply flowing from the World Bank/IMF. The policies and pressures flow from the global market and the market system. Other countries such as China and Vietnam, seeking to re-enter the global market system, have themselves also opted to implement policies including privatisation of health care and user fees, without facing any explicit pressure from the Bank or IMF.

Irrespective of how the reforms have been advocated, the results in the poorest countries have tended to be similar – an increase in inequality and exclusion of the poorest from health care. As Casas and colleagues argue in the context of Latin America, while the rhetoric surrounding reforms suggests that their ostensible purpose is 'promoting equity in health status', 'improving the quality of care', 'increasing efficiency' or ensuring 'sustainability', the reality can be very different:

> Until now, experiences both within and outside the Americas indicated that health reform processes have principally resulted in cost containment and the creation of new opportunities for gain, rather than an increase in quality and coverage of services (Casas et al 2000 p246).

The role of other organisations

'Development' Banks as policy drivers at continental level

While the World Bank is by far the biggest player, other continental-based 'development banks' also reinforce the drive for 'reform'. The Asian Development Bank (ADB) plays a regional role analogous to the World Bank in its sponsorship of market-based 'solutions' to the reform of health care systems and other social programmes.

A flavour of the ADB's ideological approach can be seen in the press release summing up a four-day conference of almost 20 nations held in the Philippines to discuss Health Sector Reform in Asia. Challenged by the Philippines' acting Health Secretary to ensure that the conference would lead to specific and recognisable improvements in people's health at grass roots level, the ADB President Mistuo Sato replied that a key element in the Bank's strategy was 'encouragement of greater private sector involvement in health care provision' (ADB 1995).

Among the other items on the agenda of that ADB conference (which was co-sponsored by 'the Washington-based International Health Policy Program') were several stock market-style proposals: decentralisation of health care systems, 'broadening health financing options to include user fees'; and 'community, social and private insurance'.

One of the ADB's Health Sector Development Programs has involved loans to Mongolia to implement reforms designed among other things to 'develop private sector delivery of health services', and rationalise facilities. The ADB is also encouraging the Mongolian government to change 'the modes of payment of health service providers to introduce market signals and incentives to improve cost efficiency' (ADB 1997).

Similar projects are sponsored in central and southern America by the Inter-American Development Bank, which is if anything even more dominated by the USA. The IADB's guidelines to member countries seeking to borrow to finance new public health programmes stipulates specifically that:

Wherever possible a fee for services rendered principle should be applied (IADB 1994).

European Central Bank

One bank that makes no claim to be a development bank is the relatively new European Central Bank, formed as part of the establishment of the single European currency. The ECB has taken forward debates originating in the OECD on the implications for Europe's economies and taxation policy of the growing elderly population (Hennessy 1995), and drawn predictable conclusions.

An important article by the ECB's Economic Policy Committee (2003) warns of the potential costs in terms of pensions and health care – and unsurprisingly rejects one possible answer to the problem which would require much 'higher inflows of immigration' and 'a lasting absorption of working-age migrants into employment' (2003:40). Instead the ECB looks towards 'reforms' which include increasing the retirement age, and a shift towards funded and privately managed pensions in place of pay-as-you-go systems.

In the health sector, the ECB urges member states to take steps to 'limit the public sector's exposure' to rising health care bills. This should include a cap on health care spending, and greater use of private finance, coupled with the use of 'market forces' to move towards 'efficient solutions', and the restriction of public health care to 'core services' for health care and prevention, leaving individuals to provide for 'non-essential health expenditure':

> Individuals could then decide to what degree they wish to seek insurance cover for such costs. Greater private involvement in health care funding can be achieved, in particular, through patient co-payments, as already implemented in a number of countries (2003:45).

Organising the reformers: the OECD

The OECD role as the body representing the world's 30 most developed economies has primarily been as an organiser, spreading practice and harmonising policies among member states:

> OECD practice papers do not themselves promote privatisation in water, energy, health or other public services, but the vehicle of harmonisation magnifies the impact of policies which do (Hall and de la Motte (2004:7).

By the early 1990s, the wider issue of health care reform had become a focus of discussion among policy-makers and academics: the OECD, representing the world's leading industrialised countries, had begun to collate information and attempt a limited comparison of health care systems among its member states (OECD 1992), and, with a first examination of reforms in seven OECD countries (Hurst 1992), debate over the trends had opened up[81].

OECD-commissioned researchers have developed detailed studies of health care systems and reforms (or the lack of them) in particular member states, including France (Imai et al 2000), Japan (Jeong and Hurst 2001, Imai 2002) and the US (Docteur et al 2003).

---

81 Influential articles included Saltman (1991) on the Swedish reforms, while left wing critics warned of the negative consequences of neoliberal reforms (Laurell 1991, Navarro 1991) and the unsustainable costs of the unreformed US system (Brandon et al 1991).

The OECD itself can express a corporate view which is far from impartial: it made clear its support for the UK government's controversial market-style reforms (Beecham 1994), and more recently expressed its displeasure at the French government's failure to contain public spending (Graham 2003).

It has also pressed member states to address longer-term issues such as the implications of a growing proportion of elderly in national populations (OECD 1995b, Hennessy 1995, Clarke 2001, Oxley and Jacobzone 2001), and within that framework counselled member states to emphasise private sector solutions and to 'curb the growth of spending on public pensions, health and long-term care' (OECD 1998:13).

The OECD has also focused on methods of assessing the performance of health care systems, launching a three-year Health Project in 2001 to 'help decision-makers formulate evidence-based policies', and convening a ministerial level international conference in Ottawa to discuss improving health system performance (OECD 2001b,c,d). OECD Secretary General Donald Johnson argued that:

> International comparisons can help us identify best practices to improve performance in
> individual countries' health care systems (OECD 2001c).

A central issue for this discussion has been the appropriate role and methods of regulating the private sector, which is implicitly assumed to play a valuable role, although Tapay (2001) argues that:

> Our role at OECD is not to come down on one side or another, or promote a particular 'ideal'
> role for private health insurance within a national health system.

More detailed studies concluded that because health care works towards different – politically defined – equity objectives in each country, and because of different methods of collecting data on health outcomes, no single measure was able to compare performance across the OECD member states (Hurst and Jee-Hughes 2001, Leatherman 2001).

These problems have not prevented an ever-expanding effort by the OECD to collate and publish its *Health Data* series annually, each carrying a 'health warning' against mechanical comparisons between the data which may well have been collected in different ways in different member states (OECD 2004). Governments have been urged to adjust their data collection methods to ensure greater consistency in comparisons (National Statistics 2003 a, b).

World Trade Organisation

The World Trade Organisation emerged in the 1990s as another global body promoting the importance of 'free trade', 'liberalising' markets and generally promoting competition and the involvement of the private sector (Moore 2000, WTO 1998).

Interestingly, given the WTO's general support for the concept of 'liberalisation', it has recognised the scale of popular opposition on some issues, and been especially eager to deny allegations that it seeks to extend this principle – or privatisation – to health care, education or water distribution. The WTO response has been indignantly to deny that any erosion of existing public services is under way, while at the same time conceding the essence of the critics' case.

A WTO document (*GATS – fact and fiction*), intended to refute allegations about the proposals, attempts to draw a distinction between allowing foreign suppliers to provide education and health services and the privatisation of public health and education 'systems'

(WTO 2001:10): but it is quite clear that the 'foreign suppliers' will be private enterprises, and that they will in most cases be taking over sections of what is currently a publicly provided service.

The WTO has denied that governments could be forced under WTO rules to open up their public services to global competition:

> It is for governments to decide which service sectors they wish to liberalise and which they do not. [...] Even for those services provided by governments on a commercial basis, there is nothing in the WTO rules which requires that they be privatised of liberalised (WTO 2002a).

However, this situation appears to represent a transitional stage rather than the end of the process of liberalisation: the sheer scale of the prize to be scooped up by the private sector from extending into health and education services means that the issue will inevitably remain on the agenda. These two public services currently account for over 13% of GDP in OECD countries, and the sizeable health sector in OECD countries[82] makes it a 'domestic economic giant', according to the WTO's Secretariat (Pollock and Price 2000).

In most advanced industrialised countries health services already involve some element of competition and some commercial provision – leaving health care open to clause 1.3(b) of the WTO's General Agreement on Trade in Services (GATS), which stipulates that to be excluded a service must be supplied 'in the exercise of government authority' and supplied 'neither on a commercial basis nor in competition with one or more service suppliers'.

GATS also allows governments to liberalise services voluntarily: the British Labour government – which once insisted that it 'has no intention whatsoever of offering to privatise public healthcare or education under GATS 2000 negotiations' (Pollock and Price 2000) – has since awarded contracts for new chains of Diagnostic and Treatment Centres to overseas private sector providers (Dyer O 2003a). The OECD, like the WTO regards public ownership and tight regulation of a service sector as an impediment to competition, and is urging its 30 member governments to remove unnecessary obstacles to competition, innovation and growth (Pollock and Price 2000).

The WTO stresses time and again that member states would be able to 'choose' and decide for themselves how to apply GATS regulations – while ignoring the extreme differences in wealth and power between the 140 GATS member states, and the enormous scale of the potential markets in services which the wealthier countries will want to open up (Joy and Hardstaff 2003). Governments in poorer countries are likely to come under sustained pressure to allow increasing levels of market competition – in which the existing multinational corporations and service providers based in rich countries will have an immediate advantage in terms of scale of operation, technology and availability of capital.

While public funding of services such as health care would continue, GATS would open up the prospect of this government funding being redirected from domestic to foreign suppliers: governments which did not seek a specific opt-out in advance would be obliged to offer the same subsidies to a multinational corporation as it would to its own public sector providers.

The WTO (2001:11) hotly disputes that as an international body it would 'review'

---

82 Estimated to reach $3 trillion by 2005 (Chanda 2002).

standards or 'outlaw' those regarded as unnecessarily restricting trade: but it concedes that such provisions may be disputed by other WTO member states – at which point they could be ruled inadmissible. Opponents of the WTO approach have warned that the application of rules similar to those that have been applied to the Telecoms industry could lead to a major challenge to the principles governing the health care systems in most advanced countries (other than the USA, which uniquely does not offer risk-pooling or social insurance):

> Governments which currently use non-market mechanisms and structures such as risk-pooling,
> social insurance funds, block contracts and cross subsidisation for the delivery of universal health
> care services could be required to switch to... market mechanisms (Pollock and Price 2000).

The WTO denies that member governments would have to submit regulations to the WTO for approval – 'unless asked to justify a specific regulation in the event of a dispute with another Government' (WTO 2001:12). And while the WTO insists that none of the principles cited by Pollock and Price has ever been considered 'or even mentioned' in the GATS negotiations, this does not mean that they could not be raised once the new framework is in place.

The process towards trade liberalisation appeared to have stalled, largely as a result of unexpected resistance by poorer and 'middle income' countries at the WTO's Cancun summit in 2003. This came despite efforts to win round opinion with the limited deal offering access to cheaper generic supplies of patented medicines for some of the very poorest countries (WTO 2003a, b).

However it is clear that for a key section of the international business community the introduction of a free 'market' in health care is more than a theoretical concept or a technical reorganisation at national level. The lure of a greater share of a $3 trillion global business is likely to bring these issues back on to the international agenda.

FTAA

The hiatus in progress towards GATS and the next round of WTO liberalisation has led the US to focus more energy on bilateral trade deals and regional agreements in the Americas. The WTO objectives have been echoed – even amplified – in the provisions of the North American Free Trade Area (NAFTA) involving the USA, Canada and Mexico, and more recently in the proposals for a continent-wide treaty to establish a Free Trade Area of the Americas (FTAA), which would explicitly include health care (and education) as services to be opened up for private sector involvement and competition from for-profit corporations (Barlow 2000).

Already under NAFTA regulations corporations in one country can challenge laws, policies or practices of an elected government in another member state, alleging that these impinge on the established 'rights' of the corporation. This challenge can include suing for compensation for current and future profits lost as a result of government action, no matter if how legal it may be or why it was carried out (Barlow 2000).

Canadian opponents of the trade agreements warn that they could endanger Canada's universal, tax-funded health care system, opening up services to competition from profit-seeking corporations in the US, which could also exploit GATS regulations to demand the right to establish a 'commercial presence' in Canada and compete with existing non-profit providers for contracts to deliver publicly funded services. The problem is worsened by the legislation already passed in Alberta which allows private corporations to tender for provision of services to medicare patients: as a result US corporations in other Canadian provinces would be entitled to sue for compensation if they are denied similar access (Barlow 2000).

CAFTA

The US has been attempting to speed up progress towards a new Central American Free Trade Agreement (CAFTA) that would sweep aside some of the protections for labour standards incorporated in the existing Clinton-era Generalised System of Preferences and the US Caribbean Basin Trade Partnership Act.

El Salvador, Guatemala, Honduras and Nicaragua signed up to the pact with the US in December 2003, and in December 2004 El Salvador's right-wing government became the first to defy popular protests and force through a motion in Parliament ratifying the Agreement.

The implementation of the 2,500-page treaty, however, requires the approval of the US Congress, where the level of opposition has delayed attempts by the Bush administration to secure ratification. CAFTA, which had been expected to be signed in May 2004, has been opposed by US trade unions as well as activists in Central American countries (where there are stronger trade unions, left political parties and social struggles than elsewhere on the continent) as an attack on trade union rights (Kyer 2002).

Opponents of the treaty also argue that it would force Central American countries to open up their markets to imports of subsidised US pharmaceuticals, and lead to the privatisation of all public services including social services, education and health care (www.cispes.org). They note that the trade liberalisation that has already taken place in the region has widened income inequality and led to the loss of 600,000 Central American jobs.

In El Salvador, the right wing government's attempts – encouraged by the Inter-American Development Bank – to pre-empt the CAFTA deal by privatising the social insurance sector of health care led to a prolonged (seven-month) strike by doctors, nurses and other health workers and a rise of popular opposition: the President was forced to declare that the privatisation attempt had been abandoned (Social Justice Committee 2002, Engler 2003).

In Guatemala, March 2005 brought thousands riot police onto the streets to repress anti-CAFTA demonstrators as the legislature voted to ratify the treaty, which has also been passed in Honduras. Accepting the CAFTA treaty required Guatemala to reverse legislation its own government had brought in to force in December 2004 which aimed to increase access to affordable generic medicines: the law was immediately to subject of a protest by the US Ambassador and the Office of the US Trade Representative (HealthGAP 2005).

Last December Costa Rica voted against the Agreement, leaving the legislatures of the United States and Nicaragua yet to pass it. A hearing on CAFTA, the first step in congressional approval of the pact, will be held in the US Senate in April (Indymedia 2005).

The World Health Organisation

Historical background

One of the global organisations which might be expected to uphold a more progressive agenda, addressing some of the genuine social and economic issues involved in the improvement of health on a world scale, is the World Health Organisation (WHO). Launched in 1946, with 61 countries signing its constitution, and 55 attending its 1948 World Health Assembly, the WHO now has 191 member countries, and is the United Nations' leading specialist agency for health (Vaughan et al 1996).

The WHO is not an NGO, and does not deliver services directly: instead it works with governments and health ministries, in a manner designed to 'avoid charges of imperialism'

(Godlee 1994a). Its Secretariat has 4,500 members of staff, with headquarters in Switzerland and regional offices in Washington (for the Americas), Brazzaville (for Africa), Alexandria, Egypt for the Eastern Mediterranean, Copenhagen for Europe, New Delhi for SE Asia and Manila for the Western Pacific.

The WHO is best known for its projects and public health campaigns reaching into the poorer countries of Africa and Asia , and for its ambitious – ultimately unattainable – Health For All 2000 project, which it launched in 1977 and promoted alongside UNICEF at an international conference in Alma Ata in 1978. HFA 2000 aimed at improving the health of the world's population by the turn of the century (WHO 1992). Linked to the HFA programme was a new emphasis on primary care as the key to developing an infrastructure of basic health care in developing countries which did not have the budgets available for a network of more advanced hospitals.

The WHO, as the global body credited by the UN in 1979 with coordinating the elimination of smallpox, and which continues a focus on preventing communicable disease in developing countries, also has the potential to be a significant force in influencing health care policies, especially among the poorest member states, although in practice its freedom to act, and even its ability to publish accurate data which may be perceived as embarrassing or damaging to influential member states can also be constrained (Murray et al 2004).

During its first 25 years, the WHO was a fairly conservative, specialist, medical-led agency, consciously avoiding political or potential religious controversy from dabbling in issues such as contraception (Godlee 1994b). However the rising number of independent member states meant that political control of the World Health Assembly, like that of the UN General Assembly, had by the late 1970s visibly slipped from the grasp of the USA and the wealthier developed countries. While the increasingly representative membership gave the WHO potentially greater authority, it also made it potentially vulnerable to 'capture' by more radical policies promoted by increasingly self-confident and independent-minded developing countries.

The Health For All 2000 policy, with its emphasis on support for the world's poorest people was followed in the same year by a WHO challenge to the profits of the pharmaceutical corporations – when it published a list of 200 cheaper 'essential' drugs, to be purchased and prescribed in preference to up to 5,000 branded drugs that were being sold at high prices to 'third world' countries (Turshen 1999). This degree of independence made the WHO an obvious target for those who valued the freedom of the market above equity in health care or access to care for the majority of the world's population.

The US government in particular objected to the WHO's attempts to regulate the private sector, and to the WHO's (far from radical) efforts, through the HFA initiative, to reduce tobacco consumption. In 1981 the US was also the only country at the World Health Assembly (WHA) to oppose the new WHO international code on breast milk substitutes, arguing that it was an interference in global trade. In 1985 the US withheld its contributions to the WHO budget (Godlee 1994b), and the WHO's central leadership has come under increasing pressure to tailor the organisation's initiatives and policies to fit within the resurgent free market ideology espoused by Reagan, Thatcher, the World Bank and the IMF.

Financial/economic pressure

As part of this pressure, the WHO's core budget has effectively been frozen since 1980, giving zero real terms growth. This has meant that any significant new initiatives have had to be funded through a rising level of 'extrabudgetary' contributions from the wealthier countries – funds and initiatives which are not controlled by the World Health Assembly (WHA). As a result of this new system, donor countries like the US, which had failed to maintain direct control democratically by winning a majority in the WHA, could now circumvent the apparatus, and decide WHO policies on the ground by granting or withholding funding (Godlee 1994a).

By 1990, the WHO had been effectively sidelined as a major player in the provision of external assistance, with its levels of spending dwarfed by NGOs such as Oxfam and Save the Children Fund, and even by direct loans from the World Bank. Godlee found that in India in 1994, the WHO's annual budget was just $7.5m compared with $100m available to UNICEF, the rival UN agency dealing with health and nutritional matters, with which the WHO was increasingly in competition for influence, despite the fact that UNICEF's rudimentary anti-HIV programme was dismissed as 'only condoms' (Godlee 1994c).

Turshen (1999) and other critics argue that the WHO's growing dependence on $1 billion of 'extrabudgetary' revenue may have steered the organisation away from the influence of the poorer member states, but has instead made the WHO increasingly subject to influence by other bodies – notably the World Bank, donor governments in the wealthier countries, and the drug companies – whose agenda can be seen as very different from the founding objectives of the WHO.

As Turshen (1999) argues, the various donors of extrabudgetary contributions are inclined to fund 'the disease of the day rather than long-term basic health care', and their contributions are given for only one year at a time, creating uncertainty and instability in any planning process. Large amounts of WHO time and resources then have to be allocated to the management of specific smaller scale projects rather than offering more coordination, international cooperation and sharing of information.

Politics and economics

WHO and health system reforms

WHO-sponsored debates reflect a rather more detached and critical approach than the World Bank to many key aspects of health care reforms, but the organisation's involvement in the process of reform since the mid 1990s has contributed to the pressure for change – at a time when the most powerful forces have been seeking to direct that change towards market-style measures.

The process of political softening within the WHO, if it has occurred, has not been an even one. But its results can be illustrated by a stark contrast. As recently as 1995 its *World Health Report* focused relentlessly on extreme poverty as the 'world's biggest killer', pointing to the way in which:

...the gaps between rich and poor, between one population group and another, between ages and between the sexes are widening.

The Report went on to warn that gains from recent immunisation campaigns were being 'eroded or even reversed by economic and social conditions'. And (without naming the World Bank or the IMF as culprits), it went on to point out that:

Structural adjustment policies aimed at improving the economic performance of poor countries have in many cases made the situation worse.

But a radically different approach could be seen five years later. Addressing the roots of ill health, the *World Health Report 2000* (WHR2000) linked ill health not to poverty but to levels of health spending, arguing:

> If Sweden enjoys better health than Uganda – life expectancy is almost exactly twice as long – that is in large part because it spends exactly 35 times as much per capita on its health system (WHR2000:40).

Navarro (2000) challenges this unsupported claim that medical treatment alone is likely to reduce mortality and morbidity levels. It seems clear from this abrupt change of emphasis that the WHO had by 2000 begun to position itself differently on issues of health care policy.

WHO meets a new line from the Bank

In part the different approach reflects an accommodation by the WHO to political developments already implemented within the more established health care systems. But another major influence seems to have been the World Bank. The changing rhetoric of its pronouncements and some of the research it sponsored at the time suggest the Bank was looking for ways to present itself as a less aggressive, more caring force on issues of social policy (Abassi 1999f).

Buse and Walt have also commented on the political convergence since the late 1970s between the UN and its agencies on the one hand and the World Bank on the other, noting that:

> ...the 1990s were marked by an ideological shift from 'freeing' to 'modifying' the market. ...most advocates of free markets have moderated their position, seeing a continuing role for the public sector, particularly within the area of health, where markets are often inefficient and equity is harder to achieve (Buse and Walt 2000a:551).

Whatever its reservations about the direction of health reforms, the WHO could play a useful role for the Bank – by promoting a debate which kept open the door for market-style solutions or for an increased role for the private sector. The influence of the WHO promoting such debates would be even greater in the developing countries, where it was more trusted than the Bank.

The WHO did so, lending its support to initiatives which attempted to steer both new and established health services – especially those in the 'third world' – in a common direction. As part of this, it supported the development of the Mexico-based International Clearing House for Health System Reforms[83], with a regular newsletter, *Informing and Reforming*. This may have been seen to encourage acceptance of market style reforms, especially when indebted countries seeking financial aid and support also faced political pressure – from OECD countries, the WB, the IMF, USAID and US-funded NGOs – to comply with market models. However there wasn't much in the way of good news about the reforms.

The International Centre, and leading elements of the WHO seemed willing to accept and work alongside market-based reforms. By Issue 2, the magazine was carrying uncritical reports, including one detailing the implementation of a full catalogue of USAID-World Bank

---

83 Funded by the World Bank and the Rockefeller Foundation in addition to WHO support (Almeida 2001).

'reforms' in Indonesia. Among the 'reforms' it listed were decentralisation, 'corporatization of public hospitals into self-reliance hospitals', promotion of public/private mix in both the financing and provision of health care, support for 'private sector services for the better off', user fees, and encouragement of 'private foreign and domestic investment.' The article reports that of the $1.4 billion that had been given to support Indonesian government spending in health care, about 75% was in the form of loans – to be repaid, presumably to the IMF or the World Bank.

Even after such 'reforms' only 12% of the population was covered by the Community Health Maintenance Assurance scheme (Suwandono and Gani 1997). It is not clear what benefit could be gained by simply exchanging information on this level without any significant accompanying comment, analysis or recommendation. The Indonesian article gets off to an uninspiring start (and gives a hint as to its limited political horizons) when it describes the (then flagging, since ousted) bloodstained Suharto dictatorship as '25 years of stable government'.

So deadpan was the reporting of potentially highly controversial policies that it was far from clear whether this, and other subsequent articles promoting some of the stock World Bank/USAID reforms were (on the model of Jonathan Swift's famous satire *A Modest Proposal*) intended to shock the reader into angry rejection, or (as appears to be the case) simply presented a confusing, agnostic, but generally supportive picture of the complex processes of 'reform' under way in developing countries.

However a number of later articles did sound warnings over attempts to transplant the seemingly ubiquitous idea of 'managed care' from the US to Latin America (Waitzkin 1997) and over other prominent elements of the 'reform' agenda, such as expanding private provision, competition, and user fees (Mills 1998). Schuftan and Dahlgren, writing from Hanoi, warned that the concept of Health Sector Reforms had 'literally been "hijacked or monopolised" by what one would call a "World Bank-led paradigm of health reforms"' (Schuftan and Dahlgren 1999). Celia Almeida concluded that the WHO had ceded political ground to the 'neoliberal hegemony' which had developed since the 1980s:

> These changes were defined and encouraged by international organisations such as the OECD and the World Bank, while the United States took the leadership role in formulating the new, post-welfare state, health agenda. To this picture we should add the loss of space within the international health policy arena by organisations charged with addressing the broad issues of health, like the World Health Organisation, which were supplanted by financial agencies like the World Bank and the International Monetary Fund, oriented towards promoting economic themes of adjustment and restructuring (Almeida 1998:3).

Evolving politics of WHO

Change at the top

The increasingly close working relationship between the WHO and the World Bank and other organisations promoting neoliberal policies developed even more after Dr Gro Harlem Brundtland was elected WHO Director General in 1998. On taking office on July 21, she was swift to appoint ten new people to a new cabinet of top-level advisors, including Dr Michael Scholz, a senior figure from the pharmaceutical industry, who was seen as providing a new 'liaison' between the industry and the WHO (Godlee 1998, WHO Press Release 1998).

Another leading light from the World Bank, the former director of its Health Nutrition and

Population (HNP) sector, Richard Feachem, took over as Editor in Chief of a remodelled WHO *Bulletin,* despite criticisms raised by the World Bank's own Operations Evaluation Department of the poor performance of HNP programmes during the time Feachem was in control. The new WHO *Bulletin* began monthly publication in 1999, and became much more overtly political and focused on the various issues of reform (Feachem 1999).

Brundtland consistently emphasised her determination to work alongside the private sector, and her quest for 'partnership' with the World Bank and other global agencies. This same 'partnership' approach with the private sector has brought the inclusion of other leading representatives of the pharmaceutical industry into the WHO's working parties, including the Tobacco Free Initiative and the HIV/AIDS campaign. During 2000 Buse and Walt discussed the emergence of Global 'public-private partnerships' in two articles in the WHO *Bulletin* (Buse and Walt 2002a, 2000b).

In March 2001, Brundtland launched a WHO/WTO workshop on differential pricing and financing of essential drugs. She appeared oblivious to the fact that the meeting took place in the midst of what was already a growing series of worldwide anti-capitalist demonstrations, challenging 'globalisation' in general and the WTO in particular. Brundtland described the WTO in wholly positive terms:

> We need WTO as an effective and fair forum for negotiating trade rules and resolving disputes (Brundtland 2001b).

And in May 2001, Brundtland spelled out an even wider and less focused agenda for partnerships with almost any global agency: she cited work with the OECD, the EU and many more organisations with very different aims and objectives, including USAID, the subsidiary of the US State Department with the most explicit proponent of private sector solutions:

> We have placed large emphasis on partnerships. […] We have stepped up our partnership with bilateral cooperation agencies like USAID, which we consider partners, not just donors. We have organised round tables with private sector industry and have undertaken several initiatives in partnership with corporations and foundations (Brundtland 2001c).

It is clear from Brundtland's speeches and personal involvement that the change of emphasis and rapprochement with the World Bank were deliberate WHO policy, not a series of accidents or coincidences.

WHO independence

It could be argued that one of the reasons why the WHO offers an attractive partner for the World Bank is because it is seen as having a degree of independence, and a concern to improve public health rather than the balance sheets of big capital. A WHO which openly embraced neoliberal policies and the World Bank's free market rhetoric would risk losing its credibility in many developing countries (Navarro 2000).

Nevertheless the WHO's *World Health Report 2000* (WHR2000) does appear to have embraced World Bank values, when it discusses ways of mitigating the problems (such as perverse incentives, exclusions and adverse selection) that can arise from the introduction of more market-based systems of health insurance. It also gave a retrospective endorsement to Margaret Thatcher's market-style reforms in Britain, by echoing the famous claim of Conservative ministers that a system is good if 'the money follows the patient' (DoH 1989).

However the most far-reaching political debate over the evolution and role of the WHO was triggered by two changes in WHO policy that were embodied in WHR2000:

- The decision to synthesise some of its routinely published statistical information into a direct comparison between different national systems
- The decision to embark on a process of building 'Global Public Private Partnerships'.

WHR2000 attempted to rank 191 health services from all over the world in a single league table – based on (contentious) calculations of 'healthy life expectancy' for the country's population, 'responsiveness' of the service to patients, and the 'fairness' of the financing system. It triggered a wave of angry responses.

While a few struggled to find positive aspects in the WHR findings or at least in the likely consequences of their publication (McKee 2001), those offended by the conclusions and/or the methodology employed by WHR2000 ranged from the aggrieved governments whose health care systems came unexpectedly low on the list (notably Brazil, which came 125th – Almeida et al 2001 to World Bank neoliberals, who ridiculed the 'counterintuitive' and 'seriously flawed' fairness indicator (Shaw 2002, Wagstaff 2002). Other critics included enthusiastic proponents of equity in health care (Braveman et al 2001).

So serious were the shock-waves generated by the WHR2000 that publication of a second, updated version, due in October 2002 (PAHO 2001) was postponed to late 2003 (Brown 2002). A full-scale debate over the methodology for any future comparisons between systems was opened up on the WHO web site.

Some of the anger arose from the very large gaps in data used for the comparisons, the use of some data as much as ten years old (Landmann Szwarcwald 2002): but the gaps in data were extremely large. Almeida et al (2001) point out that there were no data at all available for the WHO to construct its 'index of inequality' for 133 of the 191 countries (70%), while 'responsiveness' data were unavailable for even more (161, or 84%) and only 21 of the 191 countries (11%) supplied data to construct the index on 'fairness'. There were some countries for which no data at all were available on which to base a score, and therefore their ranking order was based purely on 'imputed data'. Almeida et al argue that the result was seriously flawed, and that:

> …readers deserve to know the underlying assumptions, methods and key limitations, which were not adequately acknowledged.

Navarro (2000) also condemns WHR2000's positioning of the Spanish health care system as third best major country in Europe in the overall league tables (after France and Italy), at the very time of widespread public discontent and protests by Spanish people over failures in the system. Indeed Spain emerges in the WHO's own figures as one of the least 'responsive' of all the European health services.

He also drew a link between WHR2000's selection of statistical data and lop-sided findings (in which Colombia, with its insurance-based 'managed care' health system, emerges as the 'best overall system' in Latin America) on the one hand, and political and ideological concessions by the WHO to US neoliberal economics and the World Bank on the other. Navarro also warns against seeing the WHO as apolitical or neutral, stressing that it can play an ideological role, and condemns the way in which, with no serious evidence or discussion, WHR2000 declared the long-standing WHO policy of promoting services based on primary care to be 'at least a partial failure'.

A different line of criticism argues that using statistics to measure the average level of health in a population is a reductionist retreat from the WHO's often quoted definition of health as 'a state of complete physical, mental and social well-being and not merely the absence of disease' (Van der Stuyft and Unger 2000).

Dahlgren (2000) has also pointed to the explicit World Bank input and role in these WHO debates in the form of Bank statistician David Gwatkin, and questions the extent to which the Bank's policies are compatible with the WHO's proclaimed objectives. Braveman et al (2001) argue that the WHO's controversial statistical measures of inequality are ineffective as a means to guide policy or intervention – not least because they do not differentiate between different social groups within a country, rich and poor. As a result, they argue:

> A minister of health whose country ranked poorly on the Report's inequalities measure would have no idea where to begin to look to tackle the disparities.

Critics have also questioned WHR2000's definition of health care financing as 'perfectly fair' if all households pay the same proportion of their non-food spending on health services – irrespective of how much money (if any) different households may have left over after paying for food (WHR 2000:36; Murray and Frenk 2000). Almeida et al (2001) go on to argue that under such criteria it could be deemed 'fair' if two households, one with a $500 income and one with $100,000 (each after paying for food) both paid 10% of their 'disposable income' on health care. But the low-income household would have little or no disposable income at all – and may even be forced to sell assets to raise the equivalent of 10%, while the wealthier household could easily spare its share of the health budget. So after reducing 'fairness' to the abstract question of sharing the burden of funding health services – WHR2000 appears to come down against progressive taxation as unfair to the rich[84].

WHR2000(15) also embraced the prevailing Third Way/NPM notion of a 'partnership' between the public and private sectors, explicitly criticising the 'complete omission of private finance and provision of care from the Alma Ata Declaration' and praising 'third generation' reforms which (echoing Thatcher's famous phrase about Conservative UK market reforms) try to make 'money follow the patient'. In this, as in many of the issues discussed above, WHR2000 can be seen as an indication of a growing level of convergence between the WHO and the Bank, and increasing pressure on developing countries to comply with a global menu of reforms.

'Partnerships'

A different adaptation to the pressures of the market, and an echo of the politics of the 'third way', can be found in the emerging UN and WHO concept of 'Global Public Private Partnerships' (Buse and Walt 2000a). Around 70 such partnerships have been identified, many of them involving drug companies and research projects (Buse and Waxman 2001).

This stance has been controversial among NGOs and within the WHO's own structures. Critics point out that the WHO, with its global budget of $1.7 billion, is potentially vulnerable to political and economic pressure from much wealthier drug companies and private corporations, making any 'partnership' profoundly unequal (HAI 2000). They question the altruism of the corporations concerned, and point to the potentially valuable commercial,

---

84 Its index of 'fairness' is so insensitive that on a scale from zero to one, no less than 147 countries (over 75%) score 0.9 or above.

political and public relations advantages that could be secured by large private companies that are seen to be working alongside the UN, the WHO and health NGOs.

Policies emerging from such 'partnerships' are seen as likely to revolve around the use of more costly, modern (patented) drugs and vaccines than cheaper generic alternatives, and in the case of immunisation campaigns more likely to concentrate on areas of proven success – the 74% of the target population already covered by immunisation – rather than attempting to penetrate the more needy areas, the 30-40% who do not yet receive any preventative treatment. There are also fears that the privately backed campaigns, using the latest vaccines, may result in a reduced local capacity to produce vaccines and a rejection of local generic products by a sceptical public convinced that the cheaper product is inferior.

As one critic argues:

Today vaccination policies seem to have shifted towards public-private partnerships and away from equity. [...] In vaccination programmes the focus now appears to be creating markets for new vaccines. [...] Unlike earlier vaccine campaigns, these initiatives spend little time discussing sustainability (Hardon 2000).

The ethics – and the longer term effectiveness – of the immunisation and other programmes promoted by the WHO, alongside UNICEF and the World Bank have occasionally been challenged by angry critics, often from bitter experiences in developing countries (Banerji 1999, Schreuder and Kostermans 2001). Banerji decries global programmes on immunisation, AIDS and tuberculosis in Asian countries, which he describes as 'astonishingly defective' in concept, design and implementation. Ncayiyana (2002) is also critical of the way Africans have been used to test drugs from which they will never benefit:

...either because the drugs are too costly, or because they are designed to treat conditions that largely affect industrialised nations.

Tan-Torres Edejer (1999) cites a participant in a drugs study in Guatemala, who faced the need to fund two costly drugs from a triple cocktail if he was to continue feeling the benefit he had experienced during the trial. And while arguing that 'the "scientific colonialism" that characterised earlier North-South research collaborations has slowly been transformed,' Edejer goes on to question the ethics of using placebo controlled trials of drugs in developing countries where the standard package of care did not include the use of AZT. She warns that:

Despite the good intentions of the North-South partners, clashing agendas and values persist.

Another damning criticism of the current style of WHO policy came in Lockwood's *BMJ* article reviewing the WHO's 'leprosy elimination' programme. She argues that the apparent dramatic fall from 5 million to 0.7 million in the numbers of registered leprosy patients between 1985-2001 was largely due to a change in the definition of a leprosy patient, to include only those receiving multi-drug therapy. Far from leprosy being 'eliminated', there were 719,300 new patients registered as suffering from the disease in 2000, with numbers actually *rising* in the worst affected countries (Lockwood 2002).

Lockwood goes on to challenge some of the new methods used by the WHO in tackling the disease, which involve far less patient contact and monitoring, and a halving of the length of a course of multidrug therapy from two years to one ('despite evidence that patients with high bacterial loads are at greater risk of relapse'). She argues that these changes are based on no published evidence of effectiveness – but that when they were challenged on the Global

Alliance to Eliminate Leprosy by the ILEP (the international umbrella organisation of NGOs fighting leprosy), the ILEP was excluded from the 'partnership'. Significantly the partnership still includes the drug company Novartis. She warns that the WHO rhetoric about having 'eliminated' leprosy may lead governments to wind up their own control programmes. And she asks who will pay for the drug treatments that will be necessary after 2005, or train the staff who will still be needed to care for leprosy sufferers 'for many years to come'.

Any attempt to extend to developing countries the modern medical techniques that have enabled health gains in the advanced economies would also require the additional development of modern, well equipped hospitals and specialist staff. Persuading developing countries to set their sights no higher than a primary care system – with even this minimal provision possibly underwritten through user-fees and 'cost recovery' – can be seen as a means of consolidating a global two-tier system for health care, in which whole populations and sub-continents are denied access to comprehensive services.

If this were to become the accepted model, it would mean that in developing countries, any modern and complex treatment – whether medical or surgical – would for the foreseeable future be available only to the wealthy and educated who were able to access treatment in the advanced health services abroad. For the WHO such a policy would represent not just a retreat, but effectively an abandonment of the underlying values of social solidarity and the principles of equity and access which were at the root of Health For All 2000.

Chapter four

The reform agenda

Introduction

As discussed in Chapter two above, the many pressures on health care systems in rich and poor countries offer many legitimate areas in which the right structural changes and an injection of sufficient resources could serve to enhance equity and access, accountability, professional skills, effectiveness and standards of treatment, and the empowerment of consumers. However, as this chapter will show, there is a serious mismatch between the objective problems and the policies put forward as solutions by the main groups and organisations proposing health system reform.

The question arises: has the menu of policy prescriptions been formulated to meet the needs of the sick and the poor, or to maximise the profits of the rich and the private sector? The chapter works through the main 'menu' of the most common identified reforms, analysing the context in which they are being proposed and implemented, and discussing the evidence or projections on their chances of success.

The main elements of the reform agenda in the wealthier and poor countries are depicted in diagrammatic form in Figure 2, and are also set out in Table 1. This study will argue that while some types of reform could in some circumstances be assigned to both categories, most of this menu of reforms can be categorised as either cost-saving ('market-driven') or as 'market-style' measures.

Despite largely unsubstantiated claims that they improve 'efficiency' (World Bank 2000e), cost-saving is at most a secondary consideration in market-style reforms. It may therefore be deduced that market-style reforms are driven by ideological conviction rather than economic necessity, and that questions arising from such reforms should focus on their probable consequences in reshaping health care systems around the principles of the market. For this reason it is useful to differentiate between the two very different types of reform if the underlying driving forces behind them are to be understood.

Figure 2: The menu of health sector reform in rich and poor countries

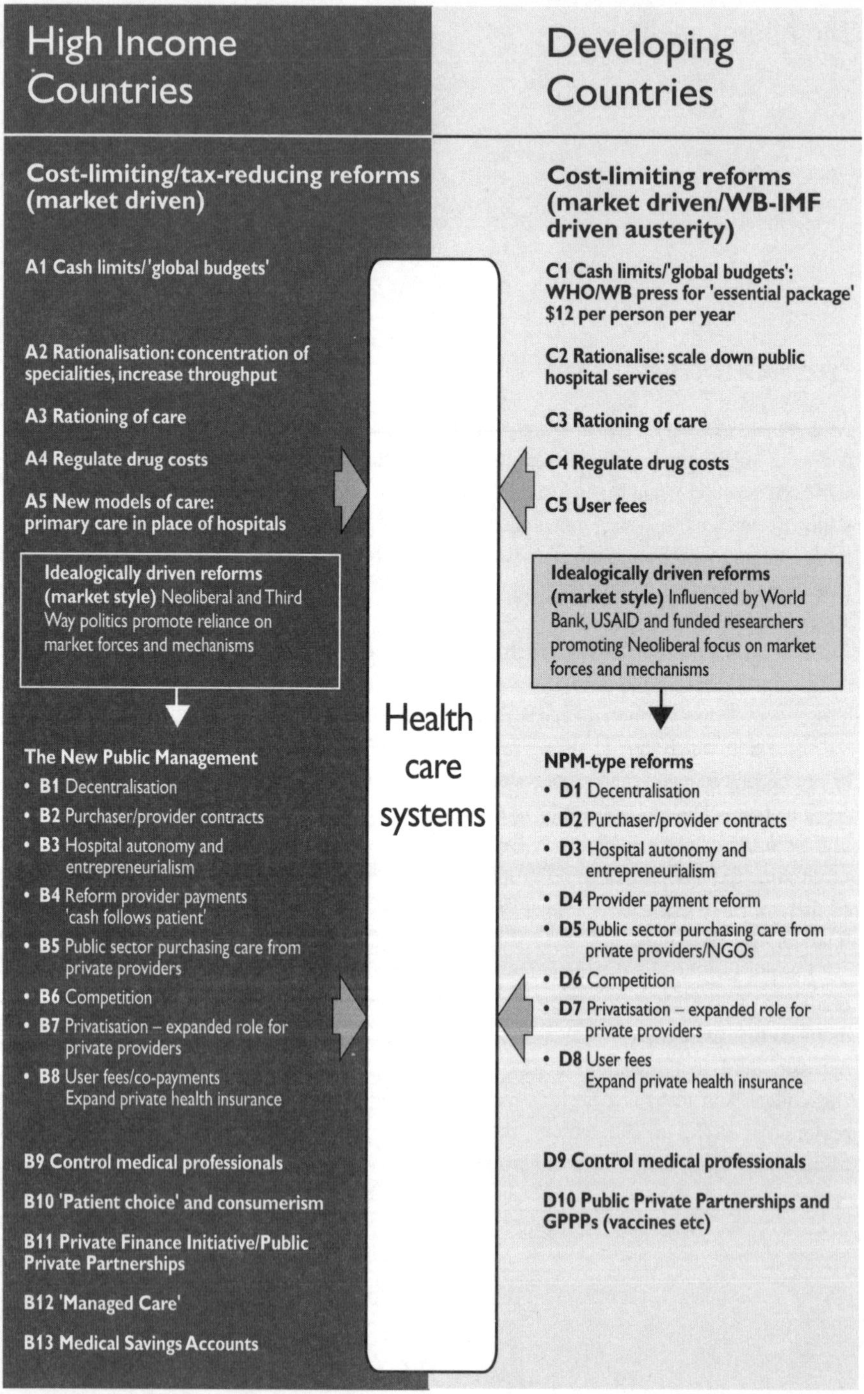

High Income Countries	Developing Countries
Cost-limiting/tax-reducing reforms (market driven)	**Cost-limiting reforms (market driven/WB-IMF driven austerity)**
A1 Cash limits/'global budgets'	C1 Cash limits/'global budgets': WHO/WB press for 'essential package' $12 per person per year
A2 Rationalisation: concentration of specialities, increase throughput	C2 Rationalise: scale down public hospital services
A3 Rationing of care	C3 Rationing of care
A4 Regulate drug costs	C4 Regulate drug costs
A5 New models of care: primary care in place of hospitals	C5 User fees
Idealogically driven reforms (market style) Neoliberal and Third Way politics promote reliance on market forces and mechanisms	**Idealogically driven reforms (market style)** Influenced by World Bank, USAID and funded researchers promoting Neoliberal focus on market forces and mechanisms
The New Public Management	**NPM-type reforms**
• **B1** Decentralisation	• **D1** Decentralisation
• **B2** Purchaser/provider contracts	• **D2** Purchaser/provider contracts
• **B3** Hospital autonomy and entrepreneurialism	• **D3** Hospital autonomy and entrepreneurialism
• **B4** Reform provider payments 'cash follows patient'	• **D4** Provider payment reform
• **B5** Public sector purchasing care from private providers	• **D5** Public sector purchasing care from private providers/NGOs
• **B6** Competition	• **D6** Competition
• **B7** Privatisation – expanded role for private providers	• **D7** Privatisation – expanded role for private providers
• **B8** User fees/co-payments Expand private health insurance	• **D8** User fees Expand private health insurance
B9 Control medical professionals	**D9 Control medical professionals**
B10 'Patient choice' and consumerism	**D10 Public Private Partnerships and GPPPs (vaccines etc)**
B11 Private Finance Initiative/Public Private Partnerships	
B12 'Managed Care'	
B13 Medical Savings Accounts	

Health care systems

Table 1: The reform agenda	
Market-driven (cost-cutting)	**Market-style** (ideologically driven, restructuring)
Cash limits (A1, C1)	Decentralisation (B1, D1)
Rationalisation/bed cuts (A2, C2)	Contracts (B2, D2)
Rationing and exclusions (A3, C3)	Provider autonomy/ entrepreneurialism (B3, D3)
Regulate drug costs (A4, C4)	Provider payment reform (B4, D4)
New models of care: primary care in place of hospitals(A5)	Public services purchase care from private sector (B5, D5)
User fees (C5)	Competition (B6, D6)
	Privatisation (B7, D7)
	User fees as market-style reform to expand private insurance (B8, D8)
	Control medical professionals (B9, D9)
	Patient choice and consumerism (B10)
	PFI and Public Private Partnerships (B11, D10)
	Managed care (B12)
	Medical Savings Accounts (B13)

Overview:
cost containment ('market-driven') reforms

Market-*style* reforms involve attempts to restructure health care systems to embody some or all of the features of a market (whether 'internal' within the public sector, or, more commonly, a 'mixed economy' public-private market) in health services.

Market-*driven* (or *cost*-driven) reforms, on the other hand, date back long before the wave of market-style reforms and the nostrums of the New Public Management became fashionable in the 1990s:

> Cost containment has been driving health policy discussions in industrialised countries since the 1970s (Mossialos et al 2002:1).

Market-driven reforms reflect the external pressures of the global market place and domestic capital on the government and the economy, and may include very basic measures designed to hold down corporate taxation by restricting expansion of the public sector – such as containing government spending on health care services through imposing global cash limits. As we have seen, this is also a part of the stock neoliberal policy agenda of 'small government', so they are not incompatible.

However in general market-driven/cost-cutting reforms do not involve substantial restructuring of the health care system: services may be rationalised, rationed or restricted, and subordinate elements of the service may be privatised, but the main driver is *cost* rather than *policy*, and as a result their organisational structure and the underlying funding system will generally remain unchanged (Collins et al 1999).

A contradiction of some market-driven policies is that by cutting public funding they may restrict the potential development of the domestic market for health care, and thus constrain the activities of private providers of health goods or services. Pharmaceutical companies in the USA, for example, normally strong advocates of neoliberal policies, have lobbied Congress against legislation that would open access to cheap imports of drugs currently sold at higher prices in the American market (McGregor 2003).

Market-driven policies involving substantial restrictions on government health spending have on occasion been forced upon the wealthier countries[85], but they are more frequently imposed upon developing countries (in various forms, including IMF Structural Adjustment Programmes).

While the rhetoric employed by those politicians and managers who implement them at national and local level suggests that the focus of both market-driven and market-style reforms is the improvement of services and maximising their availability to the patient, some critics argue that the main underlying objective is the improvement of profitability and the expansion of market-opportunity for the private sector (Vienonen et al 1999).

The main elements of market-driven reforms are set out for clarity in Table 2, though experience has shown that while many countries are experimenting with a number of these policies, no governments embarking on health system reforms have so far been persuaded to implement all of these elements simultaneously.

Table 2: The reform agenda
Market-driven (cost-cutting) reforms

Cash limits (A1, C1)
Rationalisation/bed cuts (A2, C2)
Rationing and exclusions (A3, C3)
Regulate drug costs (A4, C4)
User fees (C5)

An additional line of policy (in the diagram Figure 2, but not included in this table) was advanced as justification for a further round of rationalisation of hospitals and beds in the early 1990s in Britain, but failed to deliver results and has been little heard of since. This was the notion of substituting improved primary care services for hospital provision. The policy was always controversial, opposed not only by hospital consultants, but by some public health and primary care specialists (Holland 2000, Edwards et al 2000).

Serious doubts were raised as to whether this type of 'substitution' really does save money, or simply shifts spending from secondary care back to primary care and to individuals and their families. Coulter (1995) found that despite the increased pressures on primary care staff, there was 'little evidence that developments in primary care are reducing the demand for secondary care'.

---

85 Notably the British Labour government's 'IMF cuts', which resulted in cash limits on NHS spending from 1976: but also the more recent austerity policies in France and Germany designed to restrict spending on health, social security and pensions in order to keep the economy within the limits of the EU's 'Stability Pact' underpinning the single European currency.

Shepperd et al (1998) found that hospital at home treatment did not reduce overall health care costs in general, but actually increased them for some patients. Despite claims by Coast and colleagues (1996) that 'about 10% of admissions to general hospital might be suitable for alternative forms of care', Coulter (1998) reports research findings that undermine the central assumption that some GPs unnecessarily refer patients to hospital who might be better cared for at home, and Hensher et al (1999b) also note relatively little evidence of inappropriate admission.

The debate continues, animated above all by the need to find ways to 'manage demand for secondary care' – in order to reduce or contain costs (Edwards and Hensher 1998). More recently a new drive to switch a substantial volume of care from secondary to primary has been seen as one way to contain the vast and growing costs of a new PFI-funded hospital project in Central Manchester (CMMH 2003), although no concrete plans for achieving this objective have been published or agreed by primary care professionals.

Apparently similar policies have been advocated in developing countries by the WHO for very different reasons. Noting the disproportionate share of health spending which was going to relatively few large hospitals in big cities, while rural populations lacked even the most basic access to health care, the WHO Health for All 2000 campaign called for an increased share of resources to be reallocated to establish an infrastructure of primary care. This was envisaged as a significant way in which more care could be made available to the poor.

However if the switch of resources takes place at the expense of drastically reducing the resources for hospital care, the results can prove politically embarrassing, as Purvis (1997) argues. His analysis examines the situation at Zambia's 1,800-bed UTH hospital, which saw its allocation cut from 25% of Zambia's health budget in 1994 to just 11% in 1997, alongside a corresponding increase in primary care spending. Purvis warns that however progressive the aspirations of a policy, the politics cannot be ignored:

> Hospitals are the most visible part of the health care system and reductions in resources often result in observable deficiencies... the public visibility turns into unfavourable publicity, which becomes politically difficult... (1997:3)

The remainder of this chapter will explore some of the salient factors in the most common market-driven, and then market-style reforms.

The main menu of market-driven reforms

Cash limits (or 'global budgets')

Perhaps the crudest way of seeking cost containment in health care is simply to restrict the funds available, as a means to ensure that the providers themselves are encouraged or compelled to seek ways to cut spending, increase efficiency, and restrict (or 'manage') demand for more expensive services.

This type of policy has a long history: in theory Britain's NHS has always been cash-limited, although its very first year massively overspent the projected target (Caldwell et al 1998). The IMF-inspired 'cash limits' imposed on the NHS from 1976 were made legally binding on health authorities by the Thatcher government in 1980 as part of its 'monetarist' policies (Mohan 1995). The imposition of global budgets is clearly a much simpler process in a Beveridge-style, centralised, tax-funded system, in which the government has effective discretion to fix the level of spending. However it does carry a political price, and even the Thatcher government in Britain felt obliged to ease back its downward pressure on health care spending, which brought three successive years of negative growth in the mid 1980s, triggered a politically embarrassing series of winter bed shortages, and sent hospital waiting lists soaring (Caldwell et al 1998).

Imposing a limit on spending in Bismarck-style and other insurance-based systems, in which there is often a multiplicity of payers and providers, many or all of them acting at arm's length or even further removed from direct government control, can be much more difficult – as governments in France and Germany in particular have discovered. In general the political scope for elected governments with developed and costly health services to squeeze down spending is restricted. High-spending health services generate high levels of popular expectation of prompt and appropriate treatment.

Figures compiled by Dixon & Mossialos (2002) comparing health care spending in eight leading OECD countries[86] show that only two (Sweden and Denmark) managed to reduce health care spending as a share of GDP in the period 1988-1999, while all eight *increased* actual real-terms expenditure per head by an average of over 50%, with some governments far exceeding this increase[87] (Mossialos and Dixon 2002:Table A1).

While the rate of increase in spending may in some cases be slowed, any substantial real terms *cutback* in the public sector in the wealthier countries is fraught with political problems. Such policies tend to be more readily recommended for, and imposed upon the governments of developing countries by agencies such as the IMF and World Bank, while the richest nations in general seek other means to unload the burden of public sector funding for health care.

Levels of spending on health care also have to be viewed in the correct context. From the free market point of view, and the standpoint of for-profit health care providers, the runaway expansion of *private* spending on health care in the USA or anywhere else is no problem at all – merely a reflection of the choices made by individuals and the play of market forces (Pauly 2003). However, the price inflation which has run through the US health care system also leads to substantial increases in federal government spending – which potentially calls for tax increases, or reductions in other areas of social spending, if it is not to lead to a further widening of the US budget gap. Indeed the higher the cost of medical insurance, the greater the gap between this and the disposable income of the poorest sections of US society, and the greater the call on public funds (Hadley and Holahan 2003).

The escalation of insurance costs for the millions of Americans who are covered by workplace schemes also leads to divisions between the vested interests of different sections of employers – between those whose business is providing health care, and those for whom health insurance cover for their workforce is a substantial overhead cost, limiting their possible profits[88]. There are therefore political and economic reasons why important sections of US employers should be keen to see a more cost-effective system for delivering health care services to their workforce.

---

86 Australia, Denmark, France, Germany, Netherlands, New Zealand, Sweden and the United Kingdom

87 Deber (2000a) argues that measuring health care purely as a share of GDP leaves out any estimate of whether the economy is in recession: Canada managed to reduce its share of GDP spent on health from 10.1% in 1993 to 9.2% in 1997 as it emerged from recession, though actual spending per capita had only dropped by around 5%.

Cash limits in poor countries

While the OECD countries have in general witnessed an upward curve of health care spending since 1945, the imposition of austerity policies has been far more rigorously applied in poor and 'middle income' countries, especially those under the disciplines of IMF Structural Adjustment Programmes.

Health spending in Zimbabwe for example was reined sharply back following IMF and World Bank advice in 1988 – falling from 6.8% of government spending in 1991 to just 2.7% by 1994. The government also agreed in 1990 to introduce user fees – which eventually rose four-fold over the next five years (Kemkes et al 1997). During the 1990s the HIV/AIDS epidemic has also had an especially brutal impact on Zimbabwe, with up to 20% of the population – 1.4 million people infected with HIV by 1998, and 3,000 dying from AIDS each week in 2004 (Sapa-AFP 2004). The spending cuts brought shortages of medicines, a lack of functioning equipment and the closure of some rural hospitals: the user fees brought a sharp decline in hospitalisation, but also deterred poor people from seeking treatment for venereal diseases, thus contributing to the transmission of HIV.

Another example of the crude application of cash limits was the 'Country Assistance Strategy' for Ecuador endorsed by the World Bank in 2000, a structural adjustment package which involved slashing health spending to *half* the 1995 level[89].

When health care spending is already well below the minimal ($12 per head per year) targets set by the World Bank and the WHO for a 'basic package' of primary and preventive health services, further cuts in spending are likely to have an exceptionally heavy impact on the services that remain and those who depend upon them[90].

Meanwhile the issue in many poorer countries has not so much been cutting spending to match tough cash limits, but identifying the resources required to raise spending towards the World Bank $12 target.

Rationalisation: reductions in bed numbers

Hospital beds can be extremely expensive to run, and consume the largest share of health spending, both in the wealthier countries (Hensher et al 1999a) and in many developing countries: in sub-Saharan Africa public hospitals absorb between 45% and 69% of government health spending (Kirigia et al 2002). Hospitals require not only revenue funding but sufficient qualified medical and professional staff – resources that are generally in extremely short supply. Market-driven reforms, aimed at capping spending, will therefore

---

88 General Motors spends four times more on health insurance and pensions for its employees than it does on steel for the fabric of the vehicles it produces (Grant 2003, Mackintosh 2003, Mackintosh 2005). 'For every vehicle GM makes in North America there are $1,400 of healthcare costs and $800 of pension costs, well above the estimated $550 spent on steel for the average car. ... Each percentage point rise in the assumed rate of healthcare inflation increases costs to the company's US operations by $539m annually' (Mackintosh 2005).

89 Ecuador spent just $71 per head per year on health care in 1995, against an OECD average of $1,827.

90 More recent estimates suggest that much more needs to be spent: a WHO Commission for Macroeconomics in Health report in 2001 suggested that a set of essential interventions would cost at least $34 per head per year, while the WHO's then director general argued in 2000 that countries spending less than '$60 or so per capita' would not be able to provide even a reasonable minimum of services (Labonte et al 2004:40).

inevitably seek to reduce spending on excess numbers of hospital beds in the drive for 'efficiency'.

Where it has been driven by advances in technique and medical science, this type of change has been inevitable (though slow to take effect in much of Eastern Europe, where the underlying model of care was hospital-centred, offering little in the way of outpatient, home care or community based services, and the pace of technical change was much slower, at least up to 1990 (Kokko et al 1998).

The development of day surgery and minimally invasive techniques, together with improved anaesthetics and dressings have enabled a substantial reduction in average lengths of stay for surgical treatment, reducing the need for surgical beds. This has given a sound basis for considerable reduction of surgical bed numbers over the last 20 years (Hensher et al 1999a). However *medical* specialties have not achieved the same reductions in lengths of stay – for good reasons: most medical admissions are for emergency treatment, often for older patients[91]. In the UK numbers of bed days for *medical* admissions have since the mid 1990s outstripped those for surgical procedures[92]. Nor have the promised improvements in primary and community health services brought the expected reduction in demand for emergency medical admissions. This means that in any programme of bed reductions, a proper balance must be maintained between medical and surgical beds, if elective surgical work is not to be disrupted by emergency admissions of medical cases (Pollock & Dunnigan 2000).

For an accurate picture of current trends it is also important to ensure that more recent changes are compared with those over a longer time frame. Large numbers of acute hospital beds closed in England in the 20 years since 1982, but the closures have virtually ceased since 1994, when it became clear that hospital Trusts could not cope with peaks in demand for emergency admissions without at least their existing complement of beds. This finding was confirmed by a government-commissioned beds inquiry at the end of the 1990s, which found a shortfall in available beds (DoH 2000). By contrast, bed reductions in France began later, and have continued long after the generalised 'downsizing' of British acute hospital capacity has stopped (OECD 2003).

Though data for any detailed comparisons are hard to find, the squeeze on excess hospital capacity has had an impact around the world. In the wealthier countries the limited comparisons that can be made show that total acute bed provision over a 23-country OECD average fell by over 20%, from around 5.7 per thousand population in 1980 to around 4.4 in 1998 (OECD 2003). However the average conceals some wide variations: the largest proportional reductions in acute bed numbers were Sweden and Finland (over 40%), while acute bed numbers dropped by just 14% in Germany, and by little or nothing in Austria, Hungary, Luxembourg and Poland, while Japan bucked the trend and expanded bed capacity to almost ten beds per thousand.

The quest to increase throughput per bed

The proper objective of rationalisation is not simply to close surplus capacity, but to ensure

---

91 In Britain in 1992, 87% of medical admissions were found by the Audit Commission to be emergencies (Audit Commission 1992:57).

92 Hospital Episode Statistics for 2002-3 show 14.2m bed days as a result of medical admissions, compared with 12.4m for surgical (DoH 2004a).

that the remaining beds are used more intensively and efficiently. This often requires additional investment in equipment and training of staff. OECD data on this aspect of the rationalisation process are incomplete (only 14 countries out of 29 can be compared back to 1982), out of date, and harder to compare, but again a few issues demand attention (see Table 3). While US hospitals apparently became *less* efficient at treating and discharging patients in the ten years 1982-1992, when 'throughput' per bed dropped from 35.9 patients per bed per year to 33.7, it managed almost a 10% increase in throughput in the five years from 1992-97 – the period in which 'managed care' was seeking to regulate the market (Enthoven 1997).

Table 3: Inpatient utilisation

Acute care turnover rate

Cases per available bed: changes since 1982

Countries	1982	1997	Growth	1992	1997	Growth
United States	35.9	36.9	3%	33.7	36.9	10%
United Kingdom	31.6	55.6	76%	48.4	55.6	15%
Portugal	21.3	34.4	62%	31.0	34.4	11%
Netherlands	23.3	27.2	17%	24.7	27.2	10%
Mexico	45.6	57.0	25%	52.8	57.0	8%
Korea	22.3	23.3	4%	26.0	23.3	-10%
Japan	7.4	9.6	30%	8.2	9.6	17%
Italy	21.8	34.8	60%	27.1	34.8	28%
Hungary	25.3	36.8	45%	27.7	36.8	33%
Germany	21.6	28.1	30%	24.9	28.1	13%
France	17.8	47.1	165%	24.6	47.1	91%
Denmark	34.1	53.6	57%	48.4	53.6	11%
Austria	21.4	38.3	79%	33.1	38.3	16%
Australia	35.0	40.0	14%	41.0	40.0	-2%

Copyright OECD HEALTH DATA 2000

Similarly most of the increase in throughput in French hospital beds (which more than doubled from 17.8 patients per bed per year in 1982, to 47.1 in 1997) was achieved in the final five year period 1992-97. By contrast, most of the dramatic 76% increase in throughput in British hospital beds had already been achieved before 1992 (by which point it had risen from 31.6 to 48.4 patients per bed per year), with a further increase of just 15% in the five years to 1997. This increase in the utilisation of health care resources was therefore largely carried through *before* the market-style reforms which came into effect from 1991, and can be seen as the effects of cash limits and year-on-year reductions in real terms resources for NHS hospital services in the mid 1980s, combined with rising productivity and a rapid expansion of day case surgical treatment[93].

Rationalisation may be advocated for a variety of reasons. Centralising specialist services into fewer, larger units, to improve the training of medical and other staff and focus skills, may represent an advance in clinical terms: but it may also result in patients being treated in a larger, less familiar and friendly environment, and facing problems in access to units often much further from their homes. Maynard and Bloor (2000), reporting research findings, conclude that the efficiencies of such changes may also be debatable: unit costs may well be higher in larger hospitals, while some medical conditions may be exacerbated by long journeys to hospital. The new hospital may even act as a monopoly, preventing any wider competition.

Interestingly the USA has offered examples both of controversial cost-cutting rationalisation (with a particular pressure on HMOs to close 'surplus' and expensive Emergency Rooms) and of the proliferation of hospitals attempting high-tech (and high cost) surgery despite small annual caseload. Enthoven, arguing the US faces continuing 'market failure' in health care, notes that California had 120 hospitals performing open heart surgery, 'half of them with annual volumes of fewer than 200 cases' (Enthoven 1997:198).

Views on rationalisation are often sharply divided: different sections of the medical establishment in Britain have on occasion developed quite different policies and proposals for the future shape of services, with physicians being the least likely, and surgeons the most likely to favour the concentration of services in fewer larger units (RCS 1997:6). But the existence of even a paragraph of medical endorsement for a controversial closure can be exploited by politicians and health service management searching for protection against public anger (Lister 1998b)[94].

Rationalisation in developing countries
As with cash limits, the scope for substantial rationalisation of hospital services in many poorer countries is restricted by the inadequate infrastructure of hospital and primary care, and the lack of the technology to implement modern techniques of day surgery. The only available worldwide figures (Table 4) are from the World Bank (Hensher et al 1999a) and reflect a wider picture of the pattern of rationalisation[95]. The figures for hospital beds (right hand columns) seem to combine the totals of publicly funded beds with those of private beds, which are not available to the majority of the population[96].

---

93 Clearly these limited figures give no real picture of the effects of bed reductions on the quality of patient care – as reflected for example by growing waiting lists, increased delays in admission, pressure to discharge patients more swiftly from hospital, cancelled operations, and so on.

94 In England the medical Royal Colleges and the BMA have called for a greater concentration of specialist services in a few 'super hospitals' covering very large catchment populations, in order to facilitate the training of junior doctors and the expansion of consultant numbers. However there has been no indication that the government intends to build any hospitals large enough to meet the needs of this wider catchment (RCS 1997, BMA 1997).

95 The only available data, which offer a single total for 'hospital beds' of all types – including acute beds, long-stay beds, maternity beds, psychiatric beds and those in specialist facilities – have to be viewed with caution.

96 Hanson and Berman found that a third of the hospital beds in eight African countries were private beds, over 30% in ten Asian countries and over 20% in the 12 Latin America and Caribbean countries surveyed, in many cases 'for-profit' (Hanson and Berman 1998, Table 2).

Table 4: Health expenditure, services, and use						
	Health expenditure			Health expenditure per capita		Hospital beds
	Public	Private	Total	PPP*		per 1,000 people
	% of GDP	% of GDP	% of GDP	$	$	
	1990-98	1990-98	1990-98	1990-98	1990-98	1980	1990-98
World	2.6	3.0	5.5	561	489	3.4	3.3
Low income	1.2	3.1	4.5	74	21	1.7	1.3
Middle income	2.5	2.6	5.0	267	117	3.4	3.4
Lower middle income	2.3	2.5	4.7	190	62	3.4	3.5
Upper middle income	3.4	2.9	6.2	549	318	..	3.3
Low & middle income	1.9	2.8	4.8	179	73	2.7	2.5
East Asia & Pacific	1.7	2.4	4.2	151	43	2.0	2.5
Europe & Central Asia	4.0	1.6	5.2	326	138	10.4	8.8
Latin America & Carib.	3.2	3.3	6.5	452	272	..	2.2
Middle East & N. Africa	2.3	2.3	4.6	228	126	..	1.8
South Asia	0.9	3.8	5.1	87	19	0.7	0.7
Sub-Saharan Africa	1.7	2.6	4.3	89	42	..	1.1
High income	6.0	3.7	9.7	2,587	2,702	..	7.2
Europe EMU	6.7	2.3	8.9	1,980	2,045		7.6

* Expressed in international dollars using purchasing power parities (PPPs)

Source: World Bank (HNP statistics) 2003

It is clear from the table that while there has been a reduction in bed numbers from a much higher base in the 'high income' countries, there has also been a substantial (around 25%) reduction in beds per 1,000 population in the 'low income' countries over the last decade.

Given the mounting pressure on available hospital beds in many of the poorest countries in sub-Saharan Africa as a result of the HIV/AIDS epidemic, we can assume that the loss of these beds is not the result of a restructuring but an absolute cut in health care provision, unrelated to health needs.

Rationing services: exclusion as a cost-saving measure

One relatively unsophisticated way of reining in public spending on health care is to ration care by drawing up a list of treatments or drugs that will be excluded from coverage. This process is politically easier if it is possible to create an argument that the treatment/drug is somehow ineffective, or potentially dangerous – though ineffective or dangerous drugs should probably be barred from use by *any* patients, not just those covered by public funding or insurance schemes (New 1999).

Explicit exclusions in publicly funded health care services are politically sensitive, since the implication is that the excluded services – currently available to all – will be available only on a private basis to those who can afford to pay (Drache and Sullivan 1999). In Britain there have been various attempts at this, beginning with the Thatcher government's 1987 legislation to exclude eye tests and most provision of spectacles and lenses from the NHS. The prelude to this wholesale privatisation of what had been a key aspect of the NHS at its foundation in 1948[97] had been to limit the choice of NHS-funded spectacles to a choice from a restrictive range of unfashionable spectacle frames and lenses, while private opticians were marketing new, and more attractive lightweight versions.

The 1980s saw further attempts by particular British health authorities to exclude from the NHS a list of 'cosmetic' treatments and surgical procedures – ranging from cosmetic surgery and tattoo removal through to surgery for varicose veins, many of them non-urgent treatments with waiting lists as long as three-to-four years. Some health authorities pressed ahead and barred these treatments, leaving local patients with the choice of seeking private treatment or going without. The issue remained on the agenda of cash-strapped British health authorities during the 1990s (Klein 2000)[98].

A wider debate on rationing developed during the mid 1990s, partly in response to the perceived levels of under-funding of the British NHS, but also encouraged by American and other advocates of private medical insurance either as a 'top-up' or as a substitute to publicly funded health care (Marmor 1999). The starting point of claims that 'rationing is inevitable' (Ham 1997, Ham & Honigsbaum 1998, Smith R 1996b) is that health care demand (or, more properly, the *need* for health care) is infinite – a 'bottomless pit' (Light 1997) – whereas health care resources are of necessity finite. With only so much money and human resources to go round, the argument goes, 'hard choices' would have to be made (Lenaghan 1997)[99].

This view was challenged by Light, who argued that levels of health spending were politically determined rather than geared to measures of need (or demand) for health care, and pointed prophetically to the German health care system[100] as one example where resources had *matched* demand, and where demand had conspicuously failed to increase to 'infinite' levels. Health care is unlike most other commodities under capitalism in the sense that the demand for it is closely linked to need, and that demand is self-limiting – few people wish to prolong treatment beyond the point where drugs, surgery or other therapy have taken effect.

While there may be speculation as to levels of unmet need and undiagnosed morbidity in the wider population, the extent of health need will not be literally 'infinite' but potentially

---

97 The demand for free spectacles in the new NHS substantially exceeded the capacity of post-war factories to manufacture them, and the NHS budget for ophthalmology was overspent by 22 times the £1 million allocated in its first year (Lister 1988).

98 North Essex health authority in 1998 drew up a list of expensive treatments it proposed to ration – but eventually retreated under opposition from trade unions and local people (N. Essex HA 1998, Lister 1998a).

99 Germany, then spending up to 10% of GDP on health care was by 1997 heading towards the surplus of beds and patient care facilities which led in 2002 to German health care providers seeking to market spare capacity to other European health care purchasers.

100 In August 2003 NICE recommended that up to six courses of In Vitro Fertilisation (IVF) treatment be made available to infertile women in a designated age range who meet certain criteria. The potential cost could be as high as £300m a year, yet the NICE recommendation does not oblige the government to make additional funding available (Boseley 2003, Revill 2003).

measurable – even if the price of delivering sufficient services is deemed unaffordable or politically unacceptable. However governments and insurance funds seeking to minimise spending have an interest in maintaining systems which conceal a proportion of that need. Frankel and colleagues (2000) have challenged what they describe as a 'pessimistic' thesis of the 'infinite demand' for health care.

Alternatives to explicit rationing

Four different approaches offer an alternative to explicit rationing by exclusion: one is the establishment of an 'approved' register for new drugs and treatments. In Britain the National Institute for Clinical Excellence (NICE) was established by New Labour, as an impartial body that would assess the cost effectiveness of new drugs and treatments and advise the government. Of course such a body solves only part of the dilemma, since 'cost effectiveness' is a composite measure embodying the contradictions of use value and exchange value, leaving the question of which aspect of the treatment is to be uppermost in the decisions of NICE – the cost of a drug, or its effectiveness? A decision by NICE that a treatment should be made available, and funded by the NHS, can open up a fresh dilemma in the context of cash limits[101].

The second alternative is to establish an 'approved list' of treatments which will be funded. This was the underlying method behind the so-called 'Oregon experiment' which began in the late 1980s as a reform to the Medicaid scheme. The state of Oregon passed legislation in 1989 which offered to increase access to health insurance for some of its poorest residents, but imposed restrictions in the range of health care services that would be financed. The most controversial element of the plan was implicitly excluding the poorest people in the state from receiving treatments not on a list of 'priorities'.

The priority list was drawn up by an 11-strong health services commission, which received professional advice, research evidence, and the findings of public hearings and focus groups involving the local community. Despite fears that this would lead to a distortion of medical priorities reflecting popular prejudices over 'deserving' and 'non-deserving' patients (Dixon & Welch 1991), this process resulted in a list of 696 treatments – of which 565 were initially deemed to be priorities that should be funded. According to Ham (1998:1966) the main exclusions were treatments for 'self limiting conditions and conditions where no effective interventions were available.'

Ham's assessment of the exercise concludes equivocally:

> Whether the outcome looks like a glass half full or a glass half empty depends on your perspective
> (Ham 1998:1969).

For those who see rationing as the way forward, Oregon offers not so much proof of success as vindication that it need not lead to the horrors of populist shroud-waving and large-scale exclusions of the vulnerable. Similar efforts in Netherlands and New Zealand to define packages of care that would be funded, and effectively exclude the remainder, have also proved unsuccessful (New 1997:81).

---

101 However subsequent cash pressures arising from declining tax revenues have brought a further retrenchment in coverage for Oregon's poor: the number of services covered has fallen from 606 to 566, and at the end of 2002 Oregon's interim medical director told the Toronto *Globe and Mail*: 'We are getting to the point where, if we reduce the number of funded services even further to make the savings that are necessary, people will be living in a lot of pain' (Mickleburgh 2002b).

The spread of rationing has been limited by these negative experiences, and by strongly held disagreements even among advocates of rationing as to how it should be carried out (New 1996, Maynard and Sheldon 2001, Coulter and Ham 2000). Saltman (2002) concludes from his survey of evidence that there has been 'no explicit rationing' of publicly financed or publicly controlled health services in Western Europe.

The third alternative approach is the implicit rationing that prevails in the US and in other health services that levy charges for care – and that is to constrain demand by price. This is facilitated by the lack of any affordable health insurance policy offering unlimited cover. This mechanism, the most crude of all the market-driven devices to manage demand, clearly takes no account of ability to pay, and has most severe impact on the poor, exempting only those wealthy enough to be able to afford treatment.

The fourth and final alternative is also implicit rationing – by limiting the level of resources (money, staff, facilities) available to deliver publicly funded health care. The result when the imbalance is especially severe will be waiting lists, queues and shortages: such a policy can easily backfire on a democratic government that starves a popular public service of resources.

Rationing by exclusion: privatising long term care

One less overt form of exclusion which has been more widely adopted, and has led to a substantial shift of the funding burden from government to individuals and their families has been in the area of long-term care, especially for older people. In Britain this has centred on the 'community care reforms' introduced by the Conservative government between 1988 and April 1993, and only partly modified since Labour returned to office in 1997 (Lister & Martin 1988, Lister 1989b, Caldwell et al 1998, Leys 2001, and see above, Chapter four).

The British government has by no means been the only one to resort to such policies. Continuing care for older patients in nursing homes, frequently now simply described as 'social care' (Mossialos & Dixon 2002), has been widely seen as an appropriate area for the expansion of private enterprise even at the heart of what have until now been predominantly publicly financed health care systems in the more advanced economies. In Sweden, a system that switched financial responsibility to municipalities for care of older patients awaiting discharge from hospital has been used as a lever to speed up the discharge process – and thus free up hospital beds: but it has also led to an increased demand for nursing home accommodation, and to an expansion of private, for-profit services paid for through municipal authorities (Mossialos & Dixon 2002, Henwood 2002, Lyall 2002).

Regulating drug costs

1 Wealthy countries

'Market failure in both supply and demand' are blamed by Mossialos and Mrazek (2002:149) for the widespread intervention and regulation that governments have applied to the pharmaceutical market. Part of this market failure arises from the so-called 'moral hazard' in many insurance-based systems, under which the consumer/patient does not have to pay, or is reimbursed, the cost of the drugs they consume, so 'neither they nor the physicians have any incentive to economise'.

A large share of the profits of US pharmaceutical companies depends upon the continuation of large-scale public spending to subsidise medicines for the poor and elderly. Their political power is one reason why measures to restrict spending on pharmaceuticals have concentrated more on deterring demand and forcing patients to cover a larger share of the cost rather than on forcing down the prices of the drugs themselves.

There has also been a long-running battle over the protection of patent rights and the use of branded rather than cheaper, generic, drugs when patents have expired. In Britain, growing pressure on GPs to prescribe generic drugs for their patients has continued since the 1980s (Rivett 1998). The internal market reforms in the 1990s meant that non-fundholding GP practices were strictly monitored for their adherence to generic prescribing guidelines, while fundholders, subject to cash-limited prescribing budgets, were given the financial incentive of retaining any unspent surpluses: as a result fundholders made greater use of generic medicines (Mossialos & Mrazek 2002:158-9). New Labour's introduction of cash limits throughout Primary Care has resulted in a high profile for GP prescribing budgets in local financial reports, with pressure on 'high-spending' practices to conform to the prescribing patterns of the majority.

The contradictions of a world market in which different prices are charged for the same drug in different countries has spawned a curious trade in 'parallel imports' of drugs from low cost to high cost countries, and 'pharmacy benefit managers' – a new layer of management within the US 'managed care' industry, which seeks to secure low cost supplies of drugs. Physicians are told to prescribe the cheapest alternative from a restricted list, while pharmacists make a higher margin every time they switch to a cheaper prescribed drug.

Other mechanisms such as the use of co-payments related to the costs of the drugs prescribed have sought to enlist consumerism as a means to scale down prescribing costs and exclude unauthorised products: in Germany and Netherlands patients receiving drugs above the standard 'reference cost' pay the full difference in price in addition to the standard prescription charge of four to five euro. However the contradiction is that the price of some generic drugs which were originally below the reference price has been found to rise to the reference price level (Dixon and Mossialos 2002, Mossialos and Mrazek 2002).

France and New Zealand give no reimbursement for any drugs that are not included on the Pharmaceutical Scale (Dixon & Mossialos 2002). Other attempts to control drug prices include the establishment of a 'cost-effectiveness price' for medicines sold in Australia, Canada and Finland. In Britain the government each year negotiates a target rate of return (17-21%) with each pharmaceutical company, but allows the companies to set their prices within this margin (Mossialos & Mrazek 2002).

2 Developing countries

The pharmaceutical companies jealously guard their role in the research of new drugs, but resist any attempt to steer them towards particular areas of research. In fact numbers of new 'chemical entities' registered each year have fallen dramatically, from 100 in 1963 to just 37 in 1998. Almost half the drugs approved for sale in the USA in the 15 years to 1990 were for cardiovascular conditions or antibiotics (Mossialos & Mrazek 2002). Drugs such as Viagra to combat erectile dysfunction are proliferating, while large-scale killer diseases which haunt the African continent are all but ignored.

Drug companies make no secret of the fact that they are run for profit: but this means that they allocate little or no research work to diseases and conditions which largely affect low and middle income countries, while the drugs they develop on other diseases are often inaccessible or unaffordable in the poorer countries. This is despite near-unanimity among the various advisory agencies on the priorities that drug research should investigate (GFHR 2002:92-95).

While inflated drug costs are a problem in the established health services of the wealthier countries, they are literally a matter of life and death in the poorest countries, especially those facing epidemics of HIV/AIDS. This is the arena in which the case for generic medicines and against the exorbitant prices charged for patented drugs has been most hotly fought. As this study is completed a fresh round of talks are under way with the WTO over the provision of cut-price supplies of antiretroviral medicines to low-income countries, a price the US seems reluctantly willing to pay to open up progress on the Doha round of trade liberalisation. Washington wants cast-iron guarantees that any concessions it makes to the very poorest countries are not translated into the mass production of much cheaper generic drugs in India and Brazil (Chandrasekhar and Ghosh 2003)[102].

User fees

1 Market-driven user fees in wealthy countries

Robinson (2002), examining user charges in the context of East and West Europe, argues that user fees can be viewed as:

> ...different positions on a continuum ranging from full third-party payment (zero cost-sharing)
> to full user charges (costs met completely by out of pocket payments (2002:162).

Noting that the main claim that user fees help improve 'efficiency' revolves around their effectiveness in discouraging 'unnecessary' demand, or in some cases in generating additional revenue for funding health care when alternative funds are not available, Robinson points out that such a policy has little to do with efficiency, and is more accurately seen as 'public sector cost containment' – in other words, a market-driven measure.

Summarising surveys conducted in 1998 and 1999 (Kutzin 1998, Mossialos and LeGrand 1999), and including Russia, Central Eastern Europe and Former Soviet Union republics of Central Asia, Robinson notes that user fees are widely used by most countries in the form of co-payments for pharmaceuticals – covering as much as 35% of the drug cost in Hungary – while nine EU countries imposed charges for general practitioner consultations, and most EU countries imposed co-payments for specialist consultations. Sweden levies extensive user charges, including for children's outpatient services. However only Greece, Italy and Portugal relied upon user charges to raise more than 20% of health care funding (Robinson 2002:174).

Information on CEE and FSU countries was harder to obtain, but Robinson argues many now levied user charges as part of new health insurance schemes. The evidence of limited research shows that total revenue from user charges rarely exceeded 5% of total health revenue, while the charges had strongly reduced utilisation, and thus worsened equity of provision, having a heavier impact upon the poor. There was some evidence that charges had an adverse effect on health outcomes – and that they carried hidden costs in managerial and administrative effort (Schieber and Maeda 1997, cited in Robinson 2002:177).

A wider survey of OECD countries by Docteur and Oxley (2003) found a varying pattern, with just over half the OECD countries levying some form of charge (sometimes relatively small) for hospital inpatient treatment, and a similar number charging for consultations with a general practitioner, and slightly more imposing charges to see a specialist. While

---

102 There are also fears that the focus on procuring drugs to treat AIDS has diverted from the need to develop specialist expertise in using the drugs to ensure that patients benefit and that drug-resistant forms of the virus do not result (Kumar 2004).

supplementary private insurance schemes may cover some or all of these charges in some countries (notably France), in Australia private insurance is *prohibited* from covering fees for outpatient treatment – suggesting that this functions very much as a cost containment/demand limitation measure.

2 Market-driven user fees in developing countries

While user fees may have an inequitable impact on the wealthier countries, in the poorest countries, where the poor have even less income and resources at their disposal, the imposition of user fees, according to Newbrander and colleagues 'is a strategy that places much of the burden of financing health care on the individual patient' (Newbrander et al 2000:12). Creese (1997) argues that user fees shift the burden away from risk sharing towards payments by individuals and households:

> The higher the proportion of user payments in the total mix of financing for health, the greater the relative share of the financing burden falling on poor people (Creese 1997).

According to Gertler and Hammer there is a good reason why countries wealthy enough to do without them avoid user fees:

> Support for… use of public subsidies [is] based on the idea that nobody, regardless of income, should be denied access to basic minimal medical care. While these commitments are not boundless, they are pervasive throughout the world (Gertler and Hammer 1997, p21).

However such subsidies are not an option in many middle and low income countries, even though in many cases the sums of money raised from user fees are relatively small[103] (the fees are not so small in relation to actual incomes of the poorest). In these cases the fees are often suggested both as a means to reduce 'unnecessary' demand for services, but also act as a *market-style* reform, a lever in creating a new system of private or social insurance for the wealthy and middle classes (see below). Organisations sponsored by the World Bank and USAID, including Medical Sciences for Health (MSH), have focused strongly on securing acceptance of user fees in the market-driven context – as a means of raising resources for health care systems in some of the world's poorest countries (Collins et al 1996, Newbrander et al 2000).

Among the techniques proposed for the introduction of fees in previously free health services is to bring in the charges at a very low ('minimal') level and then increase them, 'to avoid creating public reaction':

> If there is public and political sensitivity to introducing new fees, it may be best to have a wide range of exemptions and relatively easy access to poverty waivers in the beginning and to reduce them gradually (Newbrander et al 2000:104).

Another device to soften the negative political impact of user fees is to use a different phrase to describe the charges patients must pay for treatment. According to MSH, the Kenyan government was reluctant to announce that it was instituting a system of user fees:

---

103 In Kenya, for example, which is regarded as a successful example of the imposition of user fees, the total generated was just $68 million over the 11 years 1989-2000 (Newbrander et al 2000:3).

It chose the term cost-sharing to emphasise its continued commitment to providing high quality services to its population (Management Sciences for Health 2001).

Presumably any Kenyans who had failed to spot the significance of 'cost-sharing' would have worked out that money was to change hands when they saw the networked cash registers installed as part of the MSH initiative. Indeed user fees are a blunt instrument. As the WHO (2000) has argued, payment of charges at point of use restricts services to those who can afford to pay, and is not related to the level of *need* for treatment.

Creese (1997) sums up the policy, arguing that user fees 'don't reduce costs, and they increase inequality'. Murray and colleagues point out that user fees – or 'out of pocket payments' leave service users fragmented, with no possibility of pooling risks:

> Out of pocket financing of health is the most likely reason that would characterise unfair distributions of health financing, and to generate severe financial losses and risk of impoverishment for some families. This is particularly evident in countries where other financing options are restricted to the rich, and out of pocket payments are the only option for the poor (Murray et al 2000, p4).

Market-style (ideologically driven) reforms

Introduction: reforms and the New Public Management

Much of the discourse promoting health care reforms since the early 1990s has – with little or no reservation – accepted and embodied key terms and concepts from the theories which have become collectively known as 'New Public Management' (NPM), which itself draws heavily on private sector assumptions, theories and practices (Hood 1991, Osborne and Gaebler 1992, Osborne and Plastrik 1997, Newman 2000, Preker and Harding 2003).

There is a substantial and growing literature on the NPM and on its application to health care, which there is insufficient space to detail in this study. However it is clear that within the literature there are critics as well as enthusiasts for NPM and its applicability to health care in particular. Pollitt (2000, 2003) is one of several who emphasise how partial have been the attempts to evaluate NPM policies and methods where they have been introduced, and the severe limitations of the studies that have been attempted (Pollitt 2000:187).

While there is little evidence that NPM delivers economies or increased efficiencies in the operation of the public sector (Pollitt 2000:188, 192; Manning 2000) the pro-market assumptions of the NPM approach often sit uneasily in policy documents alongside professions of concern for 'equity' and maximum access to services for the poor.

For the purposes of this investigation it is useful to note that the marriage of NPM with health system reforms has brought a steadily increasing reference to such stock panaceas as:

• Public-private partnerships

• Contracting out and various forms of increased local autonomy ('steering, not rowing')

• Competition ('managed' or otherwise)

• User choice and user empowerment

• The introduction of internal or quasi-markets.

(Osborne and Gaebler 1992:25.310)

The impact of these elements of NPM on health care services will be explored at greater length below.

Overview: limits to the health care market

Within a free market system, the main drivers are competition and private and corporate gain. In private sector enterprises, these gains generally take the form of profits and shareholder dividends. Where market-style competition is introduced within a public sector framework the gains take the form of increased revenues for providers, resulting in surpluses and the possibility of enhanced rewards for executives and other sections of staff – at the expense of the less successful providers, which may face loss of contracts, budget reductions, redundancies or even closure.

While heightened prestige may also be a by-product for the most successful public sector providers, it is clear that the introduction of a market mechanism focuses strongly on the exchange-value (money) element of health care, rather than on the use values delivered: health care is effectively commodified through market measures.

Unregulated markets therefore make no reference to equity, and represent a direct opposite to centralised planning. However, despite claims that competition necessarily leads to lower prices, and improved efficiency and cost-effectiveness, the opposite is often true. Markets which are less than perfect can encourage the many perverse incentives visible in the health care system in the USA.

It is generally accepted, even in many otherwise neoliberal policy proposals for the reform of health care systems, that the outright privatisation of existing health care systems, to replicate the dominance of private provision in the US model, is not desirable (Maynard and Bloor 2000). Indeed the US system itself – despite the failure of the Clinton reforms, which aimed to bring in a greater degree of control – evolved some time ago away from a largely unrestricted free market in health care, exhibiting what Enthoven (1997) describes as 'profound and multifaceted market failure,' towards more regulated regimes of 'managed care' (Marmor 1998, Enthoven 1997).

It is these devices intended to *regulate* the market, rather than the fraud-ridden and socially exclusive US system itself, which governments elsewhere have sought to emulate, especially as a result of the efforts of Enthoven and others (Enthoven 1985). [The US Inspector General and the Health Insurance Association of America agree that fraud is a major issue in US healthcare – accounting for roughly 14% of all insurance payments (Palast 1999).]

Over and above seeking to avoid the high and escalating costs and problems of a US-style system, World Bank policy documents in the last ten years have also tended to accept that some form of collective risk-sharing and public sector provision is necessary in developing countries – even if only to provide the most basic infrastructure of primary care and preventive services, while leaving more expensive hospital and specialist services to the prerogative of the private sector (World Bank 1993).

As a result there has been a certain convergence between the Bank and the WHO at the level of the 'essential package' of care (Buse and Walt 2000a).

It is ironic that many of the health system reforms that have been implemented in the last 15 years have *begun* with neoliberal ideology – of small government, low taxes, decentralisation, competition, privatisation and consumer power: but in many cases – perhaps all – the end result of such reforms has been *increased* state spending, and more bureaucracy (Hay 2001, Leys 2001)[104].

Countries with well-developed collectively funded health care systems may find the combination of forces ranged against market-style reforms impossible to overcome. The example of the British health care reforms – pushed through by the Thatcher government despite popular and professional opposition – is widely quoted as a model for reforms in similarly centralised systems (Busse et al 2002).

However, amid doubts over the extent to which these and subsequent market-style reforms have delivered their promised improvements in efficiency or effectiveness, relatively few wealthier countries have tried to follow Thatcher's route of imposing unpopular policies in one 'big bang' reform package (Maynard and Bloor 2000:6, Smith 2000:4, Danzon 2002).

Yet the most fundamental contradiction that ensures health care creates inevitable 'market failures' under capitalism is the inherent class division between rich and poor: while wealthier people can (and obviously do) also get ill, the main burdens of ill-health and illness are directly related to poverty 'the world's most ruthless killer' (Gordon 2002:74).

Table 5: Market-style (ideologically driven, restructuring) reforms
Decentralisation (B1, D1)
Contracts (B2, D2)
Provider autonomy/ entrepreneurialism (B3, D3)
Provider payment reform (B4, D4)
Public services purchase care from private sector (B5, D5)
Competition (B6, D6)
Privatisation (B7, D7)
User fees as market-style reform to expand private insurance (B8, D8)
Control medical professionals (B9, D9)
Patient's choice/consumerism (B10)
PFI and Public Private Partnerships (B11, D10)
Managed care (B12)
Medical Savings Accounts (B13)

Health care is therefore a commodity, the exchange value of which is least likely to be affordable to many of those for whom its use value is greatest. Those most needing health care tend to be the very old, and the very young, most of whom also tend to be among the poorest groups: so the vast potential 'market' for health care services in the developing world is largely composed of individuals and countries least able to pay for them. Health care in many poorer countries and poorer areas is correspondingly less likely to attract sustained investment by hospital corporations or by drug companies that follow purely market criteria.

The remainder of this chapter will explore some of the market-style measures that have been brought forward as part of the international reform agenda.

---

104 In Britain the Conservative government's market-style reforms increased managerial and administrative staff numbers across the NHS. Since 1997, New Labour's attempts to reduce bureaucracy have brought instead a 59% increase in numbers of senior managers, compared with a 27% increase in the NHS workforce (DoH 2003b).

Decentralisation

The call for 'decentralisation' is a theme running through most studies and reports advocating health system reform in wealthy and poor countries alike. It is 'generally recognised as a major strategy for health reform' (Rannan-Eliya et al 1996:5, Valentine 1998). From the pro-market reformers' point of view, two key factors help drive the process of decentralisation:

- It is a key element in the hotch-potch of pro-market policies bracketed under the generic label of the New Public Management (Hood 1991, Osborne and Gaebler 1992, Pollitt 2000, Osborne and Plastrik 1997)
- And, as a market-style reform, decentralisation is also embraced as a goal both by the World Bank and by USAID and other related organisations in their efforts to remodel health care systems in developing countries (World Bank 1993).

However the marketisers have an easier task in promoting this policy, since many progressive activists also campaign strongly for decentralisation, noting its potential democratic and localising dynamic, and its inclusion on the agenda of the WHO's Health For All campaign from 1978.

Support for some form of decentralisation therefore spans the political spectrum. Collins and Green, highlighting the policy's negative implications in some developing countries, point out that it has been accepted both by socialists and by the new right, by the left-leaning governments of Tanzania and Nicaragua, and by Chile's Pinochet dictatorship, as well as the World Bank and USAID. They go on to argue that:

...the value we place on decentralisation will depend upon the way we define it and its political use (Collins and Green 1994:460).

The general assumption made by advocates of decentralisation is that by breaking down centralised systems, and bringing decision making closer to local people, both as providers and consumers of health care, the reform process will improve equity of access for the poor (who can be more influential at local than at national level), improve efficiency and improve quality, since more local service providers will feel more answerable to local consumers[105].

However the decentralisation of a previously centralised service also assumes an availability of resources – including a developed planning and management infrastructure and human resources in the form of skilled health managers at local level – which may well not be available in many countries (Rannan-Eliya et al 1996, Berman and Bossert 2000). Indeed, as the same authors also show, the results of decentralisation can also prove very different from those intended:

- Control over service provision may be captured at local level by elites who are even less responsive than central government to the needs of the poor
- Decentralisation may also offer new openings for local-level corruption
- The new system may find itself struggling in the face of a lack of local managerial skills and expertise

---

105 Boyle and colleagues (2004) point out that the decentralisation in the British NHS stops far short of the level that would genuinely pass power to local communities and empower health professionals and patients.

- Decentralisation may also mean smaller scale and less well-resourced providers, which wind up delivering less training and skills for staff and lower quality care

- Smaller-scale, more local structures almost inevitably offer less scope to tackle inequalities in the terms and conditions of health workers (Rannan-Eliya et al 1996:5-6).

In countries with marked social inequalities between town and country and between rich and poor, decentralisation of services can also increase problems of equity, unless it is firmly underpinned by guarantees of adequate needs-related funding. If not, granting local hospitals and health services powers to raise local funds may liberate local entrepreneurial talent in a wealthy area, but condemn poorer inner-city and rural health services to permanent under-funding and second class status (Mackintosh 2001).

Internal market reforms which emphasise the development of autonomous and competing local hospital units can result, in countries like Britain and Sweden, in duplication of effort, wasted resources and high transaction costs. Strengthened local control can also obstruct national-level planning and any possible rationalisation of services, and restricts the ability of a health care system to offer a wider range of career options as a means to retain qualified staff (Bach 2000).

As with other facets of the New Public Management (NPM), enthusiasm for decentralisation appears to have developed and survived despite the lack of evidence to show that it delivers the promised improvements to efficiency, equity, quality or accountability (Valentine 1998). Manning (2000) argues that the whole NPM package is linked with *increased* transaction costs (that is, lower levels of efficiency) and loss of accountability, though the extent of these problems can be hard to quantify, given the general lack of evaluation of the impact of NPM policies.

Some critics go further, questioning the extent to which the commitment to decentralisation goes beyond government rhetoric. Cope and Goodship (1999) have emphasised the tightening central control over services which ostensibly have been decentralised. They say this fulfils a three-way function: distancing government from direct responsibility for service delivery ('depoliticising' control), increasing actual government control, and containing government spending. Central 'steering' agencies increasingly regulate local 'rowing' agencies, both directly and indirectly.

According to the USAID-funded Partnerships for Health Reform, the primary intended goal of decentralisation is to promote 'cost effectiveness', with a secondary objective of securing financial sustainability (Knowles 1997). It is doubtful whether those who support the progressive aspirations of locally controlled services would also embrace decentralisation as a cost-cutting measure.

Evidence to show that decentralisation improves health care remains stubbornly hard to find. Bossert argues that though decentralisation and health finance reform have been 'touted' by the World Bank through much of the 1990s, 'the preliminary data from the field indicate that the results have been mixed, at best,' and that in some cases the backlash has included moves to recentralise services (Bossert 2000:3). Decentralisation of the control over hospital services also raises difficult questions over the capacity of management both at national and at local level (Mills et al 2001).

Other World Bank researchers have come to similar conclusions. Bale and Dale (1998), while seeking to endorse the general 'success' of the sweeping New Zealand reforms, underline the specific cultural and political environment in which they were implemented (Bale and Dale 1998:)[106].

Contracts between purchasers and providers

Developed countries

For market mechanisms to come into play, a market has to be created through the separation – where they have been linked in a common centralised system – of purchasers and providers. Once the chain of command of a centralised system has been broken in this way, a new system of contracts must be put in place in order to establish the responsibilities and accountability of service providers. Contracts drafted in terms of cash, inputs and outputs, represent a first step away from notions of public service and social solidarity, and towards the establishment of health care as a commodity to be bought and sold (Leys 2001).

The replacement of an internal process of budget allocation with the development of a formal contract between the public purchasing agency and a range of providers also opens up the possibility of contracting *out* – purchasing services from the private sector in place of publicly owned and run services. Such a culture may also be encouraged at much more local level, sometimes as a precursor to wider-reaching market-style reforms. In Britain the Thatcher government required health authorities to put hospital support services[107] out to competitive tender from early 1983 – long before hospitals were given local autonomy as Trusts or the introduction of the internal market (Caldwell et al 1998:51).

Contracts can in theory be used to regulate any part of the health care system – covering not only support services, but also clinical care, again from public or private sector providers. They may be enforced either positively, through incentives for providers to meet targets, or (less frequently) negatively through the imposition of sanctions in the case of failure. In many cases (including England) the 'contracts' are better described as planning agreements – since they have not had the legal force of a normal commercial contract, and the purchasers lack any effective sanction in the case of failure, other than to seek an alternative provider (Palmer 2000)[108].

However the 'contract culture' that emerged from the 'new managerialism' of the 1980s leaves a number of unresolved problems, notably:

> ...how to be sure that when an organisation or individual is recruited to pursue the interests of the purchaser, they do not use it as an opportunity to pursue their own interests. Contracts always have 'gaps', performance indicators can always be manipulated or used perversely, and even worse, as 'contract culture' takes over from trust and good will, everyone looks to exploit these opportunities more forcefully (Ling 2000:99).

Another perennial difficulty with contracts is that they require expertise in drawing up precise specifications, and constant monitoring if they are to be upheld. In Romania, for example, where a system of contracts including an age-weighted capitation fee for each doctor's list was used to improve primary care services from 1994, purchasing authorities have been found to have insufficient capacity and experience:

---

106 In an appendix to their study, Bale and Dale point to the problems that have arisen from trying to apply the same general line of market-style reform to New Zealand's health care system (ibid 121).

107 Initially defined as catering, cleaning and laundry services.

108 In Britain new regulations making contracts between hospital Trusts and Primary Care Trusts legally binding began in the spring of 2004, amid warnings that the new system would 'throw up even bigger risks and challenges' (Plumridge and Kemp 2004).

...policymakers had to strike a balance to avoid under- or overspecifying service requirements, to set workable and monitorable performance targets, to allow the flexibility to respond to demand, and to protect the funding system against abuse and budget blowouts (Vladescu and Radulescu 2003).

Another difficulty with contracts revolves around fixing the length of the agreement: too short a period (such as the initial annual contracting round in the British NHS internal market) can serve to deter providers from any longer-term investment in capacity, whereas too long a contract can remove any incentive to innovate and effectively neutralise competitive pressures (Palmer 2000).

Contracting for care in developing countries

While the ideological commitment to market-style measures may be strong, and the market-driven pressures on health care systems may press in the direction of tighter contracts, the progress has not been even. Abrantes (2003) points to the varying levels of progress towards contract-based service provision in the Southern Cone countries of Latin America, while Slack and Savedoff (2001) identify a large variety of types of contract in Latin America and the Caribbean countries.

Nor is the mere existence of a contract sufficient to ensure control and the delivery of targets. Slack and Savedoff, examining the working of these systems, identify a number of issues that show a need for more precision and monitoring if the contract is to deliver the intended results. Examples singled out show that:

- Fee-for-service contracts with no volume restriction carry no incentive to keep costs down: Slack and Savedoff note that in Uruguay high tech services are 20-25% more expensive from private facilities rather than public units.

- Fee-for-service contracts with volume restrictions give an incentive to claim for treatments not delivered: in Brazil in 1995 an estimated 28% of hospital inpatient services that were claimed for were not delivered.

- A fee-for-service contract with volume restrictions that was not properly monitored led to increasing numbers of treatments and an overspend of more than $1 billion in Colombia in 1998 (Slack and Savedoff 2001:20).

Palmer notes that:

It is unlikely that any approach to contracting can be comprehensively transposed from developed country markets for health, which in turn are not functioning entirely as envisaged, to the different environments of a range of low- and middle-income countries (Palmer 2000:826).

Provider autonomy/corporatisation

Developed countries

The notion of going beyond decentralisation to establish local health care providers as autonomous, free-standing corporate bodies in their own right has been gathering momentum among the advocates of market-style reforms (Preker and Harding 2003). This is not new: the British Conservative government's marketising measures separated provider units from purchasers and encouraged the creation of 'self-governing Trusts', the first of which were launched in 1991. New Zealand's government also experimented along the same lines in the early 1990s, with profoundly mixed results (Lovelace 2003).

By the mid 1990s almost all NHS providers had taken Trust status, defined in the initial White Paper as 'public corporations'. Their levels of local discretion and accountability were limited, and though Trusts were in theory permitted to fix pay and conditions of their staff at local level, few did more than increase bonuses and payments to top executives. Their budget was constrained by their ability – in competition with other providers – to secure contracts from NHS purchasers, together with income from private patients and 'income generation'. Competition therefore impacted primarily in the form of a downward pressure on prices.

Any efficiencies that may have been secured through improved management in Trusts were obscured by the substantial increases in transaction costs, administration and management created by the introduction of the 'purchaser/provider split' into the NHS. This appears to be the rule rather than the exception of such policies: Manning argues that:

The successes of autonomisation in the health sector seem to be more predicted than found (Manning 2000).

In some countries the level of local autonomy has been taken further than NHS Trusts. 'Foundation Hospitals' in Spain and in Sweden, and 'hospital companies' in Portugal have gone further in floating the hospital as a free-standing enterprise, 'corporatised', with their own discretion to borrow funds and conduct deals with private sector. Britain's New Labour government has begun to copy this model in England, despite vociferous opposition from Labour backbenchers, health unions, academics and campaigners (Pollock 2003, Pollock and Price 2003, Klein 2004). This type of autonomy may prove, as with one major Swedish hospital, simply a transition point to full-scale privatisation (Busse et al 2002)[109]. The Swedish government has recently enacted legislation to forbid any further privatisation of health services. Spain's four foundation hospitals have been accused of making staff work longer hours and of 'cream skimming' the more lucrative treatments, leaving other hospitals to pick up the remainder (Nash 2003).

Hospital autonomy in developing countries

The enthusiasm for this type of reform from the World Bank's Preker and Harding (2003) cannot hide the very mixed results of the relatively limited experiments that have taken place with hospital autonomy in the poorest countries: their book collects a handful of examples from low- and middle-income countries, including Latin American (Argentina, Chile and Uruguay) Ecuador and Tunisia, not all of which have succeeded – and Indonesia, where the autonomous hospitals failed to improve financing, access for the poor, personnel management, service quality or patient satisfaction, but did succeed in raising fees and increasing revenues from patients (2003:525-6).

In other developing countries the corporatisation of hospitals has taken the form of the establishment of major teaching hospitals as 'parastatal' organisations (Kenya's Kenyatta National Hospital), and autonomous 'self governing' bodies (Ghana's Korle Bu and Komfo Anokye hospitals). One immediate difficulty in these circumstances is the disproportionate share of resources already allocated to these hospitals, which also tend to embody some of the country's most powerful medical professionals, and which governments cannot readily scale

---

109 Saltman (2002) disagrees, claiming that the majority shareholder control of this hospital is still in the hands of public sector organisations, and argues that no substantial privatisation of providers has yet taken place in Western Europe.

down. On four evaluative criteria of efficiency, equity, public accountability and quality of care, research by Govindaraj and colleagues (1996) concluded that: the experiment in Ghana had not delivered many of the hoped for benefits 'although there have been some isolated successes'.

Castano and colleagues (2004) note while the intended broad progressive effects of autonomisation ('namely resource mobilisation and an improved mix of services) were 'largely absent' (2004:14), much more common was the unintended consequence of negative impact of hospital autonomy on equity:

> The empirical evidence shows that autonomous hospitals start giving priority to paying patients, and that waivers and exemptions of user fees have been rather ineffective in reducing access barriers to services by the poor (xii).

The market-style reform agenda increasingly recognises the need to 'manage' competition and restrain the 'entrepreneurialism' of decentralised and increasingly autonomous public sector health care providers or private providers (Saltman et al 2002). Indeed it might appear that, in an increasingly decentralised system, there is only a marginal distinction between the local powers granted to what the World Bank calls 'semi-autonomous health facilities' providing contracted services to a publicly funded health care system on the one hand, and on the other the same public system buying similar services from a private provider.

Reforming provider payments

Developed countries

While Beveridge-style tax-funded systems offer their governments the opportunity to restrict individual hospital budgets through a single centralised policy decision, in Bismarck-style systems decentralised payment mechanisms have always involved a form of 'contract' between the insurance funds and the providers of care. Theoretically, this separation of functions offers more scope to constrain the increase in costs: but in practice it has been hard to control the various purchasers of health services, and even harder to control the prices charged by what is often a mix of private and public sector providers.

Despite this less than convincing experience, one argument for introducing a market-style system to Britain – and to countries which had centrally controlled health care systems – was that a combination of competition and contracts would offer new mechanisms to restrain provider-led demand and inflation, and ensure that, in the famous words of the Thatcher NHS reforms[110], the 'cash follows the patient' (DoH 1989). Following this approach, what may begin as a market-driven exercise to control costs can lead towards *market-style* policies and reforms – which may, in turn, deliver very different results.

Where provider payment reforms are introduced purely in the context of cost-cutting, the alternatives include:

*   Replacing fee-for-service payments by capitation-based funding for covering a designated population (prospective payment)

---

110 Subsequently echoed by Tony Blair's New Labour government in its controversial reform of financial flows within the NHS which could result in some hospitals having to reduce their spending by as much as £66m a year in order to conform to a new centralised pricing structure (Smith 2003).

- Replacing flexible fee-for-service payments by fixed price payments for particular treatments, on the basis of Diagnostic Related Groups or the equivalent
- Payment per diem for inpatient treatment
- Payment for designated specialist services, with fixed targets.

Market-style methods might suggest the need for systems which pay hospitals only for the episodes of treatment they deliver (case-based) or the catchment population they agree to cover (capitation-based). Case-based payment can be seen as giving an incentive to respond positively to local demand – or even to compete with other hospitals for patients – while capitation-based contracts encourage hospitals to hold down costs. The down-side to a capitation-based system is that it can create an incentive to cut costs at the expense of quality, to supply as little treatment as possible and even to ration care for the catchment population. Case-based contracts on the other hand can generate a perverse incentive to treat larger numbers of less serious cases, and to increase the numbers of cases treated – again possibly at the expense of quality.

Similar pluses and minuses can be identified for systems which fund hospitals to deliver specific designated care – setting targets for cardiac or cancer treatment, accompanied by ring-fenced allocations of revenue. While it may be possible to achieve improvements in the designated service, this may well be at the expense of diverting management and staff resources from other areas of care – and reducing any local management flexibility in achieving a balanced service.

A 1998 survey of European health care systems found that the governments seeking to pay by results were in the minority. Ten of the 16 countries examined use prospective funding systems to set budgets for hospital inpatient services, most of them global budgets, although Germany allocates prospective flexible budgets, and Sweden combines prospective payments with a further payment linked to numbers treated (Maceira 1998)[111].

While some health system reformers have seen adjustments to provider payment mechanisms as one way of reducing perverse incentives and inefficiency, Barnum and colleagues (1995) surveyed a number of existing payment systems and drew the conclusion that all of them create a mixture of adverse and beneficial effects. Despite the strenuous efforts of reformers in Europe (Saltman et al 1998), and in Latin America and Asia (Bitran and Yip 1998) it seems clear that tinkering with provider payment mechanisms can consume large amounts of managerial time and resources without offering any guaranteed solution to perverse incentives.

Provider payment reform in developing countries

In many developing countries, public sector health centres and hospitals are funded according to historic budgets, or even on the basis of numbers of staff in post, a system described by Bitran and Yip (1998) as 'the most common method of financing public hospitals in developing countries'.

---

111 The six countries allocating budgets on a service-based system were Austria (which paid on the basis of length of stay in hospital); England (in which payments related to service level agreements between local purchaser and provider); Finland (with local-level service-based reimbursement); Hungary, with a performance related payment system; and Slovakia, which paid hospitals by the bed-day for inpatients.

Not only does this replicate each year the chronic underlying lack of resources, but as the authors point out, from a management point of view the system almost inevitably promotes inefficiency, containing no incentive to alter staffing levels, reduce costs or respond to local demand for services.

Purchasing from the private sector

Developed countries

Bismarck-style health care systems, which have always had some separation between purchasers and providers, have also long accommodated a private sector in the provision of health care: in France 29% of beds are in the private for-profit sector. Italy, too, has a large number of hospital beds operating privately but in which patients are funded by the National Health Service. In Japan 80% of hospitals are in the private sector, publicly funded through a network of social insurance funds.

However some systems have historically been less flexible: the announcement by British Health Secretary Alan Milburn of a Concordat under which the NHS would purchase non-emergency treatment from private sector hospitals drew an angry response from public sector trade unions. The criticisms focused on the long-running issue of staff shortages in the public sector, which the unions argued would be worsened by any expansion in private sector capacity – creating a double problem for local NHS providers, which would lose both the funding for the work done in the private sector and potentially the staff required to sustain the fuller range of services (including emergency services) provided only by the public sector.

These issues have arisen repeatedly as further reforms create new ways in which public funds can be used to buy services from private providers. The British government is introducing a nation-wide 'patient choice' programme, beginning with a few selected specialties, which will eventually offer every NHS patient the right to choose from at least four hospitals – in either the public or private sector, home or abroad Already this is leading to a drain of resources from the public sector into private hospitals (Hirst 2003, Plumridge and Kemp 2004).

More recently, plans for the opening of a chain of new privately run Diagnostic and Treatment Centres (DTCs) have generated fresh controversy, both in terms of the threat that more NHS staff will be 'poached' to work in them, leaving existing services under-staffed, and because of the financial and caseload impact of 'cream skimming' lucrative elective work from NHS units which will be left with reduced budgets but the responsibility for the more complex and costly cases. The limited evidence so far available shows that the unit costs of the private sector units will be higher than could be achieved by expanding NHS capacity, and that doctors and consultants in the private units will be paid several times the comparable NHS salary (Dyer O 2003a).

Purchasing from private providers in developing countries

Developing countries can face pressure from global bodies and from powerful donors (notably the World Bank and USAID) which are ideologically committed to privatisation and the expansion of the private sector, which is thought to be more responsive and efficient (World Bank 1987, 1993, Skaar 1998 Mudyarabikwa 2000, IFC 2002). However the evidence to support this presumption is weak (Palmer 2000).

However, in many of the poorest countries privatisation or the purchase of services from the private sector is easier proposed than done: though public sector provision may be relatively restricted both in its scope and available resources, there may be relatively little in the way of a developed private sector either, especially if this is seen narrowly as private for-profit health care provision, operating on a scale which might compete with or even replace publicly provided services. The availability of potential providers may, as with other services, be largely confined to urban areas, with little or no provision in the rural districts. There may also be a shortage of capacity to formulate explicit specifications and contracts, and to monitor them adequately: the process may also incur heavy transaction costs without any compensating advantages (Palmer 2000).

Information on the scale and character of private sector activity in health care in poorer countries is hard to find. In 1998, Hanson and Berman attempted an analysis of private health provision in developing countries, only to conclude that the 'paucity of available information' made it impossible to generate meaningful findings on more than 25-35 countries, compared with 114 countries for which the World Bank had figures on health spending in 1993. Most of the information they collated was drawn from 1980s documents (Hanson and Berman 1998:210-11).

As a consequence, in much of the literature of health system reform the definition of private sector is widened to embrace a wide variety of non-profit providers, notably NGOs and church groups, which stand outside the funding network of the public health care system. Traditional healers, people selling pharmaceuticals (often illegally) and unqualified quacks who are paid privately in the absence of accessible health care may also be included as a part of the 'private sector' to justify a further expansion along these lines rather than the development of public health services (Brugha and Zwi 2002).

It appears that relatively little 'private' activity is 'for-profit' other than at the level of individual practitioners[112]. Skaar (1998) in an extensive survey for USAID on the extent of collaboration with the private sector in Africa, Asia, Eastern Europe and Latin America, reveals that a majority of the 'private providers' are NGOs, and most of the projects are relatively small scale, focused on health education, health promotion, family planning and reproductive health. Excluding those where the private provider is a retailer, pharmacist or outside health care altogether, of 65 schemes identified, only three schemes clearly involved 'for-profit' companies.

A case study of Zimbabwe found that non-profit missions were the 'private' health care providers for 70% of Zimbabwe's rural population: subsidies directed at this sector were found to generate more benefits for consumers than those given to for-profit private providers, which benefited only the wealthier minority of the population (Mudyarabikwa 2000).

For organisations and researchers eager to demonstrate the importance of increased private sector involvement, therefore, there is an advantage in combining together all the aspects of existing health care systems that can be regarded as 'private' – including the fee-for-service payments paid out of pocket by the poor in countries where primary care providers are largely private. While this clearly demonstrates the burden of unfunded health care on the poorest, it does nothing to show the superiority of such systems over public provision – nor indeed does it answer concerns over the uneven and often questionable quality of privately provided services (Brugha and Zwi 2002). Indeed private health care can combine higher costs

---

112 One exception appears to be Tanzania, where historically voluntary agencies have controlled around half of the country's hospital beds. Munishi (1995) reports a rapid expansion of for-profit hospital care, albeit largely concentrated in the capital, where 83% of private hospitals and 57% of private hospital beds were for-profit.

– beyond the reach of poorer households – and very low quality treatment (Mills et al 2002).

Another aspect of 'privatisation' is the use of drugs: in developing countries, spending on pharmaceuticals – the majority of it private and out-of-pocket – accounts for 30-50% of total health care spending, compared with less than 15% in developed economies (Whitehead et al 2001). In many cases the drug vendors are unqualified, and target their products at people too poor to consult health professionals.

McPake and Mills (2000:813) find that private for-profit providers seldom offer services 'of a public health nature', even immunisation: instead they 'over-prescribe in general' and tend to use excessive, unnecessary technology. They argue that there is one 'common conclusion':

> ...although the private sector can complement public health provision and provide some types of services better, it cannot lead the health sector in a direction likely to maximise its contribution to the health of the population.

In similar vein Brugha and Zwi (2002:70) question the apparent over-optimism of the WHO, which in its 1999 *World Health Report* argued that strong regulation could enable the most efficient providers to flourish and allow private providers to be brought into 'a structured but pluralistic health care system'.

Nevertheless, despite a severe absence of evidence that private provision is possible or that it delivers improvements in quality and efficiency, the World Bank (in a website briefing on Private and Public Initiatives) confusingly mingles all the different 'private' spending together, notes the varying (but large) proportions of hospital beds that are privately provided in a sample of developing countries, and the percentages of physicians in the private sector, and concludes approvingly that:

Currently an estimated 50% of all global spending for health comes from the private sector (van der Gaag 1996).

The same Bank website goes on to explore case studies of its intervention to promote greater use of private sector providers, notably Uganda, where 'improving health care is a private matter':

> To increase coverage and encourage private investment in the sector, the [Bank-funded] project will provide equipment for privately run facilities in underserved areas. [...] Another strategy that has been tested and proven in the international arena is transferring services once handled by the public sector to private providers. The District Health Project will fund studies to determine if it is feasible to contract out Uganda's blood transfusion services and to identify which hospital-related services (such as catering, gardening, cleaning, laundry) could be provided better and cheaper by private agents (van der Gaag 1996)[113].

Some of the experience of private provision in poorer countries raises questions over value for money and quality. A voucher scheme allowing Nicaraguan patients to choose which clinic they attend for treatment of sexually transmitted diseases has now excluded the public sector clinics, and pays a more generous fee to private clinics than those run by NGOs. The scheme's administrative costs 'account for a large share of total spending' (Sandiford et al 2002:4).

---

113 For an interesting retrospective look at the near-total failure of these policies 'typically written by donor-funded expatriate staff', see Okuonzi 2004.

Palmer (2000:822) notes that the promotion of contracts for clinical care rests on assumptions drawn from similar policies in advanced industrialised countries, and 'the applicability of these assumptions to health care services, especially in developing countries, must be questioned'. Munishi warns that the Tanzanian experience is not all positive, since the expansion of the private sector alongside a public sector seeking to implement full cost recovery through user fees can result in many of those most able to pay deserting the public health care system. There are also conflicts and rivalries over the recruitment of qualified nursing and medical staff (Munishi 1995) a problem also noted in Kenya by Kimalu (2001).

The situation is clearly rather different in more prosperous countries, but some of the same ambiguities remain. Slack and Savedoff (2001) in a survey for the Inter American Development Bank, have identified five distinct types of contractual arrangement between public and private sectors in middle income countries of Latin America, giving varying degrees of control on the level of financial commitment. But of their 27 case studies, more than a third are NGOs, community groups or not-for-profit providers.

Given the considerable body of evidence from developed economies, and from Thailand (Brugha and Zwi 2002) that purchasing care from the private sector serves to increase costs and thus draw resources out of limited public sector budgets, it must be at least questionable whether such a strategy could do other than worsen the crisis of health care in developing countries.

Competition

Developed countries

The World Bank's advice for health care reform, displayed on its own website, hinges on the assumption that competitive markets offer the best of all possible arrangements:

> After more than a half-century of experiments with alternative forms of economic development, the evidence strongly favours the proposition that competitive markets are the best and most efficient way yet known to organise the production and distribution of goods and services. Consensus is also forming that a market-oriented approach to development – complemented by a transparent legal and regulatory framework and government that steps in only where markets fail – can yield spectacular results (World Bank 2000e).

Despite evidence that the effectiveness of markets as a means to govern health care systems is less categoric than the Bank's assertions suggest, competition is central to the full operation of the various market-style reforms, since it represents the greatest break from traditional public service notions of planning and centralised state provision and control[114].

To create conditions for competition – and thus open up the possibility of patient choice – centralised systems must be broken up and decentralised. The policy options for those seeking to introduce competitive systems include almost the full repertoire of market reforms identified at the start of this chapter:

- Restructuring centralised systems to separate purchasers from providers
- Moves to enhance the autonomy and encouraging 'entrepreneurialism' and

---

114 Conspicuously, the promotion of competition comes as the first of the ten principles of the New Public Management as outlined by Osborne and Gaebler (1992:25.310).

competition between public sector providers

- The deregulation of public purchasers (or other measures to permit, encourage or compel them to buy services from private rather than public sector providers)
- The privatisation of publicly run services.

However competition brings with it overheads in the form of transaction costs. Modern health care systems are complex, and the requirement to formulate precise specifications and standards, and then to administer and monitor the resulting contract, means that any efficiency savings that may be generated through competition have to be offset against the overall cost increases. These are among the factors that help push the costs of administering the US health care system to over 30% of its spending (Light 2003).

Competition in developing countries

Even in the wealthiest and highest-spending countries (q.v. the USA) full-scale competition in a free unregulated health-care market is all but unknown[115]. While the World Bank sees competitive market systems as a general formula, applying to all countries and circumstances, the possibilities for establishing genuine competition between health care providers, or even 'managed competition' between rival health funds is largely restricted to the wealthier countries, where budgets are sufficiently large to allow the possibility of surplus capacity, and where there is a sufficient number of properly resourced competitors to create the semblance of a 'market'.

Even where a degree of competition exists, it by no means guarantees a positive long-term outcome for health care services to the poor. One USAID-funded study of Tanzania notes with approval that the public sector is now obliged to compete with private providers on an unusually wide front:

> …in providing a full range of curative services at all levels of care in hospitals, health centres and dispensaries, and also in providing preventive and other high-priority public health services (Munishi 1995:xvii).

Yet the same report also notes the profoundly unequal provision of competitive for-profit private health care in the rural areas. Private provision is concentrated in Dar es Salaam, and it is clear that if the private sector emerges the 'winner' in this type of competition, the end result will be to leave the public sector shouldering the costs of care for the poorest and the rural population – with resulting negative implications for equity.

As noted above, and in the case of Tanzania by Munishi (1995) competition between public and private sectors for scarce qualified staff frequently works to the detriment of the public sector – and the poor who depend upon it.

The issue is equally difficult in middle income countries. Waitzkin (1997) notes the failure of 'managed care' and competition to hold down costs or ensure universal coverage in the USA, and warns that attempts to extend it into Latin America, with the prospect of competition between large private companies, are likely to replicate similar problems.

---

115 Evans (1997:2) argues that this is inevitable: 'There is in health care no private, competitive market of the form described in the economics textbooks, anywhere in the world. There never has been and inherent characteristics of health and health care make it impossible that there ever could be'.

Privatisation

Developed countries

It is clear that any combination of the various forms of decentralisation may lead on to or include a further, more radical additional element, which is the *privatisation* of services hitherto provided by publicly owned agencies. Gilson for example (1997:2) simply adds privatisation as a fourth category of decentralisation, though this automatic connection is disputed by some including Collins and Green (1994) who argue that privatisation, by transferring power outside the public sector, goes beyond decentralisation.

Privatisation does not necessarily have to follow from decentralisation, but as another facet of the New Public Management it comes from the same neoliberal school of policy. Yet however tenuous the level of accountability between a public service and the local public, there is no similar accountability in the case of a private provider, who is not bound to serve the public interest, and unlikely to deliver any more than is required under a formal contract. Any arrangement with a private contractor is a substantial step beyond the 'new contractualism' that Schick (1998) detects as the essence of the management reforms implemented by the New Zealand government.

The international organisation of public sector trade unions distinguishes between a number of levels and forms of privatisation:

- Privatisation of ownership (of health facilities and service units)
- Privatisation of responsibility (management of public services privatised, or state provision withdrawn in favour of private sector)
- Privatisation of provision (health care services contracted out, or even publicly owned facilities leased, to the private sector)
- Privatisation of finance (the use of Public Private Partnerships, Public Finance Initiatives, borrowing private capital for public health schemes, charging higher fees for health care treatment and services, or shifting from public funding of health care to private health insurance)
- Privatisation through markets – creating conditions where the private sector can compete with the public sector for government or social insurance scheme funds – where necessary splitting purchasers and providers.

(Public Service International 1999:9)

Preker and Harding, promoting 'greater private sector participation in generating inputs and providing health services,' see privatisation as following naturally from the autonomisation and corporatisation of hospitals (Preker and Harding 2000).

Sein (2001:2), in discussing decentralisation of health care services in various Asian countries, includes privatisation as part of a general 'transfer of functions' from government to 'nongovernmental organisations, including private for-profit enterprises and NGOs in the established sense of the term'[116].

However the extent to which full-scale privatisation of health care facilities and services has

---

116 Cardelle (2000:211) notes that the number of NGOs in Chile rose by 87% after the 1973 coup 'due to the international community's growing scepticism regarding the public sector'.

been carried through in more advanced economies is very limited – even in the transition economies of the former Soviet Union and Eastern Europe, where there has been a concerted drive towards privatisation in other sectors.

In the UK, the first Beveridge-style health system to break from centralised control and introduce market-style reforms, only a part of the non-clinical support services and (later) long term care for the elderly were privatised in the hospital sector – despite the reforming zeal and neoliberal credentials of Margaret Thatcher, and a Conservative government that privatised so many state-owned utilities. The Netherlands, New Zealand and Sweden have each moved along the path of neoliberal reform in health care, only to hesitate and stop well short of wholesale privatisation.

In part these limitations could be explained country by country, as the impact of 'policy context' as described by Collins et al (1999), who point to the variety of reforms in process in a cross section of countries[117]. But the striking factor, not only in these seven countries but in almost every higher or middle income country for which data are available, is the limited extent to which the agenda of full-scale privatisation of existing publicly provided health care services has been carried through.

There have been attempts to press home a more thoroughgoing privatised model, especially in poorer countries. The model aspired to by many neoliberals was the situation in Chile, in which wholesale privatisation of the economy was driven through by the extreme right wing Pinochet junta after the 1973 coup, with advice from neoliberal guru Milton Friedman and his 'Chicago Boys'. The Pinochet regime did drastically cut health care spending, slashing per capita health spending by more than a third by 1979, and to 34% of its 1974 level by 1990 (Taylor 2003). The proportion of private beds increased from 10% to 25% between 1981 and 1992.

But such policies could be sustained only under a military dictatorship: the new government from 1990 was obliged to implement substantial increases in government spending on health care, which more than doubled in seven years in the mid 1990s. This increased spending did not reverse Pinochet's expansion of the private sector, which by 2000 collected two-thirds of Chile's health insurance contributions, and 46% of total health spending, but covered just 23% of the population, and maintained a rigorous system of risk-adjusted contributions and excluding those most likely to require health treatment. The system also imposed substantial co-payments for the public sector service, with some subsidy for the poorest. Yet even at its peak of 'authoritarian neoliberalism', Pinochet's regime pulled back from privatising the entire system, and left 75% of hospital beds in the public sector (Taylor 2003).

Privatisation in poor countries

Privatisation in developing countries is driven on by global agencies. The World Bank explains that its eagerness to privatise services wherever the conditions permit and profits can be found is based on three fundamental assumptions, none of which it seeks to explain or prove:

- The state itself is desperately short of the resources required to run a publicly funded service[118]

---

117 Brazil, Kenya, Mexico, Pakistan, Romania, Thailand and the UK

118 Of course one might conclude, as Deber (2000a) argues, that if a single-payer public service cannot be afforded, a privatised service is also financially out of reach.

- The public sector is inherently and incorrigibly less efficient not only than the private sector, but also assumed to be less efficient than the 'not-for-profit' NGOs which the World Bank often promotes as a surrogate private sector

- Public services inevitably generate inequity in access, with the wealthiest minority often consuming far more than its proportional share of services intended primarily for the poor[119].

Public sector controlled policies do not have a good track record on equity. In Indonesia, for example, the rich receive almost three times as much public health care as the poor. In Tanzania the richest fifth of the population use more than twice as many government hospital beds and more than four times as many outpatient services as the poorest fifth. In Cote D'Ivoire less than one-quarter of the rural poor who were sick received any form of medical care, as compared with half the urban rich. In Peru only 20% of the poor received care, versus 57% of the rich[120] (World Bank 2000e).

While these criticisms of publicly provided services in cash-strapped countries have at least an element of truth, such problems are not sufficient to establish a case for privatisation as the solution. The lack of state resources for public provision of health care in many developing countries flows from the three-way impasse created by global capitalism, in which:

- A very high proportion of the population is poor and/or outside the formal economy, and therefore paying little or no tax

- The government is in any event constrained by global creditors such as the IMF and World Bank to keep taxes low and reduce or eliminate tariffs which might otherwise yield resources for health

- What revenues do come through to the government are largely channelled back to the wealthier countries in the form of debt service.

(WHO 2000, Labonte et al 2004)

The 'inefficiency' of publicly provided services in these and other countries is a stock assumption made by neoliberals, with seldom any attempt at justification. By contrast the inherent 'efficiency' of private health providers is also assumed, despite abundant evidence that the overhead costs of the private sector are much higher than publicly funded systems, that the costs of private treatment are higher, and that only publicly funded systems have shown themselves able to deliver universal and equal access to services (Hart 2003, PNHP 2003a & b, Laurell 1996).

However if there are problems managing a publicly funded service, logic suggests the same weak and poorly resourced government would have just as many – if not more – problems seeking to 'regulate' the activities of a relatively powerful and autonomous private health care

---

119 It is evident that such inequality – itself the outcome of unequal power structures in dependent capitalist countries – is not avoided but compounded by health systems delivering care privately only to those with insurance or the ability to pay.

120 The shocking aspect that appears to have escaped the World Bank in this instance is that the systems in place in the poorest countries are so inadequately resourced that in some cases, like Peru, even half the rich people can't get the treatment they need.

sector – a task which has so far eluded the administration of the world's largest and wealthiest capitalist nation. In the case of developing countries, the resources to train and sustain a skilled management structure as well as front line service providers are constantly squeezed by the economic pressures outlined above.

The Bank's insistence that publicly funded services are 'inequitable' because the wealthy find ways to seize more than their share could be seen as an argument for progressive systems of taxes - though the Bank never raises any such suggestion. However, there is more than ample evidence to demonstrate that *privatised* systems, especially those involving user fees, are even *more* skewed to favour preferential access for the rich while actively excluding the poor - the majority of Chileans, for example, are too poor to afford to use the country's private health care (Taylor 2003:40).

The Bank itself admits that its objective is not a single, equitable, worldwide system, but a two tier system – with minimal care targeted at the poor, and more expensive services for the rich:

> It is perhaps futile to strive for equity in very poor countries. Yet the health prospects of the poor could be greatly improved if public resources were used to increase access for the (mostly rural) poor and to support preventive medicine and basic curative care. Greater cost recovery for tertiary care would help finance such improvements, and allowing the private sector to provide services for those who could afford them would free up public resources, which could then be used to provide better access for the poor ('Comparing Different Options' – Bank website as above).

User fees and other policies to expand private insurance

Developed countries

In the context of European health care systems, which generally offer universal coverage, it can be hard to build a substantial private health insurance market. Germany allows certain high-earners, civil servants and the self employed to 'opt out' of the statutory health system and join an alternative voluntary health insurance, and there are 'opt-out' provisions in the Netherlands and Spain: but in general private insurance has been squeezed out by publicly funded schemes.

One problem for insurers is the lack of substantial waiting lists and the high quality of public health care services in many European countries. Even in Britain, despite extensive marketing efforts by private health insurers offering swifter and more luxurious treatment, numbers of individuals covered have actually fallen, with only limited expansion in company-funded schemes for employees (Laing & Buisson 2003).

In this context the imposition of user fees in publicly provided health care services (co-payments for drugs, consultations, or hospital admission) can prove a useful spur to encourage the middle classes to take out private insurance. 'Complementary' voluntary insurance schemes to cover drug costs in co-payments are available in most EU countries, though with the exception of France (where voluntary insurance accounted for 12% of health spending in 1998 and covered 85% of people against co-payments) the business is seen as relatively marginal and not very profitable (Mossialos & Thomson 2002:129-132).

Some EU governments have attempted to pump prime private health insurance through offering tax relief: in Ireland the government spends over 79 million each year on what is effectively a subsidy that reduces the cost of premiums by 32% – though most subscribers to voluntary health insurance are high earners. The controversial British Conservative government scheme to offer tax relief for those aged over 60 who took out health insurance was shown to have cost £140 million a year, but to have attracted only 50,000 extra subscribers to private policies – and was scrapped when Labour took office in 1997 (Mossialos & Thomson 2002).

It seems that only the real and present danger of facing catastrophic bills for hospital treatment will induce large sections of the EU population to opt for private medical insurance: in Greece, despite the high level of charges faced by those who fall ill, voluntary schemes cover only 10% of the population (Mossialos & Thomson 2002).

However, after decades in which people have become accustomed to getting treatment without personal cost, there are very substantial political obstacles to imposing user charges large enough to open up a new insurance market.

User fees and insurance in developing countries
In the very different situation in Eastern and Central Europe and in many developing countries, the World Bank and other agencies have pressed for the introduction of user fees not as a means to raise serious resources, but precisely as a way of persuading the middle classes to seek out insurance schemes and a device to open up a private sector (Klugman and Schieber 1996, Shaw 1995).

While the Bank's Health Nutrition and Population division has pressed for the implementation of user fees in even the poorest countries, its International Finance Corporation has focused on developing private insurance schemes targeted at the 'lower middle and middle classes in countries without risk pooling,' which is seen as contributing 'to the strengthening of the middle class' (IFC 2002:4,5).

However, the extent of poverty in many developing countries has meant that attempts to launch self-sufficient insurance schemes have been largely doomed to remain as small-scale experiments (Musau 1999).

Patient choice and 'Consumerism'
Developed and developing countries
While publicly provided health care systems can in theory plan to meet demand, they are constrained by the level of available resources. In such circumstances a shortfall of resources will be reflected in a waiting list for treatment – which itself can sometimes become a political lever for those campaigning for additional resources.

However, the market-style/NPM approach, emphasising the role of the individual patient as 'consumer' of a commodified health service, coupled with the separation of purchaser and provider that prevails in many European health care systems, can seriously undermine planning. A shortfall in resourcing for one public sector provider which results in a delay in treatment becomes in this situation a pretext for the transfer of resources to a rival provider – whether public or private sector.

Enthoven (1997) has shown a number of ways in which consumerism could easily be utilised by a largely deregulated private sector to drive up costs (and thus profits). The key factor in his list of potential problems is:

Free choice of provider: 'destroys the bargaining power of insurers' (Enthoven 1997:196).

It was to forestall this and similar destabilising factors that health maintenance organisations and managed care were introduced in the USA: they aimed both to contain costs and improve quality by *restricting* the level of patient choice. Enthoven (1997:199) sums up the four principles of managed care as:

- Selective provider contracting
- Utilisation management
- Negotiated payment
- Quality management.

The most fundamental of these is clearly the first, the restricted range of providers with whom the insurer sets out to negotiate a package. Any return to untrammelled rights of the individual patient to seek treatment wherever they choose could generate a new round of medical cost inflation and the danger of reduced levels of monitoring and poorer quality care. Nevertheless consumerist policies are starting to have an impact in a number of countries. The 2001 decisions of the European Court of Justice that citizens of EU countries have the right to seek treatment in other EU countries if they cannot get access to care without 'undue delay' have already had substantial impact on health services across Europe (Schuppe 2002).

In publicly funded services, already struggling to supply sufficient care for a rising level of demand, the apparently innocuous suggestion of 'patient choice' can prove an impossible target, or a potentially open-ended commitment to fund private sector treatment. Deber (2000) reports that Canadian cancer patients who travel from Ontario to US hospitals to avoid long waiting lists incur bills six times higher than the cost of treating them at home.

To offer all patients a choice of where to seek treatment suggests an expansion of capacity to ensure that a surplus is always available within any provider to accommodate those who 'choose' to transfer from a competitor – or a potentially substantial and open-ended increase in budget. Patient choice thus steps beyond the general encouragement of inter-provider 'competition', and implies the development by each of sufficient additional capacity to be able to compete for a share of the workload of its rivals. Yet the public sector – increasingly as a result of market-style reforms[121] – tends to receive revenue funding only on the basis of the workload it treats, leaving little if any room for prospective investment.

Patient choice also requires breaking down the boundaries between public and private sectors, because any patient exercising the choice to seek their treatment from a private provider will also necessarily take with them the funding to pay for their treatment. In cases (such as many parts of London) where public sector capacity is constrained by shortages of professional and other staff, 'patient choice' also implies that these resources too should be made available to a private sector provider to grant the patient his or her choice – regardless of the consequences for the public sector (Lister 2003a).

Taken to its logical conclusion, patient choice, as the epitome of consumerism and the opposite of planning, counterpoises the choices of the individual to the stability of a system that has an obligation to care for the whole population. Another consequence as the policy is rolled out for an increasing range of specialties is that the public sector will increasingly wind up dealing with the more expensive or complex cases, the most elderly and frail patients – and generally those cases less financially attractive for the private sector. This problem of 'cream-skimming' is increasingly being identified as an issue confronting American hospitals (Devers 2003, AHA 2004).

---

121 Notably the new proposals to phase in 'payment by results' in the British NHS.

Another dimension of systems in which 'patient choice' is used to break down barriers between public and private sectors is the pressure from the World Trade Organisation and the General Agreement on Trade in Services (GATS). Once it is clear that private sector providers are not running parallel but competing with the public sector, there will be increased pressure for this market to be further liberalised and opened up to global competition (Pollock and Price 2000).

PFI/PPP and its extension internationally

Developed countries

The private financing of new hospital and health care projects through the Private Finance Initiative (PFI) has become a major contentious issue in the 'modernisation' of the British National Health Service – and British-based consultancy firms such as PricewaterhouseCoopers and British-led consortia are now at the forefront of efforts to promote this approach on an international level. According to the trade press[122] and other sources PFI hospital schemes are taking shape or already operational in Canada, Australia, South Africa, Italy, and Portugal. The EU early in 2004 changed the rules of the Stability Pact underpinning the euro, in order to encourage the use of PFI for public works, by excluding such investment from the total of public debts (as long as the private sector can be shown to be carrying the investment risk) (Murray Brown et al 2004).

PFI first emerged in Britain in 1992 in the aftermath of the Conservative government's market-style reforms, which established the principle of NHS hospital Trusts paying 'capital charges' on the value of their property and land assets and on any new capital borrowing from the Treasury. This policy was initially seen as a device to encourage Trust managers to sell off any unused or partially used land or buildings at the first opportunity, rather than incur capital charges: but more fundamental was the notion of the NHS as *tenant* rather than landlord, occupying buildings for which it had to pay rather than simply regard as a 'free good'.

Conservative Chancellors began a two-pronged approach, which combined a steep reduction in the annual allocation of capital to the NHS with the requirement that any substantial development (initially £5 million or more) had to be advertised and 'tested' in the market under PFI, to investigate whether any private consortium might be prepared to put up the capital, build and operate the hospital, and lease it back to the NHS for a long-term (25-30 year) contract. It was described by the Treasury as changing:

...public sector organisations from being owners of assets and direct providers of services into purchasers of services from the private sector (HM Treasury 1997, cited in Pollock et al 1997).

For various reasons the private sector could not be convinced to sign such contracts in the NHS until after the change of government in 1997, when New Labour, having first denounced PFI as 'the thin end of the wedge of privatisation', came to office pledged to 'rescue PFI', portraying it as 'a key part of the government's ten-year programme for modernisation' (Lister 2001).

Twenty-one PFI-funded hospitals have now been completed in Britain, with a total value

---

122 *Public Private Finance* magazine, and *PFI Intelligence Bulletin* are both linked with organisations promoting regular conferences exploring possibilities for international extension of new PFI deals.

of around £1.5 billion. The next ten are in the process of construction, at a capital value of £1.9 billion and a new round of PFI schemes are currently being debated around the country, three of which total £1.7 billion (publicprivatefinance 2004). The government aims to have established £7 billion worth of PFI hospitals by 2010 - 85% of all new capital investment in the NHS (and 94% of new hospitals) now come via PFI, with public funding largely restricted to smaller scale and refurbishment schemes (Sussex 2001).

As a result an increasing share of NHS property assets are being privatised. PFI also means that an ever-growing share of NHS funding is flowing straight out of the public sector into the private sector and its shareholders, for whom (despite the rhetoric claiming a 'transfer of risk') completed PFI hospitals are seen as a virtually risk-free income-stream (Lister 2001:5). NHS Trusts, once they have become PFI lease-holders, commonly retain financial control only over those services excluded from PFI – clinical services and the payroll for nurses, doctors and other professionals. Any further financial constraints are therefore more likely to impact directly upon patient care.

PFI maintains the appearance of a publicly funded, publicly provided service while in practice diverting very substantial capital and revenue resources into the private sector. The notion that PFI hospitals represent 'value for money' despite their inflated costs has been questioned. The experience of poor quality, poorly designed and inadequate-sized buildings, with poor quality privately provided support services has been highlighted in many brand new PFI hospitals: a number have been obliged to begin extensions to add extra beds and facilities not properly planned into the original building. Management in some (such as the new Edinburgh Royal Infirmary) are still attempting to solve problems of ventilation and temperature control (Lister 2003a, Lister 2003b, publicprivatefinance.com 2003).

Meanwhile the question of value for money has been overtaken in some of the larger PFI schemes by the issue of affordability. Health commissioners in Greater Manchester were warned in 2003 that the combined effects of the various capital development schemes in the area, including several high-cost PFI schemes, add up to almost £1 billion and are simply 'unaffordable'. Several projects have been scaled back and others, including the largest, a new £400m hospital for Central Manchester, have been delayed (CMMH 2003)[123].

The combined cost of health and other PFI schemes in Britain has been estimated as rising towards £30 billion per year, while the value of publicly owned assets falls back (Lister 2001). It remains to be seen how many other governments wish to follow Britain down the road of renting the core infrastructure for key public services from the private sector.

PFI and PPPs in developing countries
Few developing countries will find themselves in a position for PFI to become an option. Private sector lenders and developers know in the high income countries that they can count on top-sliced funding from substantial public sector budgets, underwritten by government guarantees. There is seldom anywhere near enough uncommitted funding available in most developing countries to offer the margins that would interest PFI consortia.

---

123 Likewise schemes to merge two specialist hospitals and a teaching hospital onto a single 'Paddington Health Campus' has escalated in cost from £370m to more than £1 billion, and is also being challenged as unaffordable. In East London the planned rebuild of the Royal London and Bart's Hospitals has also escalated in cost from £600m to £900m before the final negotiations begin.

Capital-hungry PFI and occasionally PPP (Public Private Partnership) deals for new hospitals in the wealthy countries are a far cry from the similarly titled 'Global Public Private Partnerships' which are increasingly seen by the WHO and the UN as ways of enlisting private sector help to carry through immunisation and other health programmes in developing countries (Buse and Walt 2000a). Around 70 such partnerships have been identified, many of them involving drug companies and research projects (Buse and Waxman 2001).

Critics argue that the WHO is potentially vulnerable to political and economic pressure from much wealthier drug companies and private corporations, making any 'partnership' profoundly unequal (HAI 2000).

Managed care

Developed countries

This misleading phrase has emerged as a euphemism for attempts to regulate the market in health care, especially in the USA, where private sector providers are most commonly paid on a fee-for-service basis, whether these fees are paid directly by the patient or indirectly through an insurance scheme. This type of system has a built-in perverse incentive to increase costs and maximise the amount of treatment given to each patient (Scott 2001).

Attempts to remedy these problems have focused on various forms of 'managed' care arrangement, a range of strategies to contain costs, whereby the provider receives a flat fee – either on the basis of a capitation payment for each person covered by a health plan, regardless of the amount of services delivered; or on a case-based system paying a fixed amount for each medical case regardless of its complexity and cost. By 2001 almost 90% of care in the US was delivered by one type or another of 'managed care', although this is a general category within which there is a growing variety of specific schemes offering varied levels of cover for varying premium payments: the most common are HMOs and PPOs (Preferred Provider Organisations) (Weiner et al 2001).

The emergence of managed care as a mechanism to assert (at least temporary) control over the growth in health care costs in the US has led to some advocating its extension to Britain and on a wider scale (Robinson & Steiner 1998), although others have warned that it is a 'slippery concept' that had still not been evaluated and required to be treated with caution (Fairfield et al 1997). Debate continues over controversial and highly questionable comparisons that have been made between the costs and effectiveness of one of the leading US HMOs, Kaiser Permanente in California, and the British NHS (Feachem et al 2002, Himmelstein & Woolhandler 2002b, David 2002, Tonks 2002, Talbot-Smith et al 2004, Adams 2004).

The new escalation of health care inflation in the USA is likely to reduce interest in transplanting a system which grew out of the chaos of private insurance and competition, and which depends upon modifying the actions of doctors, both at primary care level (offering inducements to act as gatekeepers restricting referrals to secondary care) and in hospitals. The basic logic of managed care is 'to give providers incentives to be judicious in the use of expensive resources' (Fairfield et al 1997). As such it appears that in a system dominated by private insurers and providers, the policy is driven not by the needs of patients or by health considerations, but by financial pressures and the quest for profit.

Medical Savings Accounts

Developed countries

This latest chosen vehicle for neoliberal reform has been branded by opposing campaigners in the USA as:

...a tax cut targeted toward healthy, affluent people that increases health insurance [costs] for the sick (Park and Lav 2003).

Medical Savings Accounts (MSAs, also known as Medisave Accounts) are personal savings accounts enhanced by tax concessions, which can be used in conjunction with low-cost health insurance schemes involving high deductibles, designed to cover the costs of any catastrophic illness. The theory is that in cases of lesser illness (incurring costs up to $1,500 or even $3,000), the funds in a patient's MSA could be used to cover costs not covered by insurance. However, any money that was not used in this way could be invested in stocks and bonds and eventually withdrawn by the individual as an additional income in retirement (Mossialos and Dixon 2002).

From the neoliberal point of view such a policy has many advantages, effectively breaking down any wider commitment to social solidarity or risk-sharing, and reducing health care provision for the well-to-do to an individual matter between them, their bankers and insurers. Jensen (2000:119) also argues that MSAs 'would give consumers a strong financial incentive to control their own health care costs':

...individuals would buy many routine medicals services with their own money, and funds not spent for medical care would be theirs to keep (op. cit. 121).

MSAs are already part of the '3 Ms'[124] system of financing health services in Singapore, where the government specifically sought a system which would curb excess demand and 'promote individual responsibility'. There they are linked with supplementary programmes designed to 'protect the poor and address potential market failures' (Taylor 2003). However per capita health care costs continued to rise in Singapore after MSAs were introduced in 1984, and in 1993 supplementary measures were brought in to curb hospital spending and restrict the prices to be charged for some services. Medisave funds cannot be used to buy a wide range of care including obstetric services, and long-term care. Medishield, which is supposed to provide cover for catastrophic costs, excludes pre-existing conditions such as stroke, coronary artery disease and cancer. The size of the out-of-pocket costs that result, often shouldered by elderly people and the poor without the means to pay, are one reason why Singapore registered so low (101 out of 191 countries) on the WHO's comparison of fairness in financing (Shortt 2002).

In Canada the recent Romanow and Senate reviews of health care financing have generated a fresh round of debate on MSAs (Gratzer 2002, Deber et al 2002a 2002b, 2002c, Forget et al 2002, Solomon 2002, Shortt 2002), in which the argument is polarised. Supporters of the policy argue that it reduces costs and can be an equitable system, while its opponents insist that the opposite is the case, and that the increase in costs would fall heavily

---

124 Singapore's 3 Ms are the Medisave MSA scheme, Medishield, which offers cover against catastrophic illness, and Medifund, a system that subsidises care for the poorest 10% of the population (Taylor 2003:3-4).

on those with greatest health needs. The strongest supporting evidence is produced by opponents of MSAs, who take a detailed look at the profile of health spending in the Canadian province of Manitoba, and from this demonstrate that while 80% of the population incur health spending well below the 'average', the sickest 1% accounted for 26% of health spending. A logical consequence of this is that the apparent financial disciplines which might result in reduced costs and health spending would be ineffective among the vast majority of the Manitoba population, who already make less than 'average' use of services – and little more effective with those in greatest need of health treatment. Instead of reducing costs, MSAs would increase health spending on the healthiest members of the population (Forget et al 2002, Deber et al 2002c).

US legislation in 1996-7 permitted limited experiments to test out the use of MSAs by self-employed people and those working for small businesses: the Bush administration has attempted to widen the use of MSAs, passing the Health Savings and Affordability Act, which is estimated to cost the federal government $174 billion in tax concessions over the next ten years (Families USA 2003c).

Savings deposited in MSAs would be tax-deductible, and any earnings from stocks and bonds held by an MSA would also be tax-free. While tax would have to be paid on any withdrawals for non-medical purposes, this only applies up to the age of 65, from which point withdrawals carry no tax penalty. The scheme has all the makings of a convenient tax shelter for the well-to-do.

Advocates of the scheme argue that MSAs would help offer coverage for the uninsured, but many uninsured workers earn too little to pay federal taxes, and cannot afford to put aside savings of $2,000-$4,000. Families USA (2003c) argue that MSAs could also increase costs for workers who currently have workplace health insurance, since it encourages employers to sign up for low-premium policies covering only catastrophic costs, leaving workers to pay out increased co-payments should they fall ill.

Park and Lav (2003:4) note that another consequence could be to push up the cost of traditional health insurance schemes. This would be exacerbated by the encouragement of healthy and wealthy subscribers to pull out of traditional schemes and opt for MSA-style coverage instead, leaving a smaller pool of older and less fit subscribers at increased risk, creating what Park & Lav describe as 'a death spiral for the employer's comprehensive coverage option'.

Chapter five

Analysing 'reform': conclusions and toolkits

Introduction

This study has a far wider scope than previously published investigations into the imposition of market-style and market-driven reforms. Few other enquiries have brought together the experience of OECD and poorer countries, while those that have done so generally consist of separately written chapters rather than offering an integrated analysis (Lee et al 2002, Sen 2003).

The experiences of the wide range of countries surveyed in the chapters below coincide in two remarkable respects:

- The standard list of 'market-style' reforms can generally be seen as compounding existing problems and creating new ones, rather than delivering the promised efficiencies and improvements in health care systems

- These new policies are most commonly introduced without regard to the availability of evidence on whether or not they deliver the intended results.

Wrong questions, wrong answers

Most of the more common reforms can be seen to worsen the situation they were ostensibly designed to improve:

1. Many of the newly established insurance funds – like some of the old-established ones in the 'Bismarck-style' systems of Germany, France and Japan – are mired in debt, requiring injections of central government funds to rescue them and pay outstanding bills to health care providers (Chapter six).

2. The switch from tax-funded to insurance-based systems, most systematically attempted in the CEE and NIS countries of Eastern Europe and Central Asia (several of which are discussed in the country summaries in Chapter six below) has proved to be socially regressive – in levying charges on a narrower range of earned income, leaving profits, wealth and dividends untouched – and if anything, less effective at delivering resources for health care. The reduction in taxation for some is more than outweighed by the increase for many in overall costs, pushed up by increased transaction costs and by the perverse incentives created by insurance systems.

3. Where the insurance system established involves multiple payers – a 'choice' of sickness funds, possibly even competing against each other – the experience appears to be even more problematic. Transaction costs are even higher in relation to the sums of money collected from subscribers, while the element of competition seems time and again to work against the long -term interests of those insured. Funds may compete by 'cream-skimming' a younger wealthier and healthier cohort of subscribers with a reduced package of services, leaving the large liabilities to their competitors or the public sector (as has happened in Chile). Others may seek less overt ways to exclude those at greatest risk in order to keep down their premium payments (Chapter nine).

4. Too many schemes can mean that smaller funds lack the expected purchasing power to drive hard deals with health care providers; or insurance funds may find common cause with a group of providers. In Poland and Estonia reforms have aimed to set up schemes despite lacking sufficient size of catchment population to ensure the viability of provider or purchaser. The Czech and Slovak republics have each seen a wide-scale bankruptcy of sickness funds and government intervention has been required to limit 'competition' between funds. The greater the proliferation of funding agencies, the more remote the prospect of being able effectively to monitor or regulate the services delivered, or work to any nationwide strategic plan for restructuring services, or exert influence over the prices charged by health care providers. Even the merger of 350 funds into a single National Health insurance fund in Korea has not ensured that the new body is ready or able to exercise any active scrutiny over the quality or cost of care in a system dominated by private for-profit hospitals.

5. The soaring costs (and inflated administration costs) and high levels of spending in the main insurance-based systems – France, Germany and the US – underline the unresolved problems even in wealthy countries which have been trying to control a system in which purchasers have for decades been divided from providers. The case argued by campaigners for a 'single payer' system to replace the ruinously expensive US system shows the extent to which even this limited reform could cut billions from bureaucracy and focus resources on patient care.

6. Competition, too, proves not to be the automatic guarantee of improved efficiency and reduced costs that neoliberals believe it to be. Competition may take the form of family doctors competing for clients by offering more generous prescribing of high cost drugs, or supplier-induced demand as over-bedded hospitals seek to ensure higher occupancy levels. Competition on grounds of price can encourage 'cherry picking' by hospitals keen to focus only on the most lucrative, predictable and least complex treatments, again leaving care of emergency cases, the frail elderly, the mentally ill and other 'high risk' cases to others. Health care providers may limit or close their facilities in poorer neighbourhoods, or seek other ways to exclude the poor and those likely to need prolonged care and attention. In each case the lower prices charged by one 'competitive' hospital are achieved at the expense of another, or at the expense of social equity in access to care.

'Breaking up' old state monopolies (especially the Semashko system, which like other post-1917 Bolshevik policies was stripped of its initially progressive dynamic under the stultifying years of Stalinist rule) raises the question of whether sufficient resources are available to fund the switch to a new system.

7. The low costs of the Semashko systems were based on the institutionalised low pay and exploitation of doctors and professional staff, which in turn led to a distinctive gender balance,

in which larger numbers of doctors, condemned to low pay, were women. To break down this system therefore raises the issue of paying market rates to staff. This means a huge injection of new funds is needed, in economies that have been near collapse. There is a further contradiction in the way in which an insurance-based system based on workplace contributions by employees has been introduced at the very time when most traditional workplaces have been shedding labour, and many have faced bankruptcy as a result of the wider 'liberalisation' and marketisation of the economy.

8. User fees have been among the more specific policy nostrums that have emerged at the centre of many packages of market-style reforms. However the experience from both high income and the very poorest countries shows – as we have seen – that user fees have largely failed to deliver the promised results.

- If covered by insurance, user fees do not reduce demand
- If not covered by insurance, user fees deter the poor
- Fees are clearly not related to health need, but to financial criteria and market pressures often outside the health care system and the national economy in which they operate
- In almost every instance user fees have been shown to raise little if any money, in exchange for the negative impact on equity of access for the poorest population
- The imposition of charging structures and their application involves substantial additional complexities and costs of administration and bureaucracy, none of which contributes to patient care.

9. Decentralisation, as has been shown above, is a policy which has potential progressive content, but which is too often applied in a way which negates this and raises new issues of accountability and equity. There is also an unresolved issue over how far 'decentralised' institutions genuinely exercise independence rather than simply responding to new mechanisms of central control. Moreover they create new problems in terms of monitoring and enforcement of standards of services provided.

10. Increasing the 'autonomy' of health care providers, for example, can result in even lower levels of local accountability, and can lead public sector organisations to maximise their links with private sector enterprises, with no clear evidence of public benefit (Pollock and Price 2003). In a context of generalised shortages of professional staff, enhancing the local autonomy of health care providers can increase the competition for scarce specialists – and may even serve to drive up costs for other providers or the system as a whole.

11. Time and again the rationalisation of services raises new problems in terms of equity: new hospitals and centralised services tend to follow the 'inverse care law', concentrating the most advanced services in relatively affluent areas where health needs are correspondingly lower. There are still relatively few examples that show governments or health care planners prepared genuinely to invest in new model of care designed to maximise access for the poorest and those currently excluded from existing systems.

12. And while the rhetoric of challenging the elitism and vested interests of medical professionals may strike a populist chord, it has often suited those carrying out unpopular rationalisation plans to 'buy in' the support of senior doctors and to then utilise this as a means of containing opposition.

Privatisation: who profits – who pays?

Despite the instinctive preference of neoliberal reformers for private sector coverage and care, there is little evidence that such systems can offer equity, efficiency or affordability – with the US example ever-present as a nightmare scenario.

Private medicine offers few serious attractions for countries which have already developed popular, publicly funded health care services with universal access. A major investigation of health care systems by a Canadian Senate committee concluded at the end of 2002 that:

> On the basis of the evidence from other countries... the Committee has concluded that no country in which a parallel private health care insurance and delivery system coexists with a public health care insurance scheme can serve as a model that should be adopted, without change, by Canada.
>
> Countries in which parallel private systems compete with publicly funded health care coverage exhibit a number of problems, including: risk selection and cream skimming; no reduction in waiting lists in the public sector; queue jumping; and preferential treatment (Kirby 2002:16.2).

Different levels of privatisation and involvement with the private sector have been discussed above (Chapter four) and below in various Country Studies, and only key points will be summarised briefly here, for completeness:

- Private (for-profit) hospitals in general offer only selective, non-emergency forms of treatment (cream-skimming) at relatively high costs: in many cases they rely on an ability to pass over more serious and complex treatment to publicly funded hospitals

- Privatised support services often rely for their profitability on reducing staffing levels, and cutting the levels of pay and the service conditions (including pensions) they offer their staff, compared with those in equivalent public sector jobs. Yet in labour-intensive services such cash 'savings' almost inevitably come at a price, in the form of questionable quality of work, problems of staff recruitment and retention, and difficulties for commissioners in monitoring and regulating standards of service provision

- PFI/PPP: the privatisation of the provision of capital for public sector projects serves to increase the overall cost of new hospitals and treatment facilities, while the experience of early PFI-funded hospitals suggests that increased cost has not resulted in high quality buildings from the point of view of either patients or staff

- Purchasing services from the private sector, effectively reducing the state/tax funding to the role of 'enabler', leaves no control over the day-to-day provision of services, or over their geographical location, which will tend to follow the 'inverse care law'. 'Enabling' will never be enough to guarantee equity as long as for-profit providers are required to satisfy their shareholders rather than meet wider social objectives.

A report on Latin America by PAHO, the WHO and the International Development Research Centre concludes that more than 20 years of attempted reforms in the Americas 'have failed, in large degree, to satisfy the critical twin objectives of effectiveness and equity':

> To generalise: while reforms of the past 20 years have been directed predominantly to cost efficiency and 'modernisation' in the health sector, policy outcomes too often have been characterised by worsening inequalities and social dislocation (PAHO et al 2001: Foreword).

Although individual health care reformers may believe that their proposals are geared to the needs of patients, the predominant influences shaping and driving these changes have been financial, political and ideological. Evidence which might moderate or contradict the reforms has been largely ignored by those shaping policy: in the case of the British Conservative government's market-style reforms, any scrutiny or evaluation of the effects of the new policies was actively discouraged.

Similar ideological and political pressures have moulded and distorted even those reforms which have had a potentially progressive, positive dynamic, such as decentralisation and the focus on primary care services. They have helped transform the WHO's notion of 'Health for All 2000' from a crusade for adequate levels of health care for all people in the poorest countries, into an appeal for a 'minimum package' supplemented by private medicine for the wealthy. They have transformed the $12 per person per year estimate for the cost of a minimum package of care into a *target* – yet to be achieved – for health spending in the poorest countries.

However the investigation into the role of international agencies in the transmission of policy ideas (Chapter three) helps to elucidate the process through which ideological concepts and policies lacking in supporting evidence can apparently win such wide acceptance in academic and government circles.

Once they become connected with the material power and political influence of leading governments (the USA, Britain) and leading global agencies such as the World Bank, abstract ideas begin themselves to carry material weight. Governments and policy-makers in other countries are more likely to take the policy seriously or, in the case of developing countries, feel under pressure to adopt a policy which also appears to be backed up by a body of funded research, and by teams of USAID-sponsored consultants and advisors.

By contrast, alternative approaches or views critical of the prevailing menu of reforms are unlikely to be endorsed or published by the leading governments and global bodies, unlikely to attract generous research funding, and therefore lack the influence that has been accorded to marketising reforms.

In other words the pressure for these reforms is not simply ideological. It flows from the dynamics of the wider capitalist system. The ideas of the ruling class are still, as Marx argued, the ruling ideas. Market-style reforms, as a reflection of the neoliberal ideology which since the 1980s has increasingly supplanted the post-war Keynesian/social democratic consensus, are very much the ideological product of the ruling class on a global level, even if they are not shared with similar enthusiasm by all sections of the ruling class or by all political leaders at a national level.

But just as these policies emerged from the background as a result of the crises of the 1970s and 1980s, it is possible that political and economic conditions could again marginalise the reform menu. This study has noted a few signs of a waning of enthusiasm for the reform package: it is hoped that the information collated in these pages will add weight to those arguing for a different way forward in health care reform.

In seeking an alternative, another famous Marxist phrase may offer a constructive way forward: 'From each according to his ability: to each according to his needs'. Health care planned on the basis of need rather than profit is more likely to focus resources on those who need them most – but cannot afford to pay market prices for health services.

A menu, not a blueprint

The influence of neoliberal ideology and the paradigm of market-style reform is more manifest in the high-income countries, where the largest share of resources for health care is also to be found. Indeed, in spite of the efforts of the World Bank to promote it, there is relatively little evidence that significant elements at governmental level in developing countries have genuinely 'bought in' to the same model[125]. Their own economic dependence (often following the collapse of earlier efforts to establish universal health care systems) together with pressure from the Bank and other agencies, have left little choice for developing countries but to embrace some elements of the new market-style model if loans are to be obtained and credit ratings secured.

However there remains the secondary question: do all of the world's various reform packages flow from the imposition of a single 'blueprint' for health care systems, a 'one size fits all' formula for market forces in health care?

Contrary to the initial assumptions of the author, the findings of this study suggest that the concept of a 'global blueprint' does not sufficiently correspond to the varying combination of policies that have been implemented. While some neoliberal ideologues may indeed have a theoretical 'blueprint' of the reforms they would like to see, as earlier chapters have shown, the neoliberal model has not proved politically acceptable in any country: even Pinochet's Chile pulled up a long way short of the full neoliberal policy for health care.

A more accurate analogy is that of a global 'menu' of market-driven and market-style policies, including key elements of the New Public Management. While the wealthier countries have been in a strong enough position to be able to pick and choose an 'a la carte' combination of policies tailored to the national appetite, the poorer countries have been under pressure to choose from a more limited 'prix fixe' range of options, one of which appears in almost every case to be user fees.

In defiance of the evidence

'Reform' packages generally purport to be a response to a defined complex of problems and shortcomings in a given health care system or social setting, but in practice frequently fail to address these problems at all. Perhaps the clearest example was Margaret Thatcher's market-style reforms, which were devised, and then imposed on the NHS, in an apparent response to a headline-grabbing winter crisis of waiting lists, bed shortages and cuts in services in 1987-88, arising from her government's cash limits: yet the reforms from 1989 imposed a more costly and less efficient system on the NHS, resulting in a large increase in managerial and administrative staff, while waiting lists grew and bed shortages continued.

Elsewhere despite its failures and contradictions in the richer countries there has been an instinctive search, not least through the World Bank's IFC and many other reform proposals, for ways of extending the system of private health insurance as a means of at least securing the health care of the middle and wealthy classes in low and middle income countries: yet as Sbabaro (2000) demonstrates, such policies are likely to compound inequalities, and the

---

125 With the possible exception of the ANC government in South Africa and other governments subscribing to the NEPAD project.

introduction of private health insurance actually represents a threat to the control of the WHO's ten basic diseases which should be the main priority.

On a national scale and around the world the underlying problems facing health care services include the mounting pressure on services from a rapidly increasing elderly population, the growing toll of mental illness, the ravages of HIV/AIDS, the need for concerted action to stem communicable disease in developing countries, the soaring death toll from smoking tobacco – again especially in developing countries – and the rising costs of medicines and health care equipment, as private companies seek to maximise their returns on the research and development they have chosen to carry out. Their jealous defence of profitable patents on anti-AIDS drugs has been accurately summed up as 'The darkest side of capitalism' (Achieng 2001).

Of course the levels of inequality in health are a mirror image of wider social inequality. The political premises of the health care system cannot stand higher than prevailing ideology or the level of material wealth in society. While some progressive reforms could be secured, a full-scale, enduring solution to health inequality is impossible in the face of a capitalist system that continually generates inequalities alongside wealth and profits.

Yet few, if any, of these problems are addressed by the imposition of market-style reforms, new funding mechanisms, or the granting of greater 'autonomy' to local providers that are then required to work as if they are commercial businesses.

These reforms are not only driving in the wrong direction: they are generally driven by the wrong concerns – and as a result yielding unwelcome and unhelpful results.

Toolkit 1: Testing the content of a health policy in context

In the course of the reading for this study it has become increasingly apparent that some of the language, and especially the terminology, that is used in discussing the various reforms proposals and the motivation for them can be profoundly ambiguous. Some 'reform' proposals, far from embracing an agenda of equity and progressive change, seek to dress up market-driven cost-cutting reforms, or market-style experiments, in language which is designed to defuse opposition.

Documents setting out national and regional policy proposals for the reform of health care systems are likely to contain a variety of potentially misleading and ambiguous terminology, catch-phrases, and formulations – language which may in some instances lead in a progressive direction, but in others back towards neoliberalism, inequality and costly market-style systems.

A focus on 'Primary care', for example, may imply either of the following:

- A courageous commitment to the progressive 'Health for All' ideals of the WHO's 1978 Alma Ata declaration, and a fight to expand and improve the infrastructure of health care for the very poorest and most isolated

- Little more than a fig-leaf covering a policy of withdrawing government support for publicly funded hospital services, and the consolidation of a 'World Bank-style' two-tier system, in which hospital care is available only to those with money for private treatment.

Since the terms are themselves ambiguous, and used not only by organisations and institutions happy to conceal their principal purpose, but also by those who are genuinely concerned with equity and universal access to care, it is only possible to gauge the significance of a given term in the specific context in which it appears.

A number of key questions can help determine the overall framework and approach of the document or paper in which potentially misleading phrases and terms appear. These questions seek out the factors that distinguish between positive proposals which are serious attempts to remedy clearly identified problems of equity and access, accountability and affordability, and those which are simply a window dressing of empty promises to disguise a neoliberal reform or a package of spending cuts dressed up as a restructuring or rationalisation of services.

The following table, drawn from experience in research for this study and the author's 20 years involved in analysing official health service documents in the UK, seeks to identify the hallmarks that distinguish a proposal for progressive reform from a rhetorical device intended to obscure an essentially unpopular proposal in the populist language of equity.

Table 6: Toolkit 1

Characteristics of plans centred on market-driven or market-style reforms	Elements that should be visible in a progressive reform agenda
Finance-driven (either by global cash constraints on health care at national level, a structural adjustment programme, or in response to price competition/market pressures)	Patient or service-driven changes
New policy centred on propositions drawn from neoliberal ideology (for example: arguing in support of the 'efficiencies' of market systems, private sector involvement or competition)	Recognises and where necessary addresses the underlying social inequalities and environmental issues that determine ill health
Policies presented without supporting evidence of success	Evidence-based policy
Policy flows from pressures and requirements outside of health care: not related to local needs	Clearly located in the current context of the appropriate national and local demographic trends and/or changing profile of hospital caseload (reduced need for surgical inpatient beds often running alongside increased requirement for emergency medical beds)
If the policy is being copied from other governments, health care systems and providers or other organisations abroad, is this change being made...	
...**under pressure** to create public-private partnership? or **under instruction**, as a condition of World Bank/IMF support?	...**voluntarily**, on the government's own initiative?
Proposals remain unspecific, with no costings of revenue or capital required	Policy and its implementation are convincingly costed, with full implications for capital investment and so on
No identified source of funding: will promised developments ever be completed?	Sufficient financial resources (capital and revenue) have been identified and allocated for the implementation of the policy
Funding has been allocated only on a short-term basis	Funding has been allocated on a long-term basis

Evasive discussion of human resource issues, or unwarranted assumptions	Sufficient human resources are in place, or training needs have been identified and incorporated into the policy proposal
Plan involves improbably quick decision-making (ultimatum) or gives no projection of future timetable	Plan includes a practicable timetable for implementation, with milestones and stages at which evaluation can take place
No identified structure of accountability	Responsible individuals, institutions or organisations are identified as accountable for implementation, with a mechanism to review and address any shortcomings
Policy being imposed by government against the express opposition of most health care professionals and their organisations, concerned over quality and accessibility of patient care	The reform addresses serious longstanding weaknesses such as: • Elitist professional power • Unequal access to care • Gaps in service provision
Where services are being restructured and reorganised, how do the new arrangements compare with the existing arrangements?	
User fees/co-payments being introduced	Levels of service/numbers of patients at least maintained or expanded
Services reduced, 'rationalised', 'centralised' or 'downsized'	

Toolkit 2: Alternative readings - the language of reforms

The overview of the policy above also suggests ways in which some of the more ambiguous terminology of health care reform, which sometimes appears deliberately misleading, should be interpreted. Policy proposals using terminology with a strong progressive dynamic and appeal can in this way result in practical reforms which head in a very different direction.

As a guide to further policy analysis, some of the more common terms used in the literature of reform have been tabulated, and referenced with examples, to show how they have been used in both their overt positive and less obvious potentially negative implications in published material.

Table 7: Toolkit 2

Common terminology: 1. Public Health	
Positive meaning	**Negative implications**
Combination of social and health care measures to reduce burden of illness, dating back to 19th century social reformers. Embraced by WHO (HFA 2000) and by other progressive reformers as an adjunct to improved health care services (Black 1980, Jarman 1993). Combined with primary care (below), free care for all, training of doctors and development of hospital system, public health has been the key to dramatic health gains in Cuba since 1959 (WHO 1998, World Bank 2003b).	Endorsed by conservatives and neoliberals as measures to curb state spending on health care and force responsibility onto individuals and their families (Baggott 2000, Farrant 1991, Whitehead 1992, Francome & Marks 1996). Central to 'essential package' underlying 'World Bank model' of health care, involving minimal public spending on hospital and specialist care in poorest countries – restricting such services to the private sector (World Bank 1993).

Common terminology: 2. 'Primary care-led' services or Primary Health Care (PHC)	
Positive meaning	**Negative implications**
Improve infrastructure of primary health care to ensure poor have access at most local level to basic services that can help maximise levels of immunisation, reduce infant mortality and (in conjunction with hospital network) ensure treatment of communicable disease and more complex illness (Tudor Hart 1994). Seen by WHO and primary care practitioners as cost-effective means to achieve HFA 2000 targets in poorer countries (Mahler 1981, Lee & Goodman 2002). The viability of the claim that improved primary care can reduce demand for hospital treatment, or substitute for hospital care has been challenged (Holland 2000). Coulter (1998) has warned that in established health services improved primary care may in practice *increase* the pressure on hospitals as a result of more effectively monitoring the health problems of local population. Good new primary care services may be more popular with patients – but more expensive than previous services (Green & Thorogood 1998).	Seen as cheaper alternative to comprehensive health care in developing countries – thus consolidating global two-tier system (World Bank WDR 1993) though available resources have lagged far behind provision of even primary care services (De Ferranti 1985). Scaled-down concept of 'selective primary health care' emerged as WHO retreated from HFA and inclusive concept of PHC (Farrant 1991). PHC has been seen as a low-budget substitute for hospital services in developed countries (Wall & Owen 2002:133). In Britain, primary care has been used as lever to weaken power of hospitals (Robinson & LeGrand 1993) even though the promised additional resources have not been transferred to GPs (Craig et al 2002). In the USA family physicians are used by HMOs as 'gatekeepers' to restrict access to more costly hospital care (Kleinke 2001, Waitzkin 2001).

Common terminology: 3. Partnership	
Positive meaning	**Negative implications**
Counterposed by some politicians of the 'third way' and social democracy as an alternative to the purchaser/provider split within public sector	Since the distinction between public and private sector is obscured by this approach, 'partnerships' can also involve linking the public sector with

health care (Robinson 2002).

The notion of getting all interested parties to work together for a common cause – at local, national or even international level – has a genuine appeal (Brundtland 1998, 2001a, Buse and Walt 2000a, Buse and Waxman 2001).

In Britain the long-term reform of the Byzantine complexities of the NHS pay structure has led to the development of a new 'Agenda for Change' which proclaims itself as a 'Partnership' between trade unions and management (DoH 2003d) though the extent of the common ground that can be found in implementing the cash limited restructuring has yet to be demonstrated. Most 'partnerships' concentrate on the consumer end of the health care system, seeking closer links at management level between purchasing agencies and providers, or between provider management and service users – commonly to the exclusion of the front-line staff who deliver the care (Lister 1999).

private sector 'partners', whether through 'Public Private Partnerships' or the Private Finance Initiative, or the purchase by the public sector of services from private sector providers (Lister 2001).

The World Health Organisation has attempted to develop 'partnerships' with pharmaceutical corporations in 'Global Public Private Partnerships', but critics have warned that the drug companies' involvement is motivated by self-interest and profit rather than partnership, and the consequences for patients and service users may be negative (HAI 2001, Schreuder and Kostermans 2001, Schulz-Asche 2000, Hardon 2000).

Heaton (2001) raises similar criticisms of what she terms 'Joint Public Private Initiatives' (JPPIs) from the standpoint of children in the poorest developing countries. The value of 'donated' drugs is often a tiny fraction of the cost of developing a system to administer them, while subsequent supplies will often have also to be purchased by the government concerned.

In Britain there have been frequent attempts to focus on 'partnership' working between health care and other public services, or between health care providers and service users, or between health care managers and front-line health care staff. Various such top-down 'partnerships' ('labour-management', 'community-government') are incorporated into versions of the New Public Management (Osborne and Plastrick 1997).

Common terminology: 4. Equity

Positive meaning	Negative implications
'The absence of potentially remediable, systematic differences in one or more aspects of health across socially, economically, demographically or geographically defined population groups…' (International Society of Equity in Health (ISEqH), in Macinko & Starfield 2002:1).	Health economists working for the WHO have devised a formula which argues that 'fairness' in financial contribution to health can be judged by assessing at the household level, and that a fair contribution is one which consumes the same percentage of non-food spending – regardless of the total household income (Murray 2000).
Serious action to tackle inequalities has to involve policies to reduce poverty and income inequality (Shaw et al 1999, Allen 2000). This runs counter to neoliberal views, and requires major political intervention which faces opposition from the most powerful interest groups (Liu 2000).	Since 2000 the WHO has also adopted the 'new universalism' – in other words, selectivism in place of universalism – which critics argue focuses on delivering a 'basic package' to the poor rather than a comprehensive service (Ollila & Koivasalu 2002). This links with the USAID notion of 'equity for the poor', which means in practice that the poor continue to receive less than everyone who is not poor (Knowles et al 1997).
Gonzalez-Block (2004) notes that out of a wide range of papers and projects on low and middle income countries conducted by 176 institutions between 2000 and 2002, studies focused on	The World Bank and many of its sponsored

equity were among the least frequent of 19 different categories and topics.

researchers have defended the imposition of user fees for health care as a means to ensure greater equity by deterring the wealthy from using public services, channelling them towards the private sector, and as a result 'freeing' more resources to treat the poor (Shaw & Ainsworth 1995:153, Leighton 1995:14). This disregards the common view that services exclusively for the poor tend to be poor services: Equinet (2000) warns that the liberalised growth of private care is *widening* the health gap between rich and poor.

Murray et al (2000) point to the imbalance in choice between rich and poor. And though 31 African countries were imposing user fees by 1997, only four of these claimed that 'equity' was an objective (Leighton & Wouters 1995, Russell & Gilson 1997).

The dangers of seeking to elide equity with efficiency are pointed out by several authors, who stress that efficiency tends to mean spending most on treating those most likely to benefit – primarily the rich – while equity should mean ensuring equal access to treatment (Marmot 2001, Defever 1995).

Scott (2001:150) argues that 'It is often more cost-effective to deliver marginal health gains to those with good rather than poor health status'.

Common terminology: 5. Decentralisation

Positive meaning	Negative implications
Decentralisation – the call for greater local control over and accountability of health care services to the communities they serve is a continuing theme running through many varieties of health system reform (Rannan-Eliya 1996, Valentine 1998).	Decentralisation was also one of the hotch-potch of pro-market policies that have been bracketed under the general label of 'New Public Management' (Hood 1991, Osborne & Gaebler 1992, Osborne & Plastrik 1997, Pollitt 2000).
Decentralisation was also embraced as a progressive goal by the WHO and its Health For All 2000 programme.	Advocates of hospital autonomy making explicit reference to NPM include Preker and Harding (2000, 2003), although Bach (2000) identifies the potential problems of 'extreme forms of decentralisation', including the establishment of autonomous hospitals and competing local providers. These can result in duplication of effort, wasted resources and high transaction costs.
However Mills and colleagues (2001) warn that decentralisation raises difficult questions over the capacity of management at local level, and Manning (2000) warns that if decentralisation results in privatisation there is a danger that what he describes as 'old public disciplines' will cease to apply.	
Bale and Dale (1998) also offer a reminder of the positive values that can be sustained within a centralised bureaucracy, but which may not be replicated in management if control is decentralised. Deeming (2001) analysing British reforms since 1997 notes the potential conflict	More local control can obstruct national-level planning and restrict the development of career options that could attract and retain qualified staff (Bach 2000). Busse et al (2002) argue that hospital autonomy can be a stepping stone to privatisation, while Manning (2000) notes that the successes of hospital autonomy in developing countries have been more predicted than found.

between decentralisation and equity between local districts.	Bossert (2000:3) argues that though decentralisation has been 'touted' by the World Bank throughout much of the 1990s, 'the preliminary data from the field indicate that the results have been mixed, at best'. It has 'often been criticised for increasing inequalities', and may have 'disrupted effective vertical immunization and family planning programs' (11). 'We have found little clear evidence of major impacts – either positive or negative' (14). In some cases the results have led to a backlash of re-centralisation.
	Hutchinson and LaFond (2004) in a survey of the literature on decentralisation in developing countries point out that the impact of such policies on more equitable distribution of resources and of better targeting of resources to the poor has been 'mixed': 'In the absence of well-functioning redistributive mechanisms, decentralisation can exacerbate existing differences' (2004:16).
	Neoliberals see the logical conclusion of decentralisation as privatisation. Others may concur from a different standpoint, so for example Gilson (1997) includes privatisation as a fourth category of decentralisation, echoed by Sein (2001).
	Collins and Green (1994) strongly disagree, arguing that privatisation goes beyond decentralisation by effectively removing control from the public sector.

Common terminology: 6. Efficiency

Positive meaning	Negative implications
'Efficiency' can be seen as the most effective use of available resources to meet health needs: in principle in many European countries it could be measured from the standpoint of the patient, who is concerned with treatment rather than price.	Proponents of user fees for health care frequently argue that it helps promote 'efficiency' (Shaw 1995).
	The World Bank (1997:7) proclaims its commitment to 'raising efficiency in the use of scarce resources'. But like other neoliberal and pro-market reformers it assumes a superior 'efficiency' can be found only in the private sector, and that the key to improving public sector efficiency is measures that replicate the competition and incentives of the private sector (Robinson 2002).
In such a context efficiency would be a measure of the most effective, speedy and sympathetic system for delivering treatment – or, in developing countries, one which increases the probability that anyone with a communicable disease seeks and receives treatment (Creese and Kutzin 1995).	
However in most capitalist systems the use of the term efficiency carries the strong connotation of cost-efficiency ('whether healthcare resources are being used to get the best value for money' (Palmer and Torgerson 1999)).	However Dunlop and Martins, weighing up the evidence for the Bank (1996:196), note that 'market mechanisms will not ensure either equity or economic efficiency, because of the characteristics of the health care market on both the supply and the demand side, which suggest

Efficiency is also an objective which in principle nobody would want to argue against: the opposite is almost indefensible in argument. 'Inefficiency is akin to a torn rice sack. If the holes are not identified and sealed/mended, it would be impossible to fill the sack' (Kirigia et al 2002).

However while the principle may be unexceptionable, the practical conclusions of the quest for efficiency may be more open to doubt.

'Efficiency' is sometimes used interchangeably with 'performance', although a debate continues over how widely or narrowly it should be applied. The 'narrow' view concentrates on the operation of the health system itself, while the wider view includes other measures and programmes (such a smoking cessation) which can make a longer-term contribution to the health of the population, and thus make health care more 'efficient' (PAHO 2001b, 2001c).

Explanations of inefficiencies also have to make reference to such issues as sufficient and timely availability of cash and other practical resources: poor utilisation of operating theatres, for example may be due to poor management and systems, awkward medical and professional staff, or a variety of shortages of support staff, equipment, drugs, anaesthetics, prostheses, ITU facilities, or beds elsewhere in the hospital (Owino and Korir 1997, Kirigia et al 2002, Kmietowicz 2003).

While technical efficiency seeks the minimal application of capital and labour to deliver the required health outcome, allocative efficiency seeks the optimal distribution of resources to deliver equitable outcomes within society (Palmer and Torgerson 1999). However the health care reform process around the world has placed a higher emphasis on technical than allocative efficiency or equity (Leon, Walt and Gilson 2001).

the presence of market failure conditions.'

As a result the reforms have not gone as expected by their proponents. A PAHO study concludes: 'To generalise: while reforms of the past 20 years have been directed predominantly to cost efficiency and "modernisation" in the health sector, policy outcomes too often have been characterised by worsening inequalities and social dislocation' (PAHO et al 2001: Foreword).

The general bias of health system reform towards greater involvement of the private sector in service provision can also be seen to mitigate against any improvement in cost-efficiency when the full costs of private care are taken into consideration: in the US, as in many other countries, for-profit hospitals tend to be significantly more expensive, and incur much higher administrative costs than their non-profit counterparts (Relman 2002).

The assumption that the private sector is unerringly 'efficient' compared with publicly provided health care is challenged by Brandon et al (1991) and others who have exposed the huge bureaucratic overhead costs of the US health care system – compared with the much lower costs of administering Medicare and Medicaid.

The World Bank's favoured formula of imposing user fees is also questionable from an efficiency point of view, given the small amounts of money raised, and assessments of the results have been skewed by omitting the costs of collecting the fees and administering the system (Creese and Kutzin 1995).

Elsewhere Diderichson (1995) warns that some of the measures to increase productivity and efficiency in Sweden's health care through user fees and the purchaser/provider split 'threaten equity in some specific respects'.

Measuring efficiency gains in health care can in itself be extremely complex, and require intensive allocation of management time and resources. Smith (2002:104) argues that despite the steep increase in administrative costs, the market-style reforms in Britain under the Thatcher government had 'little measurable impact on performance, whether defined in terms of volume, quality or unit costs'. He goes on to question whether it is possible to performance-manage the British NHS while cutting management costs.

Harvey (2001) argues that 'any meaningful analytical activity is inevitably hugely expensive'.

Hurst and Jee-Hughes (2001:17) note the

	abandonment by the British government of its controversial 'efficiency index' developed in the 1990s amid fears that 'quality was being sacrificed in the pursuit of quantity' and that the productivity measures themselves were being manipulated through 'gaming'.

Common terminology: 7. Sustainability

Positive meaning	Negative implications
Ensuring that health care (or other) systems can meet the needs of the present without compromising the ability to meet future needs.

In the context of the wealthier countries, 'sustainability' is most often discussed in terms of political support, and the political commitment to sustain a level of spending or new method of organising or managing health care in the context of established public expectations. In this sense Berman and Bossert (2000:3) can argue that 'the ambitious "managed competition" reforms of the Netherlands were not sustainable'.

However the political acceptability (or otherwise) of reform is the result of a political and economic context: the balance between social classes can be key to the affordability and the 'universal solidarity' which delivers political support for welfare state provision (Diderichsen 1995).

Similar problems can also arise in the introduction of 'targeting' of subsidies and free care to the poor in developing countries: 'Often the administrative costs of targeting are high, and the exclusion of wealthy and middle income groups can erode political support for the essential package' (World Bank 1993:118).

However even in wealthy countries the cost of publicly funded health care can rise to a level at which political opposition grows and as in Canada the question can be raised as to whether or not such a system is sustainable in resource terms (Romanow 2002).

The question is most aggressively raised by those ideologically opposed to public provision, and most uncompromisingly answered by those opposed to private for-profit medicine, who point out that if a public system cannot be afforded, a private system would be even more expensive (Deber 2000a, 200b).

In developing countries 'sustainability' is more likely to be viewed from the standpoint of the availability of revenue, capital, human resources and technical skills at the level of management or service delivery (Berman and Bossert 2000). | 'Sustainability' can be used as a euphemism for affordability, and as part of the pressure on poorer developing countries to restrict their public infrastructure of health care to the most basic World bank-style package. However the Bank itself has not got a good record on sustainable projects: its 1997 HNP strategy paper admitted that only 17% of completed Bank projects contributed substantially to local institutions, and only 44% were sustainable (World Bank 1997).

It is equally central to the argument for the imposition of user fees, and expansion of private sector provision, especially in sub-Saharan Africa: 'Raising revenues through cost recovery, with the primary goal of improving financial sustainability of health care systems, has been the focal point of financing reform in Africa' (Leighton 1995:Topic 2). Leighton also insists (Q4) that 'Willingness to pay should no longer be an issue for health care financing reform in sub-Saharan Africa,' and that user fees can ('theoretically') 'raise enough revenue to make a difference for financial sustainability in countries where most people are poor' (Q6).

Pharmaceutical companies may view the 'sustainability' of programmes based on donated drugs – such as that involving the anti-malarial drug Malarone® – in terms of the commercial sustainability of the donation, rather than the longer-term sustainability of the country's malaria control strategy (Heaton 2001:9, 11).

Khalegian (2001) reviewing the literature on immunisation projects also highlight questions over the sustainability of projects involving user fees, which deter participation by the poorest. |

Bossert and Berman (2000:2) also distinguish between reforms as 'sustained, purposeful and fundamental change' and one-off, temporary adjustments without the full political support of the policy-makers.

In many cases, donor-led pressure to develop selective areas of treatment targeted at particular groups in developing countries can make it more difficult to develop a coherent and sustained programme giving long-term access to health care (Heaton 2001).

Common terminology: 8. Accessibility

Positive meaning

'The presence or absence of physical, economic or cultural barriers that people might face in using health services' (PHR 2000c:1).

Physical barriers may include distance from suitable facilities, or restrictions on the supply of services – although discrimination on various grounds including age, sex and sexuality may also be a factor.

'Principles for health reform include universal access to essential health services, solidarity, and pluralism to allow individuals a choice of various service options. Thus the objectives of health reform are equity of access, quality of services, efficiency, and acceptability to consumers' (Bennett et al 1997:4).

Negative implications

Economic barriers in general involve the cost of seeking and obtaining health care and medicines, in relation to household income. Since at least 99% of the population in 24 of the richest 29 OECD countries were covered by health insurance (Anderson and Hussey 2001), the bulk of those facing the largest economic barriers to health care are in poorer developing countries.

The big exception is the US, where over 40 million lack insurance cover, and many more are under-insured: a 2001 study found half of all Americans miss out on some of the most important preventive services (Charatan 2001). An Abt survey found that one in four adult Americans had failed to go for a test, obtain prescribed drugs or see a doctor because they could not afford it (Abt 1999a).

However, co-payments for prescriptions or hospital treatment in wealthier countries with health insurance schemes may serve to exclude sections of the low-paid. In developing countries the user fees imposed even as part of reforms professing to promote wider 'access' can result in fewer people using services. A survey of user fee schemes in Africa, Asia and Latin America found that many did not include policies to promote health service access for disadvantaged groups (Russell and Gilson 1997).

Part II

Chapter six

Country summaries: Europe and Russia

Introduction

The four chapters of Part II (Chapters 6-9) take the concepts and policies discussed in earlier sections of this study and explore the extent to which the most common reforms can be seen to have been applied in various countries around the world – and the results they have achieved.

Inevitably this process has been subject to one overriding limitation: the uneven availability of suitable documentary information to enable a full analysis to be made of some countries. Indeed some whole continents, most notably Asia, have been much harder to research than others where international agencies have been more involved, and a greater degree of academic interest has focused.

However this is not a problem which is unique to this study: even global organisations such as the World Health Organisation have found their access to detailed information on some countries and regions of the world has been limited, and the overview reports on Latin American countries compiled in PAHO's *Health in the Americas* series contain widely varying amounts of information on the health care systems and reforms implemented from one country to the next (WHO 2000, PAHO 1998, 2002).

Having explored the basic 'menu' of market-driven and market-style reforms, and the main international agencies transmitting these policy ideas around the world, these chapters will introduce the concept of the 'country summary' – and then use this form to examine the extent to which there is evidence in the literature showing that the reforms outlined have been introduced or attempted in a number of countries.

The uneven availability of detailed literature and up-to-date information on many parts of the world has been discussed as an underlying problem facing this study. But even if much more comprehensive information were available, this study would not have the space to develop a fully detailed 'case study' exploring the health care system of each of the countries that will be reviewed: indeed in a large number of European countries, and to a lesser extent in Latin America, such detailed studies have already been undertaken elsewhere[126], though often lacking any wider comparative context.

---

126 Notably the WHO European Observatory's *Health in Transition* series, and PAHO's regular *Health in the Americas* surveys.

A recent OECD comparative survey of the experience of health care reforms also reports on the gaps in data which prevent any complete comparison (Docteur and Oxley 2003) and of course (as discussed in earlier chapters) the WHO has faced considerable problems accessing comprehensive data for its comparative 'league tables' (WHR2000).

Nevertheless, there is a substantial body of information now available on the processes of health sector reform and their consequences in many advanced and developing countries, and it is part of the purpose of this study to analyse the processes at work in the wider whole, rather than simply to focus on the constituent parts. The country summaries that follow do not therefore seek directly to compare health care systems, or to outline a complete history of their introduction, but to identify and summarise the pressures each system has faced, and compare the reforms and changes that have been implemented, and the effects achieved by those reforms.

Adopting a comparative framework

1 The advanced industrialised economies: four models

There are a number of different possible frameworks for comparative studies of health care system reforms. Some analysts have sought to define welfare states in terms of a relatively few similar 'groups' or 'regimes' (notably Titmuss 1974, Esping-Andersen 1990 and 1996, Castles and Mitchell 1991). Health care systems, too, especially in the more developed economies have most commonly been divided into three basic 'types', most often defined by their predominant method of finance and organisation: the 'Bismarck' (decentralised, social insurance), 'Beveridge' (centralised, tax-funded), and private (largely US) models (Ranade 1998:2). A further, fourth variety identified by Ranade was the 'Semashko' (highly centralised, state-funded) system which predominated in the Soviet Union from the 1920s and much of Eastern Europe from 1945-1989.

However there are other variants in the categorisation of health systems: the European Health Management Association identifies a 'mixed' type (combining elements of Bismarck and Beveridge systems) among certain EU countries[127] (EHMA 2000). The British Conservative Party employs a four-way division of health systems in its comparative study of 20 countries: these are again divided on the basis of the source of funding, with the groups comprising: Social Insurance, Mixed Finance (including the USA), Local Tax financed, and Central Tax financed (Williams 2002). Hsiao (2000) adds a further category by including the Singapore system, which is based on Medical Savings Accounts, a policy increasingly advocated in recent years by neoliberals in the US (Jensen 2000).

The OECD (1992) identified no less than seven variant systems, differentiated by the flow of patients, the flow of money and the relationships of authority, giving different levels of private market freedoms and public sector control.

However the most significant distinction in the context of global analysis is that between predominantly tax-funded systems (which, under conditions of progressive taxation, draw in contributions from – and therefore pool risk between – all sections of society, whether wage-earning, salaried, share-owning or proprietors) and systems based on social insurance, which tend disproportionately to levy contributions from – and give preferential coverage to –

127 Italy, Greece, Portugal, France and Ireland.

workers employed in the formal sectors of the economy[128].

While recognising that many 'public' health care systems incorporate a substantial and growing element of private health provision and insurance, the country summaries will refer to the four basic types described by Ranade (1998) – the Beveridge, Bismarck, ex-Semashko and private (US) systems.

2 Health systems in developing countries: a fifth model?

Each of the established comparative approaches outlined above is focused on the relatively well-developed systems in the wealthier and more advanced economies. While there are more or less rudimentary social insurance systems in place in several middle-income Latin American countries (PAHO 2002), none of the four standard categories outlined above really fits the health care systems in the poorest developing countries.

The prerequisite for the development of welfare state provision in the wealthier countries after the Second World War was not only the right political conjuncture, but also the economic strength and stability to allow such a large-scale social investment. The starting point for health system reform has been very different in the middle-income and less developed countries. The poorer countries have had less economic stability than the high-income countries, and suffered greater pressures from the world market, not least in servicing a mountain of debts to the industrialised countries. This has meant that the establishment of even limited welfare state provision and publicly funded health care has been the exception rather than the rule.

Doyal (1979) has outlined the early evolution of health care systems in a number of colonially ruled countries, and the resulting inequalities and gaps in care at the time these countries achieved independence. Many of the nationalist political parties which led the fight for independence were committed to establish affordable or free health care for their people, and in many countries in sub-Saharan Africa, health care systems involving public funding or provision were established on an ambitious basis soon after independence was achieved. Many of these schemes were able to survive in the early years of economic expansion, but had to be scaled down in the 1980s as a result of the impact of recession in the developed economies, rising debts, and Structural Adjustment Programmes imposed by the World Bank and IMF (Berman and Bossert 2000).

The social insurance system that has developed in many 'middle-income' countries covers such a small section of the population, with the living standards of the remaining population so low, that the system is very different from the modern 'Bismarck' model[129]. The majority of the world's health care systems, in the poorer countries of Africa, Asia, and parts of Latin America and the Caribbean fall even further outside the customary 'ideal types' of comparative analysis – so far outside as to require a new designation of their own. Not only did many of the poorest countries' health care systems start at a very different level and a different historical period from those in the advanced capitalist economies, but they face quite distinctive social issues, political conjuncture, resource problems, and a very different disease burden (Doyal 1979, Turschen 1999, Garrett 2001).

128 This distinction is of even greater importance in low- and middle-income countries, where formal sector employment involves a relatively small segment of the working population – see in particular the current case of Kenya.

129 The World Bank definition of 'middle-income' has a lower level of average income slightly above US$2 per day, leaving little possibility of comprehensive social or widespread individual insurance.

Almost nobody is seeking to transfer lessons from these rudimentary and under-resourced health systems to the wealthier countries: and the governments in poorer countries have been specifically urged by the World Bank and WHO *not* to aspire to the more sophisticated and expensive systems they see elsewhere (World Bank 1993).

Features of a 'World Bank' model

This study tests out the idea of a new, *fifth* 'model' of health care system, a 'World Bank model' constructed around the policies prescribed in the Bank's 1993 *World Development Report* (WDR1993), and visible in many poorer countries. These policies, if carried through, lead towards a distinctive model of health care, which is being forced upon poorer countries through the efforts of donors and global organisations. This new 'model' would result in a health care system:

- Constrained by the poverty and indebtedness of the national economy, and as a result not seeking to deliver comprehensive health services, but merely to ensure a minimal publicly funded primary health care and immunisation service for the poor

- Aiming to provide the Bank's 'essential package' of preventive and primary health care services, costed at $12 per head per year

- Focusing resources almost exclusively on primary care, and confining any public sector hospital provision to the 'safety' net services set out in WDR1993

- Imposing user fees for all treatment in public sector health facilities

- Encouraging the private sector to offer more advanced hospital and other services to the wealthy

- Decentralised, in the hopes of weakening the power of mainly urban elites and strengthening provision through local health centres.

Whether or not it is possible to bracket together the health care systems in such a wide variety of different low- and middle-income countries in a single 'fifth model', it should be clear from this brief analysis that they do not fit the standard models developed in conventional comparative literature. A starting point for the chapters to follow is therefore to widen the conventional frame of comparison, to show the social, historical, political, economic, demographic, geographical and epidemiological context in which market-style and market-driven reforms – largely fashioned in the wealthier countries – have been introduced in the poorest as well as the wealthier countries, and the impact they have had on services and patients.

Overview

The results of the research that was carried out for the Country Summaries, covering a total of 42 countries, have been summarised in table form as Figure 3 opposite. Three overall conclusions are immediately apparent:

- The agenda of reforms as discussed in Chapter four is very far from a universal blueprint – and very much more akin to a *menu*, from which most high income countries have picked policies which have seemed politically feasible and most appropriate to their circumstances. Market-style reforms may be envisaged by their most eager proponents as a 'one size fits all' package of measures (Whitehead et al 2001) – but they have not been applied in this way by any country.

Figure 3: A summary of results from 40 country studies

Advanced industrialised countries

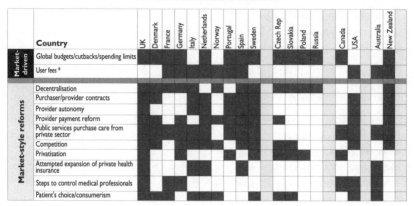

Developing and middle income countries

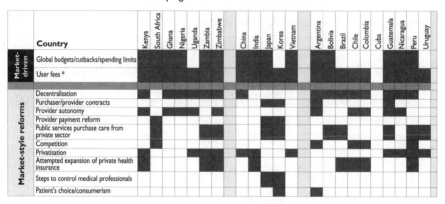

* Fees for treatment and services other than co-payments for prescription drugs, and fees for dentistry and spectacles, which are nearly universal.

- The paradigm for health care systems identified in Chapter four as a possible 'fifth, World Bank model', can only really be applied in its most basic form to the very poorest countries, which do not yet have any developed health care service.

- While most have been pressed into adopting user fees and limiting public spending, few of the poorest countries have been able to contemplate the costs and complexities of more elaborate market-style reforms, which require larger numbers of health care providers (competition, purchasing from private sector and patient choice) skilled managers and administrators (provider payment reform, decentralisation and provider autonomy), or a private sector insurance sector – which cannot function on the base of a largely impoverished population.

Even steps to control medical professionals require a firm political base, and political determination on the part of governments – factors that have generally been lacking in poor countries with real shortages of doctors and nurses.

Another feature that may come as a surprise is the relatively limited extent to which the market-style reform process has been carried through so far in Russia and Eastern Europe – although the information on Russia in particular is relatively sparse and nowhere near as up to date as other country summaries.

Fifteen years after the fall of the Berlin Wall it appears that many of the initial experiments with privatisation and with competition between insurance funds in the Czech Republic and Slovakia have served as warnings and deterrents to others, while elsewhere the inertia factor of a low-spending hospital-led system, delivering care on a tax-funded basis, has not been overcome by any zeal to establish a new health care market.

In Western Europe, however, the missionary fervour of successive British governments embarking with barely an interruption on 16 years of largely experimental market-style reforms continues to set a pace which – with the possible exception of Portugal – most other countries appear reluctant to follow.

Sweden's recent retreat from privatisation and the Spanish government's abandonment of the foundation hospital policy before its recent defeat in the 2004 general election suggest a diminishing rather than growing appetite to travel further down the road to market-style policies.

Europe's big spenders, France and Germany, both trapped in a system that has historically separated purchaser from provider, and carried the cost in the form of heavy administrative overheads, have both been seeking ways to contain health care budgets through new user fees, plus a French attempt at what has traditionally been seen as British-style rationalisation.

In summary, the problem with the neoliberal approach is that it is both unpopular *and* unsuccessful. So while the 'menu' of market-style policies has been developed by reformers, and promoted by international agencies, there appears to be a dwindling number of customers for the fare on offer.

Selection of countries

One of the findings of the study as a whole is that while the advocates of health system reforms may have been working to an ideal blueprint of marketising change (Williamson 2000, Whitehead et al 2001), the implementation in the real world has not matched the theory. Many countries have discussed and debated the full menu of market-style reforms, but none so far has implemented all of the policy options: some, even though they may have carried through market-driven reforms, have implemented hardly any market-style measures. Others (most notably New Zealand) have implemented market-style measures, only to reverse them at a later stage.

For these reasons, the common basic design of examining each country under a standard set of headings has had to be varied to match the reality of the country concerned. In some cases, the uneven availability of information has made a generalised format almost impossible to apply, and such summaries are therefore written up as additional short reports without sub-headings.

Detailed and up-to-date information on the development of ex-Semashko systems in Eastern Europe has been relatively hard to obtain, and the summaries on these countries are necessarily shorter and less up to the minute than many others. In Russia, despite the evidence of pressing need for reform, it appears that few substantial reforms of any sort have yet been implemented.

Investigation into the 'World Bank model' revealed very different problems in various developing countries. In the 'middle-income' countries with relatively well-established health care systems and rudimentary systems of social insurance for at least a minority of better-paid workers, there are issues relating to the emergence of a powerful private sector: in the poorest countries there is a general lack of even the most basic infrastructure of a health care system.

As a result it seemed appropriate to include a larger range of examples of countries that might be expected to conform to the 'World Bank model'[130], incorporating more extended studies of two sub-Saharan African countries along with some shorter summaries of other African countries, and a number of (generally shorter) summaries from Latin America to facilitate contrast and comparison, including two 'middle-income' countries, and Nicaragua, one of the poorest countries in the region, where the early health gains of the Sandinista revolution have been rolled back by years of neoliberal market-style policies.

Both Australia and New Zealand have pioneered different styles of health care reform, each with important lessons and warnings for any other countries contemplating similar lines of action, and both countries have therefore been included in the country summaries.

In Asia the process of World Bank-led reform has been more limited: the Indian system is unique in its massive reliance upon the private sector, and the resulting inequality and general absence of progressive reform. Japan and Korea have each developed their own idiosyncratic version of a Bismarck-style social insurance system – provider-driven doctor-dominated, over-bedded and riven with contradictions.

Two other key countries however have embarked upon market-style reform – with disastrous consequences for the health of their population, especially those in rural areas. The large-scale privatisation of health care in China has been largely carried through as a policy decision of a privatising Stalinist bureaucracy in Beijing, moving towards its own unique style of 'market socialism': only the deregulation and privatisation in Vietnam can be directly attributed to any intervention by the IMF and the World Bank.

---

130 These investigations show that the 'World Bank model' in its most basic form can only really be applied to the very poorest countries, which do not yet have any developed health care service. For countries like South Africa, Chile and Argentina where the technology and culture of an advanced health care service has already been established, there is no real prospect of winding back the clock to a system restricted to primary care and immunisation. The prospect in these countries is of a two-tier system based on an increasing privatisation of insurance and of hospital care, and the exclusion of the poor from all but the most basic services.

Finally, as a study of market-driven and market-style policies and their impact on health care, it seemed appropriate to include in the Latin American section the only example of a health care system that has flouted all of the rules of market-driven and market-style reform – yet delivered by what most observers regard as high quality results in terms of equity, access and health gain: Cuba. The publication of the World Bank's first-ever appraisal of the Cuban health care system as this study was nearing completion served as a further reminder that this country offers a useful comparison with the failures and misdirection of so many health care systems in low- and middle-income developing countries.

As with its unique revolution, Cuba's health care is not so much a model that could be adopted by other countries, as a reminder that another line of approach is not only possible, but in many ways preferable.

Western Europe – Beveridge-style systems

UNITED KINGDOM

Of all the developed countries, not only in Western Europe but throughout the world, the British health care system has perhaps been the most repeatedly and thoroughly subjected to both market-driven and market-style reforms over the last 25 years or so. The process has accelerated in England since 1997 with a rapid succession of reorganisations, structural reforms, and increasing levels of privatisation and sure of private sector providers – although Wales and Scotland have been able to take advantage of devolved powers to steer in a substantially different direction, looking towards the reintegration of purchasing and providing care in Scotland, and rejecting increased hospital autonomy in Wales.

The New Labour reforms revolve perhaps more than those of the Tories around the New Public Management principle of 'steering, not rowing'. Indeed it is becoming increasingly clear that the New Labour objective is that the National Health Service will become little more than a 'brand name', a centralised fund that commissions and pays for patient care, rather like the 'sickness funds' of European social insurance-based systems, while NHS hospitals compete on ever less favourable terms with private sector companies for a share of the budget and for the staff they need to sustain basic services.

Like the Tory reforms, the market-style policies introduced since 1997 have been strongly criticised both by doctors and by health unions for their negative impact on equity of access and treatment – while New Labour ministers argue that the reforms are necessary precisely to secure these objectives.

The British reforms since 1990 have been analysed here at some length[131] in order to set a comparative benchmark against which other market-driven and market-style reforms in Western Europe can be compared. While the underlying principle of a public-sector, tax-funded service has been generally upheld, and the New Labour reforms have been accompanied by a substantial increase in government spending on health, partly funded through tax increases, the British reforms are in general on the most radical end of the European spectrum.

Ministers seeking vindication for their recent reforms of course point to the sharp reduction in waiting lists and waiting times that have been achieved across much of the NHS: but they also point to the most fundamental reason for this increase in volume and pace of treatment – increased spending and increased numbers of front-line staff (nurses, doctors and support staff). Staff productivity has increased, while overhead costs of goods and services bought in from the private sector have spiralled upwards. A report by the Office of National Statistics[132] (ONS 2004) reveals that while in 1995 labour costs amounted to 57% of NHS

---

131 For a more extended analysis, see Allyson Pollock's excellent full-length account in *NHS plc* (Pollock 2004). More detailed examples and analysis by the author of this study can also be found in issues of Health Emergency newspaper at *www.healthemergency.org.uk*.

132 Misleadingly reported as revealing a 'slump' in productivity in the National Health Service. Headlines like the *Financial Times* front page 'NHS fails all tests on improved efficiency' (October 19) turn out to have been based on a press release from the ONS: and it has subsequently emerged that some journalists seeking the full report on which this press release was based were told it was 'not available'.

spending, and 'intermediate consumption' (that is, goods and services) just 40%, by 2003 this picture had completely changed: then only 46% of spending was on labour and 52% on 'intermediate consumption'. Comparing the rate of growth of spending in these two categories shows the situation even more clearly: from 1995-2003 – a period in which the NHS workforce, according to the ONS, increased by 22% – spending on labour went up just 44% (from £22 billion to £32 billion). By contrast spending on 'intermediate procurement' rose by a massive 133% – from £16 billion to £37 billion. In other words for every £1 spent on staff in 1995, just 71p was spent on goods and services from the private sector, but by 2003, for every £1 spent on staff £1.14 was spent on procurement – an increase of over 50%. Over this same period NHS output (ignoring factors which might be argued as improving the quality of care) increased by 28% according to the ONS.

The key factor in expanding health care capacity, and the most frequent causes of bed and ward closures, delays and shortages in health care is adequate levels of staff, and it is clear that the efforts of the NHS workforce have generated real gains in output and quality of care since 1995. However the ONS admits that its statistics make no distinction between the different skill levels of the NHS workforce and their contribution to patient care: everyone becomes reduced to an abstract number of hours worked. The October document admits the standard manual on measuring productivity stresses that:

> …'an hour worked by a highly experienced surgeon and an hour worked by a newly hired teenager at a fast food restaurant' should be differentiated for productivity analysis, but although desirable, this is difficult.

Without such a breakdown it becomes very difficult to work out where the increased spending on staff has gone, and whether, as the Tory leadership claim, too much is still being frittered away on bureaucracy, as New Labour recreates wasteful market-style system similar, if wider in scope, to the one that Thatcher began in 1989-90.

Market-driven reforms

1 Global budgets/cash limits/spending cuts

The first major change goes back 30 years: driven by an uncontrollable economic crisis and the falling value of the currency, the Labour government agreed to comply with IMF requirements to rein in public spending, cut aspects of funding of the National Health Service, and impose for the first time global 'cash limits' on health care budgets. These measures in 1976 were followed by the incoming Thatcher government, which made the cash limits legally binding on health authorities in 1980 (Mohan 1995, Caldwell et al 1998).

Health care spending in Britain remained at a much lower level as a share of GDP than the EU and OECD averages throughout the 1990s, and only after 2002 did the New Labour government embark upon a conscious policy of injecting substantial above-inflation increases to the NHS budget to raise it towards the EU average. By 2004-5 the NHS budget, at £67 billion was double the 1996-97 figure. Billions of this extra spending, however, are funnelled into contracts with private health providers, making profits for the private companies, whilst many NHS hospitals are still (Spring 2005) facing large cash deficits and forced to close beds and cut jobs (Hirst 2005, Timmins 2005, Lister 2004b).

2 Rationalisation

This market-driven squeeze on health spending was tightened in the mid 1980s by explicit cutbacks which created successive years of zero or negative growth in NHS spending, and prompted crisis measures by health authorities – a fresh round of rationalisation of service provision, including hospital closures. Waiting lists for treatment grew rapidly during the 1980s, and it was the resulting prevalence of delays even for the treatment of urgent cancers and child heart operations in the winter of 1987-88 which generated the political imperative for Thatcher's review of the NHS (Caldwell et al 1998).

The rapid rundown in numbers of acute hospital beds which characterised the 1980s and early 1990s has largely come to a halt, and government guidance has underlined the need for additional hospital and 'intermediate' capacity to deal with a rising proportion of older patients (DoH 2000a, 2000b). However the very heavy cutbacks in beds for older patients and mental health beds have continued, although at a slower pace than the early 1990s.

While the main drive to bed closures has weakened, and while in theory all new hospital schemes should contain at least as many beds as the facilities they replace, many plans for costly new hospitals to be funded through the Private Finance Initiative are again raising the issue of reducing numbers of acute hospital beds to hold down the size (and cost) of the project: recent examples include schemes in Epsom & St Helier, Birmingham, and Leicester (Lister 2004a; Gould 2005; *HSJ* March 24 2005).

3 Regulating drug costs

Growing pressure on GPs to prescribe generic rather than more expensive branded drugs for their patients has continued since the 1980s (Rivett 1998). The internal market reforms in the 1990s meant that non-fundholding GP practices were strictly monitored for their adherence to generic prescribing guidelines, while fundholders, subject to cash-limited prescribing budgets, were given the financial incentive of retaining any unspent surpluses: as a result fundholders made greater use of generic medicines (Mossialos & Mrazek 2002:158-9). New Labour's introduction of Primary Care Groups, followed by Primary Care Trusts has resulted in a high profile for GP prescribing budgets in local financial reports, with pressure on 'high spending' practices to conform to the prescribing patterns of the majority.

4 New models of care

Attempts to switch to a 'primary care-led NHS' in the early 1990s, with questionable levels of success (Caldwell et al 1998), appear to be undergoing a revival with new schemes seeking to restrict the size of new costly hospital projects by switching services from hospital to primary care (CMMH 2003).

Market-style reforms

1 Decentralisation

Increased hospital autonomy began with the establishment of 'self-governing' provider units as NHS Trusts as part of the Conservative government's market-style reforms in the 1990s. This was not initially accompanied by increased independence for the purchasing health authorities, which remained centrally accountable through regional health authorities to the Department of Health, which also controlled all key lay appointments to health authorities and Trust boards.

More recent reorganisations in England have scrapped regional health authorities and established 25 Strategic Health Authorities, and replaced Primary Care Groups with Primary Care Trusts, local commissioning bodies which within a few years are expected to control upwards of 80% of the total NHS budget for primary, community and hospital services.

The early promise that PCTs would exercise substantial local autonomy has been thrown into question by the Department of Health's insistence that PCTs in Oxfordshire had no choice but to agree to the establishment of a controversial private sector Treatment Centre delivering cataract treatment, despite PCT concerns that it would undermine the financial viability of Oxford's existing NHS Eye Hospital (Carvel 2004).

The widely held view that PCTs have failed adequately to establish themselves as effective purchasing bodies forcing maximum value from hospital Trusts has led to fears among some observers that these organisations, established in 2002, will in turn be reorganised and merged into new, larger and less accountable bodies after the 2005 election. One strongly critical *BMJ* Editorial on the issue notes that:

> Reorganisations are a clumsy reform tool, and research shows that they seldom deliver the promised benefits. Every reorganisation produces a transient drop in performance, and it takes a new organisation at least two or three years to become established and start to perform as well as its predecessor. Yet the NHS is reorganised every two years or so, which probably means it sees all the costs of each reorganisation and few of the benefits (Walshe et al 2004).

2 Purchaser/provider split and contracts

The Conservatives' market-style reforms were implemented from the spring of 1991. The government had rejected many of the stock proposals of the radical right, for voucher-style schemes and other mechanisms to privatise the delivery of more health care, and for the imposition of fees and charges for treatment or for 'hotel services'[133]. Instead the plans had been modified from the proposals of Alain Enthoven (1985) and built around the concept of creating an internal market, which would drive up efficiency and quality through competition between rival providers.

The kernel of the reforms was the separation of the secondary care sector, which had for 40 years been planned and run by local health authorities, into purchasers (remodelled and smaller health authorities, spending budgets allocated by central government on the basis of the age profile of the local catchment population) and providers –'self-governing' NHS Trusts.

A further key factor in the dynamics of this new 'market' was to be the encouragement of the larger group practices of GPs – who had always been independent, self-employed contractors rather than NHS employees – to see themselves and the services they delivered as a business, by becoming 'fund-holding' practices. Fundholders would receive an annual cash-limited budget based on the demographic profile of their list of patients, from which they would purchase non-emergency inpatient and outpatient care from hospitals.

They were encouraged to use this new bargaining power to 'shop around' for low prices, and high quality services for their patients (quality in many cases being linked to reduced waiting times). Fundholders would be free to refer patients to any Trust, while those smaller practices and GPs who elected not to become fundholders would be restricted to those Trusts where their local health authority had negotiated a contract. As an additional incentive to join the scheme, fundholders were given a very generous calculation of their cash allocation, and were to be permitted to retain any unspent surplus in their budgets for patient care at the end of each year. Some began to accrue very substantial amounts (Paterson and Walker 1997).

---

133 A number of these options are reviewed in more detail in Lister (1988) and in Caldwell et al (1998:54-55).

GPs were urged to opt for the autonomy of fundholding, and the government steadily reduced the size of the practice required and found new ways of drawing in groups of GPs. By 1997 a majority of patients were covered by fundholding practices.

Up until the election in 1997, Labour in opposition promised that it would abolish the wasteful and competitive internal market, and replace it with a duty of different sections of the NHS to work in partnership. However the 1997 White Paper The New NHS – Modern, Dependable fell well short of abolition: it retained the essential purchaser/provider split, and retained Trusts as the provider unit for secondary and specialist care: only GP fundholding was swept away in a curious half-way house arrangement which established Primary Care Groups (PCGs), open to all GPs in every locality, which would act as a sub-committee of the district health authority. In the event PCGs themselves were to be swiftly swept away and replaced with Primary Care Trusts, in which the role of GPs and primary care practitioners was much more marginal, and which would become the larger and less accountable bodies that still exist today through a process of mergers (Caldwell et al 1998, Pollock 2004).

3 Provider autonomy

Under the Thatcher reforms, Trusts became 'public corporations', each governed by a quango Trust Board of directors composed of executive directors and direct and indirect government appointees, conducting most business behind closed doors. Their main income would come from contracts with purchasing health authorities, for which they would be required to compete on the basis of price and quality. They were required to balance their books each year, to pay capital charges on the assets they took over, and to generate a 6% return each year on their assets.

Trusts were encouraged to generate income by whatever means they saw fit, including advertising and the expansion of their provision of private beds for fee-paying patients. They would be 'free' to vary pay scales for their staff (effectively breaking up the national pay framework), to sell surplus property assets and use the returns, and to compete for contract revenue from local or more distant Trusts, and from fundholding GPs.

The reforms were highly controversial – and strongly opposed both by the BMA and by the health unions. They required a system for pricing and billing for each item of service delivered to patients, and thus began a commodification of health care which could potentially have provided a base from which means-tested user fees could have been introduced. Once the first wave of Trusts had launched in 1991, the remaining hospitals and community services came under increasing pressure to seek Trust status.

Prior to this substantial restructuring, the Tory government had during the 1980s introduced early experiments foreshadowing the type of measures that later became known as 'New Public Management'. A new tier of general managers had been created as a result of the Griffiths Report in 1983 to replace the more traditional 'administrators' and begin the process of separating out the management of provider units from the management of health authorities.

A number of these managers were brought in from industrial and other experience outside the NHS, and the restructuring can be seen as reinforcing the hand of management in relation to the professional powers of doctors, and laying the basis for subsequent market-style reforms (Ham 1999).

There was an accompanying rhetoric promoting the idea of applying 'business methods' to the NHS, which served to divert some public and media attention from the substantial increase in bureaucracy and associated costs that resulted from the reforms. Numbers of administrative and clerical staff rose by 18% in the decade to 1991, while admin costs rose from 6% of NHS spending to 11% over the same period (Mohan 1995, Hart 1994).

4 More provider autonomy

In the recent round of reforms, 'three star' Trusts, already shown to be performing best against the government's targets and star ratings system, were urged to apply to become 'Foundation Trusts', on the model of similar hospitals in Sweden and Spain (Busse et al 2002) and Portugal's 'hospital companies' (Hospitals SA) (Guichard 2004).

Foundations are non-profit public companies (or even 'mutuals' Mayo & Lea 2002), controlled by local boards and accountable not to the Secretary of State but to a new Independent Regulator. Foundations have been promised new freedoms to engage in 'entrepreneurial' activity over and above the freedoms available to non-foundation Trusts. However the government was forced to retreat from early promises that Foundation Trusts would be free to borrow on the money markets, and free to expand private beds and services: indeed ministers insisted that private activity and borrowing will be strictly limited in Foundation Hospitals – though it is not clear how this would be policed by the Regulator (Pollock and Price 2003). The legislation eventually passed through the Commons with a majority of just 17, and only a limited number of Foundations have been established before the 2005 General Election: however the Blair government made clear very early in the process that if they are re-elected then all hospitals will be pressed to become Foundations[134].

The exceptions are Wales and Scotland, where the National Assembly and the Scottish Parliament have both exercised their devolved powers and chosen not to establish foundation hospitals.

The extent of the autonomy on offer to Foundations was thrown into question in the autumn of 2004, when one of the first wave, Bradford Hospitals, found itself facing a substantial deficit (predicting a £4 million deficit after just six months) in place of the modest surplus it had predicted in its business plan. Despite the fact that this level of deficit is modest compared with many NHS Trusts, the Regulator (now known as 'Monitor') immediately intervened, and called in a firm of New York-based business trouble-shooters to sort out the growing financial crisis. The company, Alvarez & Marsal (A&M), was chosen and called in by Monitor: but the costs of flying in the team of 'turnaround management consultants' (who had to be told that British health care is priced in pounds and not dollars) had to be paid by the Bradford Trust. One of the early victims was the Trust chair who had headed up the application for Foundation status, but was removed at Monitor's insistence. Yet even while the regulator has seen fit to intervene so publicly and dramatically, Ministers predictably washed their hands of the whole business. In the House of Commons Health Secretary John Reid has issued a statement refusing to answer parliamentary questions on any Foundation Trusts, declaring that:

---

134 One limitation to this process is the level of indebtedness of many NHS Trusts, including potentially top-performing Trusts. After apparently waving through a first wave of applicants with minimal financial scrutiny, in 2005 Monitor has so far rejected four out of nine applications in January and five out of eleven in March on the basis of concerns for their financial viability – presumably to avoid further embarrassment along the lines of the financial crisis in the first-wave Bradford Hospitals Trust.

Ministers are no longer in a position to comment on, or provide information about, the detail of operational management within such Trusts. Any such questions will be referred to the relevant Trust chairman.

5 Provider payment reform

The internal market reforms of 1991 introduced the notion of annual contracts drawn up between health authority purchasers and providers, which would be monitored to ensure compliance: additional cases above a certain threshold would incur additional payments, while under-performing Trusts could face a loss of revenue. However throughout the 1990s most negotiations and most treatment took place on the basis of block contracts, with only GP fundholders, with much smaller numbers of patients, seeking special treatment for individual cases: prices varied widely from Trust to Trust depending on the cost pressures faced by the hospital, and sometimes the skill mix of the staff and the way in which the cost of each treatment was calculated.

However as part of its new, wider-reaching marketising reform, New Labour moved to introduce a much more complex system of 'payment by results' (PBR), to be phased in for providers from April 2004. This will mean that NHS Trusts will be paid on a fixed scale of 'reference costs' for each item of treatment they deliver – the old system of block contracts will be scrapped.

The new structure seems designed to create a new framework within which Foundation Trusts can secure a wider share of the available contract revenue in a competitive health 'market', while Trusts less well resourced, or whose costs for whatever reason are higher than the reference price, could lose out (DoH 2002c). However it is also the case that by effectively commodifying health care at such a basic level, the PBR system facilitates the New Labour objective of breaking down the barriers between the public and private sectors, and making much greater use of private sector providers. NHS Trusts therefore have increasingly to compete not only against other NHS Trusts, but also against private hospitals which have a much more selective, purely elective, and thus much less complex and costly caseload. And the pace of this competition has been forced by putting the responsibility not on to Primary Care Trusts, but on to individual patients, who will be offered a progressively wider 'choice' of where they want to have their treatment – at first to include at least one private hospital.

By the end of 2005 Primary Care Trusts will be obliged to offer almost all patients a 'choice' of providers – including at least one private hospital – from the time they are first referred but eventually (from 2008) any patient will be allowed to choose any hospital which can deliver treatment at the NHS reference cost. Irrespective of what patients may choose, ministers have made clear that they want at least 10% of NHS elective operations to be carried out by the private sector in 2006, rising to 15% by 2008 (Ward 2005).

This policy has been strongly criticised, not least by the BMA, but also by studies produced by London NHS managers for Health Secretary John Reid, which warned that the plans were 'problematic, unaffordable' and of 'no benefit' in London, since they would have serious impact on the financial stability and viability of NHS Trusts (Smith 2005, McGauran 2004). The Commons Public Accounts Committee has warned that the policy could result in private sector providers 'cream skimming' the most straightforward and lucrative cases, leaving NHS hospitals with reduced resources to cope with the chronic, the complex and the costly patients: it could also give GPs perverse incentives to refer patients to hospitals which did not have adequate facilities or medical support (Coombes 2005).

There has been growing concern that hospitals which lose out as patients choose to go elsewhere could be forced to close departments or close down altogether: ministers and senior NHS officials have said that they are willing to see this happen, arguing that it would not be their policy, but patients who made the decision (Timmins 2004a, Smith P 2003). However it is not only this factor that could push hospitals into difficulties, but also the problems faced by hospitals where for whatever reason operations are currently costing above the NHS reference cost, which will face a substantial cut in revenue under PBR.

Even where hospitals have been charging less than the new reference cost, and would stand to make windfall gains under the new system, the Primary Care Trusts which buy services from them would find their budgets cut. Estimates of the mis-match in funding are as high as £1 billion a year across the NHS, with some Trusts set to lose very heavily.

This new market-style system makes no reference to social and other inequalities, and runs the risk of funnelling an ever-larger share of the NHS budget to the best-resourced and largest Trusts and GP practices at the expense of those struggling to cope in more deprived areas. But the new system also represents the end of 30 years of efforts to equalise allocations of NHS spending on the basis of population and local health needs. Now PCTs in areas where Trusts are currently delivering services below the new NHS reference costs will require extra cash to pay an increased fee – which will become a 'surplus' for the Trust. Conversely PCTs whose Trusts currently deliver relatively high-cost treatment will see their cash allocations reduced.

None of this bears any relation to social deprivation, the age profile or relative health of the population: the new market system emerges as the enemy of equality. The prospect of widespread financial instability has forced a delay and a phased introduction of the new payment system, which was to have applied to 70% of treatments by April 2005, but in the run-up to the General Election has already been postponed by 12 months[135], and may well be postponed further (Conrad 2005).

6 Purchase services from private sector

New Labour's commitment to buying an increasing volume of NHS treatment from the private sector began with the signing of a Concordat with the private sector hospitals in 2000, and, more recently, the signing of contracts for the establishment of a new network of privately run for-profit Treatment Centres that will deliver certain types of elective care to NHS patients. The government is determined to forge ahead regardless of the mounting evidence that many of the private units are neither needed nor welcome. The case of the private treatment centre specialising in cataract operations, to be foisted upon Oxfordshire's Primary Care Trusts despite the evidence that it will cut the ground from below the well-established Oxford Eye Hospital has achieved national notoriety.

Early in 2005 the government invited private tenders to deliver a further 250,000 operations a year, worth an estimated £500 million annually: in addition another £400 million worth of X-rays, scans, blood tests and pathology tests will be hived off to the private sector. These moves will almost double the number of private sector operations to be purchased by the NHS, pushing the government's total spend in the 'independent sector' up towards £1.5

---

135 Also postponed until after polling day is a twice-delayed report on the financial health of the NHS by the National Audit Office and the Audit Commission which could emerge with damaging findings (Day 2005).

billion – two-thirds of the total £2.3 billion turnover of the private medical industry in 2003. Among the companies hoping to cash in on this new bias in favour of privatisation are Swedish private health firm Capio and Nuffield Hospitals.

It is clear that in some areas, especially those where private hospitals are few and far between, PCTs could find themselves obliged to meet their targets for increased private sector referrals by effectively denying patients the option of NHS care. Critics are also warning that if large numbers of individuals are encouraged to opt for a private sector provider they could trigger the financial collapse and even closure of local health services or even whole NHS hospitals – even those which are doing well under the current system.

Hospitals which lose a slice of their elective care will see their unit costs go up, as existing capacity is used by fewer patients, and as they are left to deal with the cases which the private sector does not wish to treat. The BMA has warned that even hospitals losing less than 10% of their patients to private sector or other NHS Trusts could be forced to close. Even where public capital has already been invested in state of the art NHS-run treatment centres there is no long-term guarantee that these will remain viable or operational. Some are already in trouble.

The blatant bias that is being shown in favour of private providers and against the NHS is exposed by the problems faced by one of the pioneering NHS-run treatment centres, the Ambulatory Care and Diagnostic (ACAD) unit at Central Middlesex Hospital. While the privately run treatment centres receive long-term guaranteed income on a 'play or pay' basis, and have up to now been allowed to charge higher than NHS reference costs, none of these conditions applies to NHS treatment centres.

Elsewhere NHS consultants have been instructed by managers to pass over a share of their waiting list workload for treatment in private sector units – but no such pressure exists to maintain the flow of patients to NHS units. By the winter of 2004 ACAD, like other NHS treatment centres, reported having spare capacity to treat thousands more patients: instead partly used NHS facilities result in rising costs and poor productivity – giving ministers a ready-made pretext for favouring an apparently cheaper and more efficient private sector. University College London (UCLH) has warned that it may have to scale down its treatment centres if the odds remain stacked against them: but it seems that the government's fixation with expanding the private hospital sector could lead them to ban Foundation Trusts like UCLH from bidding for the provision of the next round of treatment centres in the January tendering process. Ministers want to take every opportunity to convince private firms of the government's commitment to privatising an ever-increasing share of clinical care.

An underlying difficulty for those arguing in favour of a greater 'partnership' between the public and private medical sectors is the chronic and worsening shortage of suitably skilled professional staff, all of whom in Britain are trained by the NHS. The relatively small scale of private medicine and the long-standing under-occupancy of private hospital beds has meant that any additional caseload diverted from the NHS to private hospitals must result in intensified competition to recruit and retain nursing and medical staff.

7 Competition

Although competition on the basis of price has now been ruled out, with the phased introduction of Department of Health reference prices for specific treatments, competition for contracts seems set to be fiercer than ever once the PBR system is phased in. Ministers appear to be set on a course of building up sufficient capacity in the private sector to generate a real fear that failing NHS Trusts will be allowed close down, with services delivered from alternative private providers. What this scenario does not address is the wide range of emergency and other services which are currently available only from NHS hospitals, and which the private sector has shown no interest in providing.

8 Privatisation

During the last two decades the UK has been characterised by the World Bank as one of the world's most active privatising governments (Bach 2000), although in health care this has largely centred on non-clinical services. From 1984 onwards hospitals were required to put their main ancillary services (catering, cleaning and laundry – later followed by portering and security services) out to competitive tender, with evidence of mounting government pressure to accept the lowest tender regardless of quality (Whitfield 1992).

Even where this did not result in the outright privatisation of services, this early exercise in 'steering, not rowing' served to introduce the notion of partial private provision within a publicly funded service, separated off these 'hotel' services from the clinical services in each hospital, and resulted in a large scale reduction in jobs, pay and conditions for the lowest-paid staff, with questionable effects on levels of hygiene, patient care and staff morale (Bach 2000).

The first wave of PFI hospitals were delivered on contracts which included the privatisation of the core non-clinical support services: subsequent PFI schemes incorporate the privatisation of the management of these services, with support staff seconded to the private contractor – a system which has yet to demonstrate any evidence of success in the improvement of quality or efficiency.

9 User fees

The rapid, above-inflation rises in prescription charges which characterised the period of Conservative rule from 1979 have ended, but prescriptions for the 20% or so of patients who are not exempt have continued to increase with inflation. No additional user fees have been imposed: the NHS remains largely free at point of use.

In Wales, the National Assembly has made use of its autonomous powers to freeze, reduce and eventually eliminate prescription charges, which generate little revenue but serve to deter the working poor from fully accessing the treatment they require.

10 Steps to control medical professionals

A dimension of many of the reforms since 1990 has been the attempt by successive governments to control the cost and quality of services delivered by hospital consultants and by GPs[136]. Conservative reforms attempted to discipline consultants by incorporating them as directors of departments that would be obliged to work to fixed budgets.

Those who opted to become GP fundholders from 1991 were the first primary care doctors to be subjected to the discipline of cash limits: this regime has now been extended by the New Labour government to cover the whole of the NHS (DoH 2000). Since 2000, a succession of new contracts have been used in a bid to curb the amount of private work that can be undertaken by consultants, and stipulate a minimum number of hours that must be worked for the NHS, while a new GP contract has also stipulated new tasks and duties.

---

136 Unlike hospital doctors (who are salaried NHS employees) almost all GPs have remained as self-employed contractors outside of NHS employment since Bevan's settlement that established the NHS in 1948.

11 Patient choice

As discussed above, a key factor driving a new round of market competition and also drawing more NHS spending into the private sector is the new system of 'patient choice', which began with a scheme under which patients waiting six months or more for treatment were entitled to transfer to another NHS – or private sector – provider (Pollock and Price 2002, Lister 2003a).

Health Secretary John Reid now insists that patient choice is a more fundamental principle than maintaining local access to NHS hospital services, following a line from Tony Blair in October 2003:

> Choice is not a betrayal of our principles. It is our principles (Knight 2004).

12 PFI/PPP

Ironically the payment by results system will cause the biggest problems for new hospitals funded under the Private Finance Initiative (PFI) – which are saddled with high, fixed overhead costs for non-clinical services, in the form of legally binding, index-linked payments to the PFI consortium, while lacking spare beds and capacity to take on additional patients. Since the non-clinical costs are largely fixed and non-negotiable, the only area of activity capable of variation is clinical care – resulting in the £120 million Queen Elizabeth Hospital in Woolwich running with wards closed to save on staffing costs.

The attempts by the Tory government to privatise the provision of capital for major hospital development projects through the private finance initiative (PFI) was a part of their market-style reform of health care. Although the policy was introduced from 1992, alongside year-by-year reduction of allocations of NHS capital, but the concerns of private sector companies that their investment may not be secure in the context of Trusts struggling for financial viability meant that the Conservatives were unable to finalise any PFI schemes, and no new hospitals were built under PFI until the New Labour government legislated new guarantees for private consortia after 1997 (Pollock 2004, Lister 2001).

By spring 2004, 21 new hospitals, capital value £1.5 billion, were complete and operational, with ten more new hospitals, capital value £1.9 billion under construction. A further three new hospitals, total value £1.7 billion, were still in negotiation, with more lining up for approval. Nine-tenths of all new hospital projects were being funded through PFI, with only one major hospital funded through capital from the Treasury.

More PFI hospital projects, worth £4 billion, were given the go-ahead by John Reid during the summer of 2004, many of them reflecting the massive cost inflation of PFI schemes since the first wave was rubber-stamped back in 1998. While the average cost of a new hospital project in the first wave PFI was £75 million, there are now a series of schemes under consideration costing over £500 million, raising serious questions of affordability and value for money[137].

---

137 These include the new Royal London Hospital and redevelopment of Barts (£1,100 million); Paddington Health Campus (£800 million), Liverpool Royal and Alder Hey Hospitals (£835 million), University Hospitals of Leicestershire (£761 million, despite comprising 328 fewer beds than the earlier plan costed at £286 million in 2001), and University Hospital Birmingham (£521 million). The combined payment for the £420 million Central Manchester PFI was to begin at £47 million a year, index-linked, suggesting that the Leicestershire scheme could come in at around £85 million annually for 35 years or more, index-linked.

Despite the soaring costs and less than satisfactory performance of many of the PFI hospitals, most of which are already mired in debt long before PBR is implemented, there has been little attempt at ministerial or Department level to learn from the failures in the design and build quality of the first wave of PFI hospitals, many of which proved difficult and uncomfortable places for staff and patients alike[138] (Lister 2003b, 2003c).

More detailed critiques of the theory and practical experience of PFI as a method for financing health care facilities have been set out elsewhere (Lister 2001, Pollock 2004): but the government's commitment to establish upwards of £7 billion of privately owned facilities to be leased by the NHS is equivalent to the privatisation of a third of the NHS property asset base when New Labour took office. PFI-built hospitals and other assets are themselves now being traded as risk-free profit streams in the financial markets.

SWEDEN

Market-driven reforms –
Global budgets/Cash limits/spending cuts

Cutbacks led to a loss of 128,000 full and part time health care jobs in the four years 1990–94, while the increase in workload for reduced numbers of staff remaining have caused concern over possible overload and 'professional burnout' (Saltman 1998).

1 Rationalisation

Capacity problems continue to reflect themselves in long waiting times for health care in Sweden: waiting lists are reported to have grown again to the levels of the early 1990s, despite the reputed success of the Adel Reform of 1992 (a version of which has since been copied by Britain's New Labour government) which placed the responsibility on municipalities to resolve the long-standing problem of 'bed blocking' in hospitals. Municipal authorities (which, unlike their UK equivalents, own and run nursing homes) were required by law to accept patients deemed ready for discharge within five days of being required to do so: and for every day they failed to find suitable accommodation for the patient they would be obliged to pay the full cost of their inpatient hospital care (Saltman 1998).

2 Regulating drug costs

Sweden operates a national system for distributing prescription drugs: the patient has to pay the full cost of drugs up to 99 euro per year, and then a decreasing proportion of the cost up to a ceiling of 472 euro (a co-payment limited to 198 euro per year) (Dixon and Mossialos 2002).

3 New models of care

The innovative Adel Reform (see above) has been reported to place a heavy strain on relatively weak systems of municipal community care. Patients have to pay higher out-of-pocket charges for community care than for hospital care (Dixon and Mossialos 2002).

---

138 Among them the architectural award-winning £220 million Norfolk & Norwich Hospital, a low-rise building with the kitchens in the middle, and most office space housed in converted storage areas without windows or air-conditioning, resulting in sweltering temperatures (Lister 2003b).

Market-style reforms

1 Decentralisation

Unlike Britain, where the control of the NHS has always been in the hands of unelected local health authorities controlled centrally by the Secretary of State, Sweden's health services have always been decentralised, with most public sector hospitals still owned locally, by county councils.

2 Purchaser/provider split and contracts

Internal market reforms launched (like the British reforms) in 1989 meant that by 1999 three-quarters of county councils had established separate purchasing bodies. Before the wider spread of market-style reforms, Sweden was described as 'perhaps the Northern European country that is farthest along in the design of planned market models' (Saltman 1991). Early proposals to base the new system around patient choice and a 'primary care-led' system of purchasing – with money following patients, and the potential to force the closure of any hospitals which failed to secure sufficient contract revenue in the new marketplace (Saltman 1991, Saltman 1998) were abandoned in 1996 (Dixon and Mossialos 2002).

The first market reforms were implemented in only a minority of counties, while the improvements that have been noted in hospital productivity apply to nearly every hospital, suggesting that the productivity gains flow largely from budget cuts and other more general pressures and incentives (EHMA 2000).

3 Provider autonomy

Two-thirds of the counties' expenditure on health comes from county taxes, and the local level of control by elected bodies has led to the possibility of political shifts, as when the victory of right wing parties in several counties led to them adopting more market-style policies, including the contracting out of hotel services and the floating of hospitals as publicly owned companies. In Stockholm one hospital, St Goran's, was sold in 1999 by the county council – against the wishes of the central government – to a private company, Capio, which operates in other Scandinavian countries, Poland and the UK. St Goran's is now described as 'Sweden's largest private emergency hospital' (Sectra 2003). In 2001 the government legislated to prevent further public hospitals being privatised in this way. Despite early claims that the privatised hospital had cut costs and increased caseload (Taylor and Blair 2002) the experience in this and other corporatised hospitals has been of failure to achieve cost savings or productivity increases (Lyall 2002, Dixon and Mossialos 2002).

4 Provider payment reform

Sweden combines prospective payments with a further payment linked to numbers treated (Maceira 1998). The 'money follows the patient', despite the lack of a 'quasi-commercial market as in the UK' (EHMA 2000:33).

5 Purchase services from private sector

In 2002, 8% of state insurance funds to reimburse hospitals for treatment went to Sweden's handful of private hospitals. Now the coalition government has passed new legislation that will prevent any new private hospitals that start up from treating state-insured patients (Burgermeister 2004).

6 Competition

Competition between the providers has been identified as a factor in increasing costs and activity levels (while counties were prevented from raising additional taxes) and in plunging levels of public satisfaction in the years 1996-98. This in turn led to a 'tempering' of the purchaser/provider split (Diderichson 1993, Freeman 2000, Dixon and Mossialos 2002).

7 Privatisation

Early in 2004, new legislation was brought in to prevent any further privatisation of hospitals, which had begun in two right wing-controlled provincial authorities. Companies will no longer be allowed to run hospitals that treat both private and state insured patients (Burgermeister 2004).

8 User fees

Swedish patients pay relatively high user fees for treatment:

- To see a primary care physician
- To see a specialist in hospital
- A daily charge for inpatients staying in hospital.

The national parliament has fixed a maximum ceiling of €99 on out of pocket payments, excluding inpatient care (Dixon and Mossialos 2002). Patients may have to pay more if they choose to receive their outpatient treatment in a hospital rather than a primary care centre, or if they choose to consult a private doctor of clinic, only part of whose fee is subsidised by the public sector.

9 Steps to control medical professionals

With no private medical cover offering an alternative to the National Health Service, and a negligible number of the population covered by voluntary private medical insurance (the market leader having just 30,000 people, 0.13% of the population insured) there is little scope for professionals to move in to private practice. Any NHS patients who go to a private physician or clinic are only partly subsidised by the public sector.

10 Patient choice

Sweden maintains a firm dividing line between the public and private sectors: however patients have a choice of hospital, a choice of GP, and waiting list guarantees.

11 PFI/PPP

No movement reported on these lines.

Shorter country summaries – Beveridge systems

SPAIN

The current National Health Service in Spain came into operation relatively recently, in 1986, although the General Health Service Act's provisions for decentralised management across the country's 17 autonomous regions still had not been fully implemented in 1999 (Freeman 2000, Reverte-Cejudo and Sanchez-Bayle 1999). The final decentralisation was eventually completed in 2002, with the central health ministry retaining only limited powers, and budgets totalling £6.4 billion transferred to regional control (Bosch 2002).

The system has been very effective at reducing waiting lists: numbers waiting over six months for treatment have been slashed from almost 54,000 in 1996 to just 510 in 1999, when the average wait was just 60 days. But Spain has a chronic surplus of doctors and nurses, with the second highest per capita number of doctors in Europe (4.2 per 1,000 population), and over 24,000 doctors unemployed in 1999 (Rico 2000).

The launch of the National Health Service was accompanied by a concerted programme of hospital building, which resulted in 60 new hospitals being constructed between 1983-1996, meaning that almost the whole population lives within 60 minutes of a general hospital, and that the capital stock of health facilities is very modern (Rico 2000, Nash 2003). However, capacity constraints may underlie the substantial use of private not-for-profit providers for some 15-20% of hospital provision.

The funding formula for allocation to the regions controversially included preferential allocations to those areas which already had centres of excellence and teaching hospitals: critics complained that this meant more money went to better-resourced areas (Reverte-Cejudo and Sanchez-Bayle 1999). The same authors point out that devolution of control appears to have resulted in duplication of functions and a growth of regional bureaucracies.

However the decentralisation measure which seems to have attracted most international interest recently has been the provision for 'foundation hospitals' to gain a large measure of autonomy from government, and run as a private enterprise. As such they are free to borrow and to issue shares.

British Health Secretary Alan Milburn visited Madrid's Alorcon Foundation Hospital in 2001, and has since announced a scheme to promote similar autonomous hospitals as not-for-profit companies in England. Yet a year before Mr Milburn's visit, the Spanish government had stepped back from its promotion of foundation hospitals after encountering strong opposition from unions and public health organisations, who were critical of the unfairness of allowing foundations to borrow money or do deals with the private sector, since this would lead to inequalities in access to care. Only four hospitals had launched as foundations before the scheme ceased to be a priority of the right wing government (Bosch 2001).

Unions have also complained that staff at foundation hospitals work longer hours than elsewhere: doctors at Manacor hospital in Majorca were reportedly working 32 hours without a break (*The Guardian* 2003). Subsequent criticisms of foundation hospitals have also pointed to the fact that they focus heavily on short-stay treatment and younger patients, and deal with fewer long-term and elderly people, who wind up being treated in other hospitals. This in turn can skew the statistics to make foundation hospitals appear more efficient (Nash 2003).

With the costs of prescribed drugs reaching 25% of national health care spending, the highest in Europe, government attempts to rein in spending on drugs have included the introduction of a system of co-payments which ended the tradition of free drugs for pensioners, obliging them to pay up to 10% of drug costs, in proportion to their incomes. Employed and unemployed health care users had always been obliged to pay 40% of the cost of most drugs (Bosch 2000).

ITALY

The National Health Service (SSN) was established as late as 1978, and was modelled on the 1974 structure of the NHS in Britain, later adding general managers along the lines proposed in Britain by Sir Roy Griffiths in 1983. Italy also appears to have followed the British government into market-style reforms (1993) in which large hospitals were encouraged to 'opt out' of SSN control and become NHS-style self-governing Trusts independent of health authorities (Bevan et al 1992, Coopers and Lybrand 1993). These changes, which led to 98 trusts being created by 2000, were accompanied by a limited internal market, with hospitals competing for caseload on the basis of fee-for-service financing (Donatini et al 2001).

Yet although the SSN was set up after the imposition of cash limits on British health spending, there was initially a very loose control over health care budgets at regional level, where authorities regarded their unrealistically small allocation as a valid reason for overspending. Relatively large numbers of charitable and private hospitals also remained outside the SSN, but continued to sell services to the public system, resulting in a high level of health finance being spent in the private sector in the early 1990s (Bevan et al 1992, Freeman 2000). Out of pocket payments for prescriptions and for outpatient treatment have also grown in scale over the last 20 years, rising from 20% of total health spending in 1980 to 33% in 1999, although inpatient care and primary care are free at point of use (Donatini et al 2001).

The relatively loose financial controls were further loosened by a very generous provision for patient choice to avoid long waits: any patient required to wait longer than four days for outpatient care could choose to go instead to a hospital outside the SSN – or even, in the case of high-tech medicine outside the country, and the SSN would pay most or all of the bill (Bevan et al 1992).

However this type of system led to an escalation of health care spending and despite attempts between 1997 and 2000 to tighten controls, by 2000 it had resulted in a cumulative debt to suppliers equivalent to 36 trillion lire, 1.8% of Italy's GDP. Public health spending was running 8.8 trillion lire a year above the limit set by central government, and legal requirements to balance budgets were simply being ignored in the knowledge that central government would eventually cover any deficits. This drew stern criticism in an IMF study which described 'weak enforcement of unclear rules' and 'decentralisation without fiscal responsibility'. As such the Italian style of decentralisation is seen as 'allowing regions to be irresponsible on the expenditure side,' even while waiting times for treatment had grown longer (Reviglio 2000). It ran the danger of expanding the size of government rather than decreasing it, demonstrating that the formulae of New Public Management can misfire and produce very different results from those anticipated.

Perhaps the biggest crime in the eyes of the IMF analyst was that 'weak cash ceilings and a lack of incentives for controlling suppliers make it possible to ignore the struggle for cost effectiveness' (ibid p15). Italian authorities are urged to take 'steps that are socially and politically unpleasant,' such as firing redundant staff, controlling wage increases, and making general practitioners responsible for the public funds they receive. The document concludes that:

> Today Italy's physicians and health program managers do not face hard budget constraints, therefore their incentives to limit costs are weak (p25).

The lack of control also affects the for-profit private insurance sector in Italy, which has expanded rapidly over the years from a premium income of 71 million euro in 1982 to 1.14 billion euro in 1998: but its rate of expenditure has also risen rapidly, and its overall deficit for 1998 was estimated at 61 million euro (Donatini et al 2001). Almost 40% of hospitals in Italy are private, many of them carrying out services funded by the SSN: however many of them are very small, and 81.5% of beds for ordinary admissions are public sector.

Italy and Greece are unique in Europe in having fewer qualified nurses than doctors, with a level of nurses per head which has barely changed since the mid 1970s.

DENMARK

Denmark's hospitals are owned and run by 14 elected county councils, and the counties also finance general practitioner and other primary care services, while nursing homes and community health services are the responsibility of 275 municipal councils. Services in each case are funded from taxation, with funds allocated through global budgets.

The counties have a large degree of autonomy to plan health services, but are expected to work within the framework of priorities set by an annual budget negotiation with central government. And since 1993 patients have had the option of seeking treatment not offered locally in other counties, with their home country being obliged to pay for it (Vallgarda et al 2001).

Remarkably, in view of the short waiting times and comprehensive care available free at point of use through the public sector, and the lack of serious private sector capacity, some 28% of Danes have some form of voluntary health insurance (Vallgarda et al 2002). User charges have been discussed, but are payable only for physiotherapy, dental care and spectacles as well as co-payments for prescription drugs, which reduce according to the individuals' growing need for medication.

Hospitals are mainly funded through global budgets which have proved successful as tools for cost containment (Vallgarda et al 2001). Supplementary contracts for hospitals were introduced by some counties in 1993 as a means of increasing activity and focusing on costs, and not as a competitive mechanism. In 1999 it was agreed that treatment outside a patient's home county should be paid on the basis of Diagnostic Related Groups – which tend to represent an increase on the previous rates paid, and was thought likely to generate a degree of competition to attract additional patients. However only around 2% of patients requiring hospital admission have been taking advantage of their right to choose to go elsewhere.

Denmark's health services operate a waiting time guarantee for life-threatening conditions which ensures a maximum wait of two weeks for investigation and two weeks for treatment. Otherwise a general guarantee of a maximum two-month wait has applied since July 2002 to all types of non-urgent treatment. If public sector hospitals cannot meet this timescale the patient is entitled to seek private treatment or to seek treatment abroad, paid for by the county council.

NORWAY

Like the Danish and Swedish health care systems, Norway has had a decentralised, but tax-funded service, run at local level by elected county and municipal councils. But there have been concerns that this high level of decentralisation created problems in achieving equity in access to services and in coordinating services between hospitals and community and primary care (Furuholmen and Magnussen 2000).

Spending has been declining as a share of GDP since 1992 (OECD 2000), though Norway's own national statistics show health spending at 8% in 1996 and 9% in 1998 – slightly above the European Union average.

Patients pay charges up to a maximum ceiling each year to cover a part of the cost of outpatient treatment, laboratory tests, X-rays and visiting a GP or a specialist outside the hospital and for some prescriptions. There are some exemptions for specific diseases and groups of patients. However dental care and spectacles are largely paid for out-of-pocket by service users, and there is also a substantial private market in dental care, which in 1993 was larger than the public dental service (Furuholmen and Magnussen 2000).

Until the end of the 1990s there was a negligible private medical sector in Norway, though some centres have opened up more recently to offer high-tech treatment on an outpatient basis otherwise only available in hospital. Small private hospitals in Oslo, focused on the typical areas of surgery favoured by private medicine the world over[139], have just 1% of the country's acute beds and 5% of outpatient services. Their custom hinges on relatively long waiting lists in public sector hospitals, which have been seen as a serious problem over the last ten years.

In 1998, more than a quarter of patients discharged had waited over 90 days for admission. Attempts to manage down the waiting lists by targeting additional resources created perverse incentives for hospitals to keep their lists high in order to attract additional resources. While Norway has for some time had a system that facilitated cross-county flows of patients, with a pricing mechanism for charging their home county for treatment elsewhere, this was altered in 1997 to include a cost per case payment to counties designed to encourage hospitals to treat more patients. Hospitals now receive a combination of a global budget and cost per case, which is based on the Diagnostic Related Group system (Furuholmen and Magnussen 2000).

Norway has a relatively high number of doctors per head, but this is not evenly distributed and there are problems in persuading physicians to practise in some of the more remote areas of the country. There is also a shortage of qualified and specialist nurses. In 2000 Norway offered contracts to 50 specialist doctors from Hungary, arranging intensive language courses and allowing them also to treat private patients (Kovac 2000). The specialists will be welcome in Norway, but left a mounting crisis in Hungary's under-funded hospital system that was already desperately short of key specialist medical and nursing staff.

Norway was among the most energetic countries at rationalising both acute bed capacity and psychiatric beds in the two decades to 1990: a switch to day surgery and outpatient treatment brought reductions of 35% for acute beds and 66% in psychiatric hospitals, though this rate of closure has slowed for both sectors in the last ten years (Furuholmen and Magnussen 2000).

The decentralised service tends to be especially sensitive to local pressure, especially when there have been proposals to rationalise hospital services or centralise specialist units.

> Regardless of location, the proximity of fully fledged hospital services, including acute and specialised elective care, is seen as an acquired right by large segments of the population (Furuholmen and Magnussen 2000:69).

To get round this obstacle to restructuring, the government in 2002 created five new regional offices, which would take over the ownership of all hospitals, previously owned and run by 19 counties. The hospitals had in most cases already merged to form larger trusts, and the new arrangement further separates them from the control of the counties – opening more scope for rationalisation and centralisation of services (Lien 2003).

Other changes ushered in as the government attempts to unleash the consumer power of patients to force an increase efficiency in Norway include the enactment of a bill of patient rights, which allow patients to choose which hospital they should attend within the category of

---

139 Open heart surgery, hip surgery, and minor surgical procedures such as hernias, cataracts and varicose veins.

hospitals selected by their GP – although most psychiatric hospital referrals are exempt, with only specialist psychiatric care included (Furuholmen and Magnussen 2000:71). The objective of these changes is to increase the flow of patients being treated in hospitals outside their home county, and thus to trigger a competitive drive to increase capacity and reduce waiting times.

However Lien (2002) points out that despite the allocation of extra funding and an 'augmented political focus on mental health,' the various reforms appear to ignore or work against an improvement in mental health services, which he sums up as:

> ...to increase the community mental health care capacity and to build up easy accessible district
> mental health care service with polyclinics, ambulatory services, day care and short and long term
> beds in all local hospital catchment areas.

The switch to cost per case funding for acute hospitals could result in the transfer of resources away from psychiatric services, which are still funded through global budgets regardless of caseload. And there are real doubts over the appropriateness of pricing mental health services on the basis of DRGs, not least because of difficulties in predicting the likely length of stay of an individual admitted for treatment. Drawing up market-style contracts for mental health has been shown to be the most difficult, costly and least likely to result in genuine competition (Lien 2003). To attempt this type of reform in Norway would require diverting scarce and skilled staff from their main duties.

But Lien also argues that any introduction of market-style pricing is also likely to result in pressure to treat more patients in hospital rather than develop more appropriate services in the community. It can also lead hospitals to discharge people more swiftly, with an eye to norms and targets rather than to the needs of the patients. There could also be an upward pressure of supplier-induced demand, 'as long as the government does not cap total expenditure'.

PORTUGAL

The Portuguese National Health Service was formed as a tax-funded, Beveridge-style public-integrated service following the country's democratic revolution in the mid 1970s, through a series of nationalisations of hospitals and medical facilities owned by religious charities (1974), local hospitals (1975) and medical units and health posts (1977) (Bentes et al 2004). It replaced various Bismarck-style workplace insurance schemes under the old Salazar regime, and gave all citizens the right to health protection and a guaranteed right to free health care through the NHS regardless of economic and social background.

However the system that was taken over lacked adequate outpatient and primary care services (around 1 million people, 10% of the population, are still waiting to enlist with a GP), and proved unable to meet demand for care, resulting in extraordinarily long waiting lists (123,000 people, over 1% of the population was waiting for treatment in July 2002 – with an average waiting time of six years) (Guichard 2004).

By 1990 the problems of an under-staffed and under-resourced NHS were met by new legislation seeking to stimulate private sector health care, including private management of NHS facilities. User charges replaced the principle of treatment free at point of use in 1990, with exemptions for the poor and high risk groups. These 'reforms' were followed by an explicit adoption of policies based on 'New Public Management', in particular the encouragement of 'public entrepreneurism' in the first three public hospitals (1996) and the introduction of a purchaser/provider split, with regional contracting agencies established to decide the allocation of resources (Bentes et al 2004).

The years from 1993 were characterised by growth on health spending, constantly outstripping the allocated global budget by an average of 7.5%, culminating in a massive 19.6% overspend in 2002. That year despite the soaring waiting list, Portugal's hospitals ran at below European levels of occupancy, and longer than most European average length of stay. Many were plagued with enormous levels of debt, with the top performing hospitals singled out as those with debts below 35% of total expenditure (Guichard 2004).

After 1997 hospital payment systems have been partly changed from retrospective to prospective payments based on DRG-style reference costs. More recently almost a third of the country's NHS top-performing hospitals (34) comprising 50% of available public sector beds, were transformed into 'hospital companies' ('Hospitals SA') analogous to Foundation Trusts.

Ministers followed this with the announcement that ten new hospitals would be constructed by 2010 as 'Public Private Partnerships' – combining private investment, public finance, private management of all services, and public ownership. More controversial plans have also been proposed for the reorganisation of health centres, either as professional cooperatives, social non-profit organisations or private for-profit (Bentes et al 2004). Staff in the new hospital companies were offered the chance to switch to individual contracts incorporating a performance-related element, but to the surprise of the OECD's Stephanie Guichard 'very few employees changed status in 2003' (Guichard 2004:25).

The first year of Portugal's 'Foundation Trusts' appear to have succeeded in increasing activity faster than costs, implying greater efficiency, but there were big variations between the 34 units. The remaining public sector hospitals also managed to increase production but their costs increased, along with their level of debt 'by about 60%'. New financing arrangements are expected to be applied to these hospitals during 2005 to treat them more like the Hospitals SA.

Within a very short space of time (30 years) Portugal has implemented the type of nationalisation that established the British National Health Service, and begun rapidly to reverse the process, reverting to a familiar menu of market-style reforms. The period of investment in health care for the whole population since 1974 has borne fruit in a dramatic increase in life expectancy and a spectacular reduction in infant mortality: whether the ongoing reforms will yield further positive results remains to be seen.

Western Europe – Bismarck-style systems

GERMANY

Market-driven reforms

1 Global budgets/cash limits/spending cuts

Like many other countries, Germany tried to rein in spending on health care in the late 1970s: a new Health Insurance Cost Containment Act was passed in 1977 which limited the level of contributions to sickness funds (and by implication the scale of charges imposed by health care providers) to the level of salaries – preventing any real terms increase. However the imposition of legally binding cash limits on health care providers did not take place until 1992, after reunification of the country. This reunification pushed up health spending as a share of Germany's GDP since it led to higher investment and spending in the east, where productivity has been lower (Busse and Riesberg 2000)[140].

The reforms in the 1992 Health Care Structure Act attempted to combine the introduction of cash limits and fixed case and procedure fees for hospital care (to begin in 1996) with more market-style measures to create a degree of competition, which included a new freedom for almost all insured people to choose which sickness fund they should contribute to; a limited weakening of the ambulatory physicians' monopoly on outpatient treatment – to enable day case surgery in hospital, new restrictions on opening new ambulatory care practices and increased user fees for pharmaceuticals.

A reform that would have allowed individual sickness funds to decide whether or not to include certain treatments and services in their list of benefits to members was defeated under strong opposition from the funds themselves. Those lobbying against the change pointed out that if sickness funds were allowed to exclude certain services, this would in turn enable them to offer a reduced premium to attract younger and fitter contributors who may be confident they would not require such care – and effectively pass over older, poorer and less healthy clients (and the costs associated with them) to more generous funds (Busse and Riesberg 2000).

In December 2002 a cash crisis forced an unprecedented halt to operations at a German university hospital: it had already treated the total number of patients covered by the sickness fund budget, and was unwilling to treat up to 1,400 more, for each of which under the new arrangements it would be paid only 15% of its actual costs. The hospital was already €2.7 million in debt, and expecting further shortfalls in 2003 (Tuffs 2003a, b, c).

One other response to the rising cost pressures has been a substantial increase in recent years in the average rate of contribution to the sickness funds, up from 13.5% of gross earnings in 2001 to 14.3% in 2003 and 2004 (Busse and Riesberg 2004).

2 Rationalisation

The net reduction in hospital bed numbers that has taken place in Germany since 1990 has been largely at the expense of public sector beds (down almost 30% by 2002), and not-for-profit sector beds (down 8% by 2002) leaving a substantially increased share of beds in the private sector (up by 84% to 42,000 between 1990-2002, representing over 8% of general hospital beds) (Busse and Riesberg 2004:56).

Since German figures combine 'general and psychiatric' bed numbers, it is not clear to what extent this decline reflects the changes towards more community-based services to replace the previous heavy reliance on inpatient care. Psychiatric bed numbers have more than halved from 150,000 in 1975 to 69,000 in 1995 (Busse and Riesberg 2000).

3 Regulating drug costs

Reforms aimed at capping the rising level of spending on pharmaceuticals have included more than halving the medications that will be funded by sickness funds, from 45,000 to 20,000, and seeking to cap physicians' prescription drug budgets. The first 5% of any physician spending above their fixed ceiling would be shared between the relevant physician association: any spending more than 15% above target would have to be covered by the overspending physician (Garcia 2001).

---

140 The dramatic health gains, and especially increases in life expectancy, experienced in Eastern Germany after reunification are an unsung result of this substantial investment in health care, alongside other social spending and improved living standards (Busse and Riesberg 2004).

The most recent measures include incentives to sickness funds to promote ambulatory care, giving increased rebates for drugs dispensed in that setting, and a change in the method of reimbursing pharmacists, from a profit margin related to the cost of drugs (an incentive to promote more costly medication) to a fixed fee per item.

4 New models of care
The new user fees are designed to reduce the heavy use of primary care and prescription medicines.

Market-style reforms

1 Decentralisation
The long-standing division of responsibilities in Germany's health care system does not result from decentralisation: rather, the Länder have retained powers which pre-date the Federal government, and the sickness funds have maintained their role as set out under the nationwide health insurance scheme brought in 120 years ago by Chancellor Bismarck, partly to defuse trade union strength and tie workers more closely in to the developing capitalist system (Marrée and Groenewegen 1997). The Federal government only sets the general framework of the health care system, addressing issues of policy and finance.

2 Purchaser/provider split and contracts
Germany is a good example to show that the separation of purchaser from provider in a health care market, which has prevailed since the system was first established in 1883, is no guarantee of genuine competition – let alone of cost containment. The system is commonly described as 'top-heavy', wasteful and carrying excess capacity (Garcia 2001, Williamson 2003).

Indeed at around 11% of GDP, the €270 billion a year German health care system is the most costly in Europe, despite more than two decades of attempts at cost-containment (MSI 2000, Busse 2002:54). It is a system with a large degree of localised control in the hands of the 16 states (Länder) which retain responsibility for planning and investment in hospitals and health care facilities, as well as a variety of purchasing agencies – 300 competing sickness funds which finance the care for the 88% of people covered by Statutory Health Insurance.

3 Provider autonomy
Hospitals were given greater managerial freedoms in the 1990s, including a loosening of the requirement to document daily the nursing hours allocated to each patient (EHMA 2000). Hospitals are allowed to make profits.

4 Reform provider payments
Hospital funding was until 1996 effectively based on per diem payments, which clearly encourage longer stays and higher bed numbers: Germany has the sixth highest rate of hospital admission in Western Europe and, with Switzerland, the longest average length of stay (Busse and Riesberg 2000:65). Unlike the UK, where spending restrictions during the 1980s applied predominantly to the hospital sector, allowing increased spending by primary care services, Germany saw the costs of inpatient treatment rise by 16% between 1995 and 1999, compared with an overall increase of just 4% in health spending and a 7% rise in outpatient costs (MSI 2000).

Nevertheless Germany has retained a level of hospital bed provision 50% above the EU average, leaving an excess of capacity that has not only ensured the Germany has no waiting list, but recently forced health care providers to tour Europe seeking to sell spare capacity to patients from overseas (Agasi 2001, Garcia 2001, ref). Instant access to hospital care close to home means that Germany is unlikely to face major problems as a result of the liberalisation of health care markets in the EU. Proposals in the 2000 Reform Act for all hospital services other than psychiatry to be paid for on the basis of a fixed scale of case fees began on a voluntary basis in 2002 and has applied to all hospitals since 2004: the effects of this on the system as a whole are not yet clear (Busse and Riesberg 2004, Busse 2002).

5 Purchase services from private sector

Within a general 14% reduction in hospital beds 1990-1999, non-profit hospitals increased their share of the total even though 1% of beds closed, while for-profit private hospitals have witnessed an astonishing growth, with a 66% increase in beds since 1990, almost doubling their share of available beds from 3.7% to 7.1% in 1999.

However, the requirement to generate a profit on the hospitals' assets must exert an upward pressure on fees. Elsewhere in the system the private sector can be seen to be more expensive: in the ten years to 1999, fee-for-service payments for privately insured patients visiting ambulatory care specialists rose by an average 40% above the equivalent payments for patients covered by SHI. The longer-term impact of the reform of hospital funding may also reveal more obvious differences in cost between the public and private sectors.

6 Competition

Germany has competition between purchasers (the sickness funds) as well as between providers. Longer-term and controversial changes including steps to increase competition and private sector involvement in health care were discussed in a government policy document at the end of 2002 (Simonian 2002). But as Busse and Riesberg (2004:212) point out:

> True market competition is not possible, since the sickness funds have to offer nearly the same benefits for very similar contribution rates: in addition the range of providers is also the same since they are contracted collectively. In this situation it is not surprising that funds – particularly the more successful ones in terms of gaining new members – are demanding greater flexibility for selective contracting.

7 Privatisation

Privatising hospitals in Eastern Germany has resulted in double the level of private hospital beds in the East compared with the West. Busse (2002) argues that because most private hospitals have established contracts with the sickness funds and Länder, and are therefore regulated to ensure equal access and financial sustainability, the individual service user has no reason to draw a distinction between private and public hospitals, and may not even know which is which (Busse 2002:57).

Hospitals seeking to ride out the squeeze on prices from the sickness funds and utilise their capacity have been searching for private patients from Europe and beyond. In 2001, amid revelations that 20% of German hospital beds were empty, a new private company GerMedic visited Ireland, Denmark and Sweden offering 'package deal' operations in a network of 80 hospitals and clinics (Payne 2001).

More recently luxury hospitals in Berlin have focused efforts on drawing wealthy patients from Kuwait and Saudi Arabia who can pay €10,000-€15,000 for treatment, with foreign patient numbers increasing by up to 30% per year (Williamson 2005).

8 User Fees

1996 legislation looked to raise substantial new resources for health care through increased user fees for inpatient treatment, rehabilitation, drugs, dentistry and ambulance transport: but two years later almost all of these changes were reversed by the Act to Strengthen Solidarity in Statutory Health Insurance 1998 (Busse and Riesberg 2000). The attempts to cap spending on treatment and drug costs proved ineffective: fixed budgets were widely exceeded in 1996, creating a £3.7 billion deficit across the health insurance industry (Karcher 1997).

However, new fees of €10 for a first visit to a GP in any quarter have been imposed since January 2004[141]. The same reforms have also introduced co-payments for spectacles and prescriptions (10% of the cost of the drug up to a maximum of ten) and a ten daily co-payment for inpatient treatment. However co-payments are limited to 2% of annual gross income, or 1% for those with chronic illness (Riesberg and Busse 2003).

The implementation of the fees had been a controversial issue, with doctors protesting at the costs and time involved: but the new regulations were pushed through with the backing of both the Social Democratic-Green government and the Christian Democrat opposition, united in an attempt to generate savings beginning at €9.8 billion in 2004 (much of it from shifting costs to service users, with relatively small savings to be drawn from health care providers and drug companies), and rising to €23 billion by 2007. Only children under 18, pregnant women and preventive services are now exempt from charges: the previous exemption for the poor has been abolished (Busse and Riesberg 2004).

The regressive user fees are an attempt to deter patients from unnecessary visits, but will also help insurance companies pay off collective debts estimated at €3 billion (Tuffs 2003b, 2004a, 2004b).

From 2005, dentures will be excluded from the state health insurance scheme, and will require separate mandatory insurance – expected to save €3.5 billion. From 2006 employees' contributions (but not the employers') will increase to raise a further €5 billion (and shift the balance of contributions from 50.50 to 54% for employees and just 46% from employers) (Riesberg and Busse 2003).

9 Steps to control medical professionals

A variety of vested interests – 'a coalition of physicians, sickness funds, media and health product companies' (Busse and Riesberg 2000:16) have repeatedly been able effectively to repel or scale down the few attempts there have been to reform or control the system.

The system is also characterised by a weak primary care system, which does not have any 'gate-keeping' role, though the latest reforms include attempts to change this, with the development of incentives to persuade patients to seek a referral from a family doctor or paediatrician before visiting a specialist.

A dominant factor is the fundamental division between the office-based specialist ambulatory physicians, the most dominant section – on the one hand, and the hospital sector on the other. Since 1931 the ambulatory physicians have been able to maintain a near-monopoly on outpatient treatment, leaving the hospitals to deal purely with inpatient (and more recently some day-case) treatment (Busse 2002).

---

141 After a rush to see doctors throughout December before the charge came in.

10 Patient choice

There is no 'gate keeping system' of referrals into secondary care in Germany: patients are free to go to the provider of their choice (EHMA 2000).

11 PFI/PPP

No proposals for such schemes yet announced.

12 Privatisation

An area of private sector growth and domination is in the provision of intermediate and rehabilitation services, where more than two-thirds (69%) of the available beds are in for-profit private nursing homes, and just 15% in the public sector. Despite the implementation in 1994 of reforms designed to ensure that long-term care of the frail elderly would be covered by the sickness funds, these services are therefore not subject to public planning in terms of capacity. There have been attempts to create competition between providers on the basis of price and quality (Busse 2002:58-59).

The private insurance sector in this situation serves not to improve efficiency but to further complicate any process of reform. Fifty-two private health insurers, organised in the Association of Private Health Insurance Companies, share the largest voluntary health insurance market in Europe, with almost 14 million subscribers (Busse 2002:48).

An Arthur Andersen study in 2000 examining options for the next 15 years looked to a substantial reduction in the numbers of both hospitals and beds (down 25% and 40% respectively), an even bigger reduction in average length of stay in hospital, and the privatisation of much of the current public sector provision (Tuffs 2000). However, German hospital doctors pointed angrily to 'cherry picking' by the private sector, selecting the most profitable treatments, leaving the public sector to cover the harder and more expensive cases.

FRANCE

Market-driven reforms

1 Cash limits and spending cuts

The French health care system, consuming 10% of GDP (141 billion euro) in 2000, ranks just below Germany as the most expensive health care system in Europe (Dixon and Mossialos 2002). The share of spending has grown rapidly, from 7.6% of GDP in 1980 to 8.9% in 1990 (Imai et al 2000).

The 1995 Juppé Plan, much of which continued even after the electoral defeat of the government that enacted it, introduced a new tax – 0.5% of income – and instituted a system in which Parliament has been obliged each year to fix spending targets for each sector of health care.

Hospital staff staged protests and strikes against the 1997 budget cuts which attempted both to reduce hospital spending and make allocations fairer, with smaller cash increases for areas such as Paris and Ile de France which were seen as already over-provided (Eiro online 1997a, Bilous 1997). The resistance to these cutbacks brought a partial retreat by ministers, and a smaller cutback than had been planned in Paris. The differential allocation of spending continued in the following three years, with Paris and Ile de France receiving much smaller increases in hospital budgets than the country as a whole (Volovitch 2000a). The new Socialist government remained committed to the main features of the Plan, especially to holding down costs and cutting the numbers of hospital beds (Dorozynski 1997b).

The rate of growth in spending slowed for two years, but by 1998 reimbursements for health treatment were again rising well above the underlying rate of inflation (Imai 2000:20). The targets set by Parliament have also been routinely exceeded: in 2000 health spending for the first six months rose by double the rate agreed by Parliament (Dorozynski 2000b).

2003 began with the revelation that the sickness insurance fund was again deep in deficit, and likely to run further into the red, with a shortfall of €6.1 billion in 2002 rising to €8.2 billion in 2003. Despite a Parliamentary limit of 3.8%, spending growth for 2002 had been 7%. Concerns began to be expressed that the government strategy to tackle the soaring level of spending could be to break the link between 'top-up' insurance and the charges most patients have to pay to obtain treatment and prescriptions.

In May 2004 the health minister unveiled the 14th attempt since 1975 to rein in health spending, to reduce the annual 12.9 billion euro overspend and clear the accumulated 32 billion euro debt (Spurgeon 2004). The measures included new charges for visits to a GP and a new system effectively making GPs into gatekeepers referring patients for specialist care.

2 New sources of funding

In the autumn of 1997 the Socialist government announced plans to switch the funding of health insurance from salary deductions to income tax, meaning that income from investments and savings would also be taxed towards the cost of health care (Eiro online 1997b, Dixon and Mossialos 2002).

In 2000 this was followed by the introduction of a new system of Universal Health Insurance (CMU) which provides free health care to all those on incomes of less than £350 per month, many of whom may have not been properly covered for user fees prior to the scheme. Six million became eligible for free top-up health insurance (Volovitch 2000b).

3 Rationalisation

As a system rated top of the WHO's controversial 2000 'league tables' (Kmietowicz 2000), and generating high levels of public satisfaction, French health care has also proved a problem for those seeking to contain costs through reforms and rationalisation: no other system in Europe has been subjected since the 1990s to so many strikes by health workers opposing government reform efforts. Disputes on a variety of grievances arising from the reform agenda have involved hospital staff, junior doctors, general practitioners and midwives (Herbert 1996, 1997, Bilous 1997, EIRO online 1997, Dorozynski 1997a, 2000a, 2002a, Volovitch 2000a, 2002a, Dufour 2001).

The longer-term effect of the caps on spending from the 1990s eventually made itself felt early in 2000 in a wave of hospital bed closures and staff shortages, which in turn led to a series of strikes by hospital workers, again including large numbers of doctors. Up to 20% of hospital posts were vacant, with shortages of nursing staff combining with a loss of up to 80% of newly qualified medical graduates to private practice (Dorozynski 2000a). Staff shortages and low pay also triggered strikes by doctors, nurses and other health workers in 2002, while emergency and maternity services in parts of the country were struggling to cope with high levels of demand at the same time as a lack of nurses and doctors (Dorozynski 2002a, 2002b).

Partly as a result of generally successful rearguard actions by health workers, but also partly because of the extent to which the hospitals are embedded in the local political structures (with the local Mayor chairing each hospital board), the rate of change has been relatively modest. But this also means that there are vast disparities in levels of health care provision, especially hospital services.

Acute bed numbers average 4.2 per 1,000 population across the country, while local provision ranges from 2.5 in some *départements* to 6 in others and a massive 9.8 in Paris (Dixon and Mossialos 2002:41). Access to certain types of care, and waiting times for treatment vary widely between different parts of the country. Efforts to reduce local inequalities in access to hospital services have been hampered by the fact that improvements in under-provided areas imply a reduction in existing services in areas which have retained more generous provision, and which often carry more political influence [142] (Imai et al 2000).

In the mid 1990s a government drive to reduce bed numbers by 22,000 was accompanied by a report from the Inspectorate General of Social Affairs exposing a range of financial irregularities and abuses of their position by senior doctors. Yet the report also revealed the obstacles to any rapid rationalisation of hospital services, pointing to the experience in one hospital where it had taken 67 staff meetings, totalling 17 days, to close just nine beds (Dorozynski 1994). In the event, 17,000 hospital beds were cut in the years 1994-1998, though it appears that many of these were available beds rather than beds in daily use. In 1999 the government announced a target of closing another 24,000 beds from a total of 275,000 (Volovitch 2000a).

With such entrenched opposition to bed reductions, and with funding arrangements that effectively encourage demand-led growth, and enable producer-led demand, France has the second highest provision of beds in Western Europe, the highest rate of admissions to hospital care, and the highest consumption of pharmaceuticals.

Attempts to hold down spending date back to the early 1980s, when levels of expenditure rose more rapidly than insurance payments received: in 1983-4 global budgets were imposed on public hospitals, while there were also attempts to control prices charged by ambulatory care doctors and for prescription drugs.

These measures failed to contain the rising costs of the system: by 1995 the health sector of the insurance funds was facing a total deficit of almost £11.5 billion, forcing new measures at national level to generate the funds to pay it off (Dorozynski 1995a, Imai et al 2000:17). As a result of this the 1995 Juppé Plan was developed, which set out both to remedy the deficit through an injection of tax funding, but also to hold down overall spending and costs of treatment. Funding would be allocated on a new basis to hospitals by regional authorities, while numbers of hospital beds were to be reduced (Dorozynski 1995b). The proposals triggered strikes by doctors whose unions united against the Plan's call for doctors to face penalties if medical spending exceeded targets set by parliament (Dorozynski 1996).

4 Regulating drug costs

The new reforms make no new proposals to regulate drug costs: a study a few years ago found that more than 10% of 8,000 listed medications were ineffective, and they were to be removed from the list of reimbursable drugs (Dixon and Mossialos 2002).

5 New models of care

The new plan for a €1 charge for each visit to a GP, and for consultations on tests and x-rays, is intended to give people a 'sense of responsibility' – and raise €1 billion a year.

---

142 Successive British governments encountered similar difficulties when they tried to implement the 1976 RAWP exercise which attempted to equalise resources for different areas while restraining overall·spending (Caldwell et al 1998).

Market-style reforms

1 Decentralisation

French health care remains strongly centralised.

2 Purchaser/provider split and contracts

As a mixture of public and private provision, largely financed through a system of compulsory insurance topped up by additional insurance schemes, French health care has a long history of separating purchasers from providers: the additional spending arises not from the lack of this element of a 'market system', but from the perverse incentives and 'market failure' common to insurance-based schemes.

3 Provider autonomy

In 1991 a Hospital Reform Act brought regional planning of hospitals and gave greater local management autonomy (Freeman 1998).

4 Provider payment reform

While public sector hospitals are still largely funded through global budgets which give little incentive to increase performance or quality, the private sector is free to 'cherry pick' the most lucrative and least demanding specialties, leaving emergency treatment, psychiatric care, major operations, life-saving treatment and research to the public sector hospitals. It is frequent for private sector providers to transfer more complicated cases to public sector hospitals. Imai and colleagues argue:

> The French health care system is thus a blend of an entirely public system like the British NHS, and a private sector which operates on market principles as in the United States. [...] The financial distortions in the system have resulted in a segmentation of supply by type of care but without any price competition (Imai et al 2000:24).

The same authors warn that any new system of payment based on Diagnosis-Related Groups could worsen rather than resolve the problems of cream-skimming, leaving the public hospitals dealing with the (more expensive) care of the chronic sick and disadvantaged groups, while the private sector could concentrate on those areas of care where it enjoys a relative advantage: it could even press some public hospitals to seek ways of selecting which patients they would prefer to treat.

5 Purchase services from private sector

The private sector may appear to charge a lower rate than the public sector for some hospital care, but its selective provision and its incentive to drive up demand for care mans that it can still exert a constant upward pressure both on prices and on costs, intensifying competition for scarce qualified staff.

As health spending lurched out of control in the first six months of 2000, the largest increase was in private practice (Dorozynski 2000b). In the spring of 2000, the government agreed to pay an annual 'public service commitment bonus' beginning at £2,500 to hospital doctors who had no private sector work, to compensate for their lower level of earnings. In 2001 private clinics staged a two-day strike complaining against 'unfair competition' from public hospitals, which had led to some clinics beginning to lose money – and secured a £300 million subsidy from the government: this followed a £400 million financial boost for public sector hospitals voted by Parliament earlier the same year (Dorozynski 2001).

However, the problem is not just at the hospital level. Two-thirds of French doctors are in private practice and paid on a fee-for-service basis (Durand-Zaleski et al 1997), and no French government has attempted to control their escalation of costs by instituting a system of capitation funding analogous to the funding of health care providers in Britain (Dixon 1997).

There is already evidence of some doctors, mainly specialists, charging above the reimbursement rate for consultations and treatment, while doctors' organisations continue to lobby for 'free pricing'. From a government point of view the easiest way to seek to restrain overall costs would be a 'reform' which secures the support or acquiescence of the medical lobby, leaving individual patients to pay an increasing share of the cost of their own care.

6 Competition

Freeman (1998) has argued that both France and Germany are prime examples of health care systems that could be improved and made more efficient by the introduction of a degree of competition and market forces. However there is little sign that a political coalition seeking to impose such a regime could prevail in France over vested interests which include not only a large public sector, but a large and influential private sector that continues to profit within the system as it is presently organised.

7 Privatisation

It might seem that the different factor driving spending upwards and inducing producer-led demand in France is not moral hazard but the relatively large scale of the private for-profit sector, which accounts for almost a third (29%) of hospital beds and employs 300,000 staff (Volovitch 2000a). Dixon and Mossialos (2002) point out that France and Germany can offer patients a free choice of health care provider 'because of a surplus of providers' – but all of these providers carry a cost.

8 User fees

Since the early 1990s the various attempts to bring spending under tighter control by increasing user fees have largely failed because virtually all costs are covered by insurance. Patients have been largely shielded from each increase in user charges, most of which are subsequently reimbursed: some are even reimbursed at a higher level than the original charge[143], and Imai and colleagues argue that this inevitably creates a situation of 'moral hazard' in which excess health services are consumed:

> Any insurance plan that lacks adequate safeguards will encourage individuals to alter their behaviour and ask the insurer to bear the consequences of decisions they would probably not have made had there been no insurance (Imai et al 2000:26).

It is not clear however why this objection should apply so dramatically to the French system and not, for example, to the Danish system, which also provides very prompt and generous coverage to all, without levying at point of use.

9 Steps to control medical professionals

French medical interns staged prolonged angry strikes in the spring of 1997 against the

---

143 Most of the voluntary health insurance schemes which reimburse patients for charges pay 150% of the official rate for a basic dental prosthesis. Ten percent of schemes reimburse more than 285% (Dixon and Mossialos 2002:32).

prospect that doctors could face fines as high as £1,550 a year if spending limits were breached (Dorozynski 1995a)[144].

When French ministers tried to bring in a new system establishing a network of 'referring doctors' to act as a form of gatekeepers, limiting the right of patients to seek consultations with a variety of GPs and specialists, it received a limited response, with only 10% of GPs signing the new contract. The incentive for patients is that they pay only a third of the standard £11.50 consultation fee to see a 'referring doctor' (Dorozynksi 1998c).

A further step towards a GP system took place in 1998, when the major union representing family doctors agreed that patients should be encouraged to join the list of a single GP for treatment and referral: while the patient would no longer have to pay the doctor for each consultation, the 'subscribing GP' would be paid a capitation fee for each patient on their list, plus a £12 fee for each consultation up to a maximum of 7,500 a year. However the scheme was immediately denounced by other GP unions and by organisations representing specialists, who feared a decline in consultations (Dorozynski 1998b).

In the summer of 2000 the unions representing independent doctors which took the hardest line against the government's policies gained ground in elections, while those most sympathetic to the reforms lost out (Volovitch 2000c).

10 Patient choice

Chambaud (1993) summed up the political pressures that have helped to shape today's contradictions in the health care system:

> In France there is widespread support for the three principles on which the national healthcare system is based: funding through social insurance which covers all health and social care; the co-existence of publicly and privately owned hospitals; and the public's almost total freedom to choose a doctor, whether generalist or specialist (Chambaud 1993:24).

11 PFI/PPP

No reported movement.

Western Europe – the Hybrid system

NETHERLANDS (shorter country summary)

The complex health care system that has evolved in the Netherlands has been described as a combination of the German system of social insurance and the US system of private insurance: 'few countries have so much private activity where the government is simultaneously omnipresent': the result has been a high-cost system of questionable quality (Schippers 2002).

Successive efforts at reform, beginning in 1987 with the Dekker Committee's attempts to implement ideas from Alan Enthoven (Van de Venn and Schut 2000) have attempted to inject 'regulated competition' and incentives for efficiency into a system which has maintained a largely private, not-for-profit provider network since the middle ages, and which first introduced forms of health insurance in 1850, with the main outlines of today's system

---

144 Eventually in 1999 the imposition of collective fines on doctors was ruled unconstitutional, and had to be abandoned (Dorozynski 1999).

imposed on Dutch citizens by the Nazi occupation in 1941 (Reilly 2001).

The Dekker proposals, later modified under health minister Simons, set out to introduce 'managed competition' into a highly regulated system in which a very large minority (31%) of the population on relatively high incomes (£18,700 a year in 2001) is required by law to buy private insurance cover for their day-to-day health needs, while most of the rest, other than civil servants and local government staff, are covered by compulsory social insurance 'sickness funds', supplemented by universal compulsory insurance against 'catastrophic' risks such as costs of long-term care, severe mental illness and mental handicap.

Despite the division of the population into different schemes, everyone uses the same hospitals, doctors and clinics, at least 90% of which are in the independent sector, although for-profit hospitals are forbidden by law (Reilly 2001, Van de Venn and Schut 2000). The main difference is that members of the 30 sickness funds are treated under contracts which they have been obliged to negotiate with all interested local providers, thus delivering treatment free at point of use: by contrast those with one of over 50 private insurance plans are obliged to pay for their care on a fee-for-service basis, and then claim back the costs afterwards.

Eighty-five percent of funding for Dutch health care comes from 'public' sources (social insurance, mandatory private insurance and tax subsidies) while general taxation contributes just over 4% and patient co-payments amounted to over 8% of health spending in 1998 (Schippers 2002). There are elaborate arrangements to ensure that private insurers will accept older and high-risk patients at a legally set premium, with insurers compensated from a surcharge on others with private insurance: however there remain concerns that sickness funds and private schemes could be tempted to evade the various regulations and attempt 'cream skimming' younger, healthier subscribers, while seeking to deter the elderly and those with greater health needs (Den Exter et al 2004).

Attempts by successive governments to balance greater competition and the expansion of large-scale private insurance with ensuring equity and access have been hampered by EU legislation which effectively forbids any measure that would compel a private insurer to accept any individual who would be predicted to generate a loss.

The outcome of various reforms since the early 1990s has been to open up competition between the sickness funds, lifting restrictions that limited them to their original geographic region, and allowing them to recruit subscribers nation-wide. Funds have also been made responsible for managing an increasing level of financial risk, which has risen from just 2.5% of turnover in 1995 to 36% in 2000. Their main funding comes through the Healthcare Insurance Board (CVZ) drawn from workplace taxes, with employees paying 1.75% and employers contributing 6.35% of pay up to €25,000. The funds receive just 90% of their costs, and are allowed flexibility in how they cover the remaining 10%, much of which will be collected as flat-rate per capita premium payments by members.

New freedoms for funds to negotiate with hospitals and providers on what had previously been fixed prices – including for the first time an option for sickness funds to negotiate selective contracts with providers in place of their 50-year legal obligation to offer contracts at standard prices with any provider seeking to offer services – brought a reduction in the cost of some treatments by up to a third, while the lowest sickness fund flat rate premium was a full 30% below the highest in 2000.

However the competition has also resulted in the diversion of resources from front-line health care into administration, with 'increasing investments in cost-accounting systems by hospitals and others health care institutions' (Van de Venn and Schut 2000), while Rutten

(2004) notes the failure of the reforms to contain a 'healthcare cost explosion'.

There is also evidence of a growing market concentration as funds and providers seek ways of working more closely together to maximise their surpluses and minimise risk. And where the government explicitly sought to contain costs and ensure access, as in the case of cover for 'catastrophic' risks, there have been moves to eliminate competition and regulate prices and provision.

The Netherlands system has continued to create major anomalies: as a relatively high-cost system, it has nevertheless imposed global budgeting limits on hospitals which have resulted in growing waiting lists and capacity problems (Reilly 2001), while even after government intervention to reduce bed numbers, bed occupancy levels remain astonishingly low, at 58.4% by far the lowest of any in Western Europe other than Turkey (den Exter et al 2004).

While the funds and providers have been moving closer together, governments have dropped the initial centrepiece of the reforms, which was the notion of a single national health insurance scheme. This was dropped without explanation in 1995 (Van de Venn and Schut 2000), although a version was resurrected by health minister Els Borst, in her 2001 plan which would scrap the division between sickness funds and private health insurance, and would offer additional choices including the option to pay lower premiums in exchange for accepting limitations in the range of providers that would be available. A contentious element of the scheme was the introduction of a universal co-payment of €100 per year. Since then repeated changes of government have left the shape of future reforms in doubt.

Den Exter and colleagues (2001) note that the division of the population into two separate insurance regimes creates noticeable effects, especially at the margin, where:

> ...one euro income above or below the threshold determines whether a person pays an income-related contribution or a (health) risk-related premium, and whether spouses and children are covered (almost) free of charge.

Robinson (1998) and den Exter (2004) note the coalition of interest groups that have obstructed the drive for market-style reforms in the Netherlands over the last 18 years: Robinson identifies no fewer than six major groups opposing the reforms – employers' associations concerned over labour costs, trade unions concerned over equity and access, hospitals and service providers worried about the squeeze on prices, medical professionals, sickness funds and private insurance companies: interestingly the wider public, as consumers of health care services, and their elected political representatives are not included, although their support for market-style reforms could hardly be assumed.

More recent efforts to push through reforms have seen the introduction of a controversial 'no claims bonus' system which will effectively land higher costs on those who suffer most ill-health and therefore make most use of health care services. The scheme is designed to deter excessive use of health services, and will refund the difference to patients whose use of hospital and pharmacy services add up to less than €255 per year. Even though GP services have now been exempted from this scheme, after attacks from the Dutch Association of General Practitioners, it is expected to save around £1 billion a year. Patients are expected to receive an average €20 refund each year, while around half the population are expected to lose out, among them those facing chronic complaints, the elderly and people with disabilities (Sheldon 2004a).

At the end of 2004 a manifesto opposing the extension of market forces into health care from January 2005 (involving the negotiation of prices for elective treatment such as knee, hip and cataract operations) attracted the support of almost 40 professors, doctors and hospital managers concerned that the result would be a new downward pressure on prices and quality of care (Sheldon 2004b).

Eastern Europe and Russia – Ex-Semashko systems

Overview

The fall of the Berlin Wall in 1989 led to most of the former 'Eastern Block' countries of Central and Eastern Europe (CEE) and the Newly Independent States of the former Soviet Union (NIS) beginning a process of political and economic transition, in which full and partial privatisation of previously state-owned and centrally controlled services has been widespread. As we have noted in earlier chapters this process has been systematically encouraged by the active involvement of the World Bank and its related organisations – perhaps most conspicuously in the former Soviet republics of Central Asia, which were perceived as easier to persuade of the merits of more rapid and far-reaching market-style reforms (Staines and Lovelace 1999).

In all of the CEE and NIS countries, where the main productive forces had been nationalised and under centralised control, health care systems had essentially been based on the Soviet Semashko model. But although they have all been urged in the same basic direction of reform by USAID, the World Bank, and in many cases their own domestic advocates of private medicine and private health insurance, not all countries have looked in precisely the same direction or moved at the same pace when it has come to the process of reform.

Nor have the arguments for reform been identical or completely straightforward. Afford (2001) argues that while the ostensible aim of the reforms that have taken place across the various countries has been to improve quality of care and make services more locally responsive, the need for what have in many cases been collapsing economies to cut costs and rein in government spending has been a key motivating factor.

Of course a reduction of government spending and collective provision can also be seen as offering new openings for private sector medical services: one organisation promoting investment in private medicine in CEE countries sums up the situation, noting approvingly:

- Change of method of financing from central control to insurance-based systems
- The gradual introduction of market principles between providers of care
- A general recognition that the public system will remain under-funded and therefore will be complemented with private funding and insurance.
(oresaventures.com 2003)

As one of the pioneering private medical firms sums up:

It all adds up to an unprecedented opening for daring entrepreneurial companies willing to brave the waters (D'Amato 2000).

Most CEE countries have looked to create, or in some cases resurrect, Bismarck-style systems (Marrée and Groenewegen 1997). Indeed the candidate countries for EU membership have 'experienced "market forces" to a considerably larger extent than have the EU member states' in the years since 1990 (EHMA 2000).

The Semashko system, established in 1918 in the early days of the Soviet revolutionary republic, was based upon the principle of delivering free health care for the entire population, funded from the central state budget. It was distinguished not only by the extent of centralised control and by a heavy reliance on hospitals and large numbers of relatively low-paid doctors, (reflecting an overriding early concern with treating and containing communicable diseases (Tchernjavski 1998, Afford 2001:5)) but also by the lack of a functioning primary care system based on generalist family doctors. Under a Semashko system, primary care is delivered by specialists based in outpatient polyclinics covering each area. In the Soviet Union this structure was also supplemented by extensive occupational health facilities for industrial workers (Marrée and Groenewegen 1997).

Another aspect of the Semashko system which is still reflected in the various health care systems emerging in Eastern and Central Europe is the undervaluing of medical staff, who in a curious inversion of the elitist attitudes that have emerged in western capitalist societies, have been regarded as part of the 'non-productive' sector, and are often amongst the lowest-paid employees. Semashko systems imposed on CEE countries after the Second World War characteristically broke up professional organisations of doctors and incorporated them instead into generic trade unions of health workers. In 1995, Russian surgeons were typically earning just £45 per month, while 70% of Russian health professionals were paid below the official poverty level (Ingram 1995).

Prior to the Second World War, limited social insurance schemes had operated in many east European countries including Czechoslovakia, Hungary, Romania and later Poland and Bulgaria. And although the basic system installed under Soviet influence in all of the post-war 'socialist' states was based on Semashko, there were variations in a number of countries: Czechoslovakia developed district and regional level 'institutes of national health', Hungary established local district doctors as the gateway to outpatient and hospital care. East Germany, which had previously experienced the original Bismarck system, retained a small private sector of physicians and allowed the church to own and run some hospitals. Poland too retained a private sector, while it also developed a more integrated model of service (Busse 2000, Gaál et al 1999, Karski et al 1999, Hinkov et al 1999).

From 1990 onwards, as evidenced by the WHO European Observatory's *Health in Transition* series, new governments, aspiring to market-style economies and encouraged by loans and advice from the World Bank and the EU, began to remodel health care services. The common features have been:

- Decentralisation
- The move from tax funding towards insurance-based schemes (which fall most heavily on working people, leaving wealth and other unearned income relatively untaxed)
- The privatisation of dentistry, pharmacy services and a variety of other professional services (though hospitals – many of them over-sized and dilapidated after years of under-investment – have in general remained within the public sector).

However, the pattern has not been as consistent and complete – nor the information as accessible – as in previous country studies, and in many cases the reform process is still incomplete. The two country summaries in this section therefore focus on a reduced list of the better-documented reforms that have been taking place.

POLAND

Market-driven reforms

Rationalisation

By 1997 numbers of hospitals had remained largely unchanged since 1980, with levels of hospital admission slightly higher and average length of stay slightly reduced (Karski 1999). The controversial 1999 reforms also involved a rationalisation of hospital services, with the loss of up to 30,000 jobs in 2000 (PAP 2000). Opposition to these changes was muted by the fact that they came at a time of plunging union membership in Poland and many CEE countries: in 2002 just 20% of Poland's eligible health workers were in a trade union (Vaknin 2002).

Market-style reforms

1 Decentralisation

Poland has been an example of rather hesitant and faltering moves along the lines of market-style and market-driven reforms. Early moves towards decentralisation of health care in the early 1990s left catchment populations of less than a million, which were too small to sustain the planned network of tertiary level specialist hospitals. The World Bank pointed out that such 'extreme decentralisation' had therefore created new inefficiencies (World Bank 1993:163).

2 Purchaser/provider split and contracts

The Health Insurance Act introduced in 1997 and ratified in amended form in 1999 set out to create an internal market system through the introduction of regional health insurance funds, but proved highly controversial, and forced the government to look towards a reinstatement of strategic planning – to the horror of those seeking greater freedoms for the private sector and a free market involving competition between insurance funds (Medicover 2003).

According to Marek Balicki, chair of the Polish social policy and health committee:

> Accountability has become fuzzy, there is a lack of stewardship, a lack of contracting procedures and talk of corruption that has been growing steadily (Lyall 2002).

3 Privatisation and private health insurance

The 1999 reforms aimed to open the way for private health insurance to compete for subscribers against the regional funds: but this scheme was delayed as a result of public opposition. The regional funds ran up deficits in 1999 and 2000, forcing the government to increase the payroll tax, while the funds imposed limits on outpatient treatment, creating waiting lists, and squeezed payments for hospital care.

This has prompted the hospitals to establish a two-tier system, with preferential care for those prepared to pay an additional fee over and above the scale paid by the insurance funds: and this has helped create a market for private health care and insurance (Tapay 2001, oresaventures.com 2003).

The privatisation of health care provision is still on course to reach levels higher than anywhere else in Europe. By 1999 an estimated 90% of dentists and two-thirds of doctors were working privately, though most hospitals were still in the public sector (Karski et al 1999). The expansion of private medicine has been held back by the generally low levels of incomes: one estimate in 1998 suggested only 15% of Poles could afford private dental treatment (Hunter 1998) [145].

Forty to forty-five percent of total health care is expected to be delivered by private providers by 2005, in a health care market expected to be worth a total of 17 billion euro annually. This would be just 450 euro per head of Polish population, a figure seen by the private sector as evidence that 'healthcare in Poland is under-funded and is likely to remain under strong budget pressure for years to come' (oresaventures.com 2003).

The World Bank subsidiary the International Finance Corporation has funded efforts by the private company Medicover to expand its operations in Poland, though Medicover insists that its goal is not to attempt to undermine or replace the public hospitals but to:

> ...help foster an appropriate mix of private and public health care systems in a period of dramatic sectoral reforms (D'Amato 2000).

The private sector claims to 'promote cost-consciousness and better care', but laments the residual opposition to privatised services in countries used to care free at point of use:

> Perhaps the biggest hurdle facing Medicover and other commercial entrants in the region's health sector is the fundamental lack of a popular consensus regarding the role of private money in financing health care and the widespread expectation that such services lead to improperly unequal outcomes (D'Amato 2000).

RUSSIA

Market-driven reforms

Cash limits and spending cuts

A growing crisis in Soviet health care had been noted by analysts from the mid-1980s, but the turning point in triggering far-reaching reforms to the original Semashko system came with the fall of the Berlin Wall in 1989 and the rapid unravelling of the Soviet Union and its relations with the CEE countries and the states that were to achieve independence from the Russian Federation at the end of 1991.

Between 1991 and 1998 public spending on health shrank in real terms by 33%, while levels of contributions raised by the workplace insurance scheme were just over a third the amount required to fund its basic entitlements. The decision to institute a health insurance system, as a way to pump additional resources into health care at a time when the slump in GDP was putting a huge strain on government resources, was made in 1992-93. But as critics of the reform pointed out, introducing a payroll tax at a time when many businesses are struggling even to pay wages simply moves the problem from one part of the economy to another (Ingram 1995). Many employers simply failed to pay the contributions: others were already filing for bankruptcy.

---

145 Meanwhile Polish doctors have been existing on salaries averaging just £4,200 per year. Poland's accession to the EU in 2004 is widely expected to trigger an exodus by doctors and health professionals in search of higher pay and better resources elsewhere in Europe (Burgermeister 2004b).

Many regions by 1998 were facing a collapse of investment in new equipment and seeking cash savings through wholesale closures of local hospitals and beds. In Kursk (near the Ukraine border) 14 out of 63 district hospitals had closed, while primary care had been 'devastated'. In Yaroslavl (close to Moscow) there was funding for only 40% of inpatients' nutritional needs; and in Saratov (south of the Volga) the budget would not even stretch to buying enough bandages (Tchernjavski 1998).

There are few up-to-date overviews of the evolution of the Russian health care system, but it seems that the chaos continues. Dmitriev and colleagues (2000) reported to the IMF that in the absence of sufficient money to pay for the promised benefits there was a choice between cutting the cost of health care services or imposing 'co-payments' from patients. As for the attempt to create competition, supposedly one key reason for introducing the insurance scheme in the first place:

> It is difficult to make reliable assessments of the existence and extent of competition between and among insurers. A general opinion is that there is no such competition (Dmitriev et al 2000:2).

In March 2002 Interfax reported that 41 of Russia's 89 regions owed back wages to their health workers, while Russian health minister Yuri Shevchenko announced that 500 medical workers were under investigation for offences ranging from accepting bribes through issuing fake medical certificates and reselling medicines for-profit (Vaknin 2002).

Early in 2003 a World Bank document summed up the situation in Russia's health sector:

> ...a complex picture of weak governance at the federation level, inefficient allocation of resources despite financial constraints at the regional level, inequities across and within regions, as well as underperformance in terms of aggregate health status (World Bank 2003d:5).

While an unstable economy limits government funds and limits possibilities for increased public or private financing of health care, Russia faces a dual epidemic of drug resistant TB and HIV/AIDS which, if left unchecked, could reduce GDP by over 4% by 2010 and by over 10% by 2020 (Cullinan 2001, World Bank 2003:5).

The most recent survey for the European Observatory's Health Care Systems in Transition series concludes that although the reforms were drawn up aiming to preserve universal access to a basic package of care, the expected efficiency savings have not been achieved, and that 'a de facto rationing now takes place without scrutiny'. Increasing out-of-pocket payments mean that equity is 'clearly being compromised' (Tragakes and Lessof 2003).

A *BMJ* correspondent has reported a renewed attempt at a 'root and branch reform' of the health care system 'that could see half the country's medical professionals given the sack'. The plan would close upwards of 500,000 hospital beds and axe 300,000 doctors and health workers (Osborn 2004).

Market-style reforms

1 Decentralisation

Tchernjavski (1998) points to localised experiments in decentralisation and new funding systems in Leningrad and Kemorovo going back to 1988. Kemorovo was one of the first areas to pilot a compulsory health insurance programme which in 1992 began collecting income-related payroll tax from employers, and subsidies from local authorities and competing with private insurance schemes.

The scheme permitted primary care practitioners to retain any savings made through reducing referrals to hospitals, and succeeded in reducing admissions and hospital bed numbers (Tchernjavski 1998).

The abolition of the power of central bodies to plan and set targets for local and regional health care provision appears to have been the signal not for a constructive development of decentralised planning but for a chaotic descent into localism, with growing levels of inequality, while the expected market discipline arising from competition between insurance companies and providers has either not developed at all or failed to deliver the expected advantages.

2 Privatisation

Extremely low levels of spending on health care (estimated by the WHO at just 2.2% of GDP in 1997), and the context of rapid economic decline during much of the 1990s has left little scope for the expansion of a private sector even while the state-run system has been increasingly discredited. By 1998 hospitals were still 'exclusively' owned by the public sector, while privatisation had been largely restricted to the usual front-runners: pharmacies, dentistry and ophthalmology (Tchernjavski 1998).

3 Patient choice

The promised expansion of consumer choice has not materialised, except for those wealthy enough to pay privately, who can choose freely. According to Tragakes and Lessof (2003) the only sector in which quality of care appears to have improved is the private sector.

Shorter country summaries – ex-Semashko systems

CZECH REPUBLIC

In both the Czech Republic and in Slovakia the health care system (which had been separated into two ministries of health after 1968) was decentralised to create a partly privatised Bismarck-style social insurance system with competing sickness funds, each bidding for subscribers on the basis of offering more generous benefits, and with subscribers allowed to change fund as often as every three months. In the Czech Republic primary care was privatised, as were ambulatory specialists and later some hospitals.

Patients were free to choose any provider, who would then be reimbursed on a fee-for-service basis. As the EHMA point out, this, perhaps the most extreme marketising reform in Eastern European health care, soon led to a crisis of provider-led demand, which forced all but nine of the 27 new sickness funds into bankruptcy – and this in turn rebounded on hospitals and providers, who were not paid for services delivered. The government was forced to step in and restrict the competition between providers, imposing a uniform list of benefits. The reform also changed the system of provider payment to introduce prospective capitation-based payments (EHMA 2000:57)[146].

The Czech reforms, including decentralisation and privatisation, have nevertheless led to an increase in spending on health care, rising to above 9% of GDP in 2001 (Medicover

---

146 Slovakia, too, allowed a proliferation of competing sickness funds, all but five of which then collapsed, although only a few hospitals have been privatised (EHMA 2000: 57).

2002a). The four-fold increase in spending and the substantial increase in the share of GDP spent on health (from 5.2% in 1990) has run alongside a reduction in the proportion funded publicly, although the public share of Czech health spending is still higher than every EU country other than Luxembourg (Marrée and Groenewegen 1997:12, Busse 2000).

Perhaps surprisingly, after a reduction in the early 1990s, the Czech Republic has seen an increase since 1996 in the number of acute hospital beds, hospital admissions, and hospital admissions per head of population, with a larger number of frail older patients being admitted to hospital for lack of suitable alternative care in what will soon be the world's oldest population, with as many as 41% aged over 60 (Busse 2000, Afford 2001, Kalvach 2001).

Although most health care providers are now privatised, only 9% of hospital beds are in private hospitals. A limiting factor in any further privatisation of hospitals is the lack of funds to purchase or invest in facilities, which generate at best limited surpluses, as well as a lack of public and professional support for any further extension of privatisation.

SLOVAKIA

A sombre assessment of the pitfalls of the reform package adopted underlines the contradictions in many market-style policies. Six years after the health insurance system had been introduced the insurance companies were facing debts totalling over 12% of their total resources. The switch from tax funding to payroll-based insurance suffered as a result of the economic downturn, in which many employers closed down without paying off contributions owing, and a decision by the government to cut its share of contributions to just a tenth of the amount indicated in the Act on Health Insurance (Hlavacka and Skackova 2000).

The proliferation of health insurance funds, far from improving efficiency, led to an increase in transaction costs. The aim of a shift towards primary care was not achieved: and the impact of patient choice on health care providers was to persuade them to compete for clients by prescribing more and more expensive drugs.

Hlavacka and Skackova conclude that a 'pluralist' health insurance market may be affordable in the wealthier countries with more advanced economies, but is a model requiring 'a great deal of financial resources' and offering few incentives for efficient behaviour by hospitals. They also note that workplace insurance implemented, as in Slovakia, proportional to income but with a ceiling on contributions is a regressive method of funding health care: the new system has left health workers on very low pay while not delivering the promised cost containment or cost-effectiveness (up. cit. 69-70).

HUNGARY

Hungary too has moved to implement far-reaching reforms that re-established social insurance as the basic method of funding health care, supplanting the National Health Service that had been established in 1975. By 1989 the Hungarian government was spending 4.6% of GDP on health care, though this was supplemented by a systematic use of gratuity payments, unofficial payments equivalent to as much as 0.6% of GDP. The government elected in 1990 developed a policy based on the 'right to health care on the basis of insurance', establishing a free choice of doctor, an expansion of primary care, a reduction in hospital care (but an expansion in long-stay beds) and encouraging greater privatisation. Almost 7,000 family medical practices were privatised in 2000.

The switch from tax-funding to insurance served to hold down public spending as required by the IMF, but at the expense of increasing costs for working people. A survey at the turn of the century found 82% of households could not afford the health care they need – possibly because of the continued increase in gratuity payments (Marrée and Groenewegen 1997:82-3; ILO 2001:5, Lewis 2001). However, private sector organisations have expressed impatience at the slow progress towards further reform and privatisation (oresaventures.com 2003).

As with other CEE and NIS countries, Hungary's health system reforms began at a point where GDP was falling in real terms, leading to an increase in the share of GDP spent on health care. However, the growth of unemployment in Hungary has had an impact on a system based on workplace insurance, resulting in deficits in the social insurance fund. Gaál and colleagues (1999) calculate that real terms health spending fell by 21% between 1989 and 1996, and spending per head in 1997 was just over a third of the EU average.

Numbers of acute hospital beds have been reduced by 19% since 1990, though few hospitals have closed and many of the beds were not fully operational – resulting in relatively few savings and loss of jobs. Numbers of hospital admissions have proportionally increased, giving Hungary the second highest rate of hospital admissions in the WHO's European Region, and average lengths of stay have remained high, increasing in 1996-97 (Gaál et al 1999:49).

Most privatisation has been confined to pharmacy services and primary care: the growth of privatisation in the hospital sector has been hampered by the limited spending power of the majority of the population. Some hospitals have created private wards with enhanced facilities for a supplementary fee, but by 1999 just 6% of hospital beds were privately owned, including church-owned hospitals.

The absence of any substantial private health insurance system means that the gradually rising share of private funding for health care (17% in 1996) consists entirely of out-of-pocket payments, part of the increase driven by reductions in the package of benefits covered by compulsory health insurance and by payment for medicines, which have increased six-fold since 1991 (Marrée and Groenewegen 1997:91, Gaál et al 1999).

BULGARIA

As late as 1999 the Bulgarian system was still based largely on the Semashko system – tax-funded, largely publicly provided and hospital-led – though legislation in the early 1990s permitted private medicine and devolved responsibility for health services to municipalities. A new Bismarck-style insurance system, though with a single National Health Insurance Fund receiving compulsory payments from a payroll tax, was initiated by legislation in 1998, but due to be phased in by 2001. Privatisation was largely confined to pharmacies laboratories and dental treatment, with just 16 private hospitals by the end of 1998, though a dozen private health insurance schemes had been established (Hinkov et al 1999).

The reforms have restructured the health care system, but follow a decade of falling real terms spending on health care, with inflation-adjusted health spending in 1997 running at just 26% of the 1990 level rising back to 41% in 1998, and per capita spending in 1997 estimated to be less than 10% of the EU average. The country's heavy reliance on imported pharmaceuticals meant that the proportion of the health budget allocated to drugs almost doubled between 1990 and 1998 (Hinkov et al 1999:22-23).

The number of hospitals increased almost 10% during the 1990s, though numbers of hospital beds fell sharply towards the end of the decade as rationalisation brought the closure of some TB hospitals and psychiatric hospitals (Afford 2001).

ROMANIA

Decentralisation, along with privatisation of dentistry and pharmacy services and a new health insurance system have run alongside a limited rationalisation of hospital services, closing 10% of beds (Afford 2001) though numbers of beds per head and rates of hospital admission have remained virtually constant.

Most health care providers are now no longer state employees, and the ministry of health is no longer the controlling and financing body for health services, but a regulatory body supervising 'Romania's emerging health care sector'. By 1996 almost a quarter of health spending went through private health care enterprises. However only a few (smaller) hospitals are privately owned. Romania is also unusual in its plan to increase health care spending both on a per capita basis and as a share of GDP, after a prolonged period of low spending prior to 1990 (Vladescu et al 2000).

ESTONIA

In Estonia the post-independence government switched from a tax-funded health system to one based on social insurance, again levied at workplace level, coupled with privatisation of health care providers, which was further urged along by legislation in 1997. Side-effects of these reforms had included rising unemployment among doctors (Hunter 1998).

There were also concerns that the 1991 decentralisation of health care to 15 counties and 17 sickness funds had – like the early decentralisation in Poland – gone too far, leaving purchasing organisations too small to bargain with providers or secure improved efficiency. Private sector critics argue that a country with such a small population as Estonia should restrict itself to three to four sickness funds (Medicover 2002d).

GEORGIA

As with the Russian Federation, a fundamental problem confronting health care services in Georgia is a lack of funding, with government health spending running at around $8 per head of population per year in 2001, and the basic package of care covered by state insurance is now described by health minister Amran Gamkrelidze as covering only 20% of the needs of the population. However, his answer is to restructure the hospital system so that the hospitals freed up:

> ...could be turned into private clinics and the money resulting from their sale could be reinvested into further development of the healthcare sector. This process is actually already under way right now (AIHA 2001:116).

A rationalisation of hospital services has brought the closure of almost 60% of hospitals (down from 480 in 1990 to 280 in 1999) though many of those that closed had fewer than 100 beds. Staff numbers have been cut back, though those still working in health care are struggling to survive on low pay (Gamkrelidze et al, 2002, Afford 2001). Heavy user fees for treatment led to a reduction in demand for services, though the government has proposed a system of social insurance and specified user fees.

World Bank-aided reforms from 1993 brought a decentralisation of the system, and the introduction of a payroll tax to help fund a 'semi-public social insurance': the new system was also planned to include user charges and co-payments, alongside support for privatisation (Gamkrelidze et al 2002). Privatisation as normal began with pharmacies and dental services. Health care providers were to be paid on a fee-for-service basis in the hope that this would stop them levying unofficial payments – but this did not go to plan. It was soon clear that these changes had not yielded the expected health benefits:

> One of the main challenges has been the overall very low allocation of funds to the health budget and consequent high levels of individual direct payments by patients with inadequate risk sharing (Gamkrelidze et al, 2002).

Chapter seven

Country summaries: Africa and Asia

Overview: Sub-Saharan African countries

The study will focus centrally on the Kenyan experience because it epitomises the consequences of the 'World Bank model' of health care, and embodies many of the issues affecting other African countries as they have come under pressure to implement the same basic package of reforms that has shown itself so ineffective in Kenya. The more neoliberal policies have been adopted, and the more the advice of World Bank-sponsored researchers and consultants has been heeded, the worse the state of health of Kenya's growing and impoverished population has become.

While the debate still continues over the impact of IMF's Structural Adjustment Programmes (SAPs) on the health of populations in developing countries and the level of health care available to them, it is clear that many researchers have come to negative conclusions, and there are few unambiguous advocates of the IMF/World Bank approach (Samba 2004, Breman and Shelton 2001). It might be concluded from this study that it is not necessarily the SAPs alone which have done damage to the health care provision of poorer countries, but a combination of market-driven austerity, and market-style reforms, often promoted by academics from a safe, long distance [147].

The general line of World Bank-style 'reforms' lies behind many of the changes in health care systems in other countries of Sub-Saharan Africa (SSA). For the Bank/IMF it appears that no matter what the question, the answer must always involve privatisation. An IMF seminar in 1998 heard of the problems in shifting public health spending towards primary care: the IMF's Sanjeev Gupta responded by arguing for a series of policies that have been shown to fail time and again:

> ...better intrasectoral allocation to benefit the poor; shifts in geographical targeting to benefit the poor; stronger civil services reform; devolution of spending to the lowest levels of government; and a bigger role for the private sector (IMF1999).

---

147 Public expenditure in health has fallen during the 1990s in 29 of the poorest African countries. Meanwhile Structural Adjustment Programmes (SAPs) have opened up developing countries to Foreign Direct Investment, including the expansion of private health care systems in Latin America (Labonte et al 2004).

Despite the lack of supporting evidence that these policies work, many countries – often under the persuasion of the World Bank or other donors and agencies – have struggled to introduce user fees for health care in publicly funded hospitals. By 1995 no fewer than 31 African countries were seeking to recover all or part of the cost of treatment through user charges imposed as a result of health sector reforms (Leighton and Wouters 1995). While around 40% of the Bank's Health Nutrition and Population projects included the introduction or increased use of user fees, almost 75% of Bank projects in SSA involved fees (Dunne 2000).

As will be seen in the case of Kenya the standard Bank reform package involves:

- User fees
- Attempts at some form of health insurance
- Encouragement for increased private sector provision of health care
- Moves to decentralise control and planning of health care provision, and
- Steps towards the autonomous running (or 'corporatisation') of hospitals.

Often those involved in the full package of reforms will also have been working with one or more of the agencies most closely linked to the World Bank model – USAID and its sponsored research bodies Partnerships for Health Reform and Health Finance and Sustainability, and/or Abt Associates, the private sector consultants who have made a big business out of reforming health services in poor countries.

The attempts by the World Bank (IFC), USAID and other reform proposals to find ways of extending private health insurance in low- and middle-income countries has been shown by Sbabaro to compound inequalities:

> The introduction of private health insurance does represent a threat to the control of, and care for, the WHO's ten basic diseases, especially if the insurance plans are accompanied by new technology and treatments (Sbabaro 2000:14).

Since there is not scope in this study (or sufficient comparable information available) to explore in detail the situation in more than a sample of countries, this chapter will examine Kenya, which has attempted to implement many of the World Bank model reforms, and South Africa, which is perhaps the most glaring example in the continent of a system in drastic need of progressive reform, but where the inequalities of a heavily privatised system continue to restrict any improvement of health care for the majority of the population.

Africa

KENYA

Background: population and pressures on health care services

Kenya achieved independence in 1964, and now has a rising population of 30 million, 42% of whom are aged 14 or under, with fewer than 3% aged over 65. UN statistics suggest that as many as 15% of the population have AIDS or HIV, and 500-700 will die from AIDS-related causes each day in 2003. Around 50% of hospital beds are occupied by AIDS sufferers[148]. In

---

148 Official figures show 16.5% of the urban population and 12.5% of the rural population to be HIV positive in 2002 (Central Bureau of Statistics 2003).

2001 Kenya had half of the East African total of 4.2 million HIV-infected people, with 500 more contracting the disease each day (Achieng 2001).

The new government elected at the end of 2002 announced a change of policy towards prevention of the further spread of the virus, centred on a mass distribution of 300 million free condoms, to be funded through the World Bank (Wax 2003).

Kenya's total GDP was $46 billion in 2000, but the very large informal economy and low levels of earnings resulted in total government revenue of just $2.9 billion per year, and external debts of over $6 billion. Debt service charges have run at more than 15% of the country's export earnings throughout the 1980s and 1990s: these payments are prioritised by the government above spending on health care (Kimalu 2001). Seventy percent of the labour force is unemployed, and government estimates suggest that 56% live on less than $1 per day. Only 50% of health spending in Kenya is publicly financed. Forty two percent is paid privately, while the remaining 6% comes from international donors and NGOs (Kimalu 2001:7).

In the period immediately after independence, Kenya's economy grew rapidly – averaging just over 6% a year for the first decade, a rate exceeding Malaysia and Indonesia – and the government began to implement its 1963 election pledge to develop a health care system offering free basic treatment, introducing free outpatient care in 1965. It achieved reductions of almost 50% in mortality among the under-fives in the years to 1993. Life expectancy increased from 40 to 60 years (Colgan 2002, Gatheru and Shaw 1998). Rural health centres were set up, and there was an expansion of the renamed Kenyatta National Hospital, which enabled the launch of a programme for training Kenyan doctors.

But during the 1970s the emerging system was swamped by the demands of a rising population while the economic growth faltered, stretching resources. Although bed numbers have grown more than four-fold since 1963, they have not kept pace with the rapid growth of the population. It is common for beds to be shared by patients, and for patients to sleep on the floor (Kimalu 2001)[149].

The service was never able to grow on a sufficient scale to confront the major endemic threats to health. Diseases that could be prevented or contained are still among the major causes of illness and death: malaria (23%); respiratory tract disease (26%); skin diseases (7%); diarrhoea (5%); and intestinal worms (4%). These could be tackled through improved primary care, preventive health policies, clean water supplies and enhanced nutrition (Gatheru and Shaw 1998).

Another aspect of the decline in Kenya's health care system has been the reduction in coverage for immunisation from 79% in 1993 to just 65% in 1998 (Kimalu 2001:11). Despite the prevalence of disease, Kenya still spends 75% of its health budget on curative (mainly hospital) care (Kirigia et al 2002), and just 11% on health promotion and preventive health measures.

The 1980s brought the end of economic growth, and with it pressure from the IMF and World Bank to implement 'structural adjustment' programmes, including cuts in public spending (Amrith 2001). Government health spending fell sharply in the 1990s, from $10 per capita in 1990 to just $2.90 in 2000 (Heaton 2001, Achieng 2001).

---

149 The most recent official figures show a slow increase in numbers but uneven distribution of hospital beds, ranging from just 14.2 per 100,000 population in North Eastern Province, to 21.6 in Nairobi and 31.4 in Coast (Central Bureau of Statistics 2003).

Infant and child mortality rates which fell so dramatically in Kenya's first 20 years both rose by around 50% in the years 1992-1998, bringing fears that many of the gains recorded in the 25 years after independence could rapidly be lost (Kimalu 2001:10). Maternal mortality rates also doubled in the period 1993 to 2000 (IFC 2002).

WHO/World Bank model reforms

Switch resources from secondary to primary care

Aspects of the World Bank's model of health care for developing countries have also been tried and largely failed in Kenya, as have WHO policies to build up and improve primary care services.

The public hospital sector is dominated by the Kenyatta National Hospital in Nairobi, which in 1993-4 received no less than 13% of the entire Kenyan government health budget and treated up to 30,000 inpatients, while just 26% of the budget was allocated to primary care services for the remainder of Kenya's population (Hsiao 2000).

A strategic plan designed to shift more government resources towards primary care (Wang'ombe 1997) has not been implemented, partly because of political pressure exercised by consultants and others in the hospital sector. As in the case of Zambia's UTH Hospital (Purvis 1997), the Kenyatta is too visible and politically sensitive for major cutbacks to be politically acceptable. Funding for primary care has increased, but not in real terms (McEuen 1997).

Market-driven reforms

1 Cash limits and spending cuts

Kenyan government spending on health care has not kept pace with the growing population and the need for preventive medicine and health promotion, which even with rural health care receives less than 20% of the budget. Kenya is caught in the classic bind of a poor capitalist economy in a harsh global market: the major constraint on government spending is that 'devoting more resources to health would compromise overall growth and employment goals' (Kimalu 2001:18). However, constraints also apply to the private sector: high domestic interest rates exceed the margins of the not-for-profit hospitals, making it impossible to borrow money for investment in new technology or improved capacity (Stenton 2002).

2 User fees

Since 1989 the government has – largely at the behest of the World Bank – imposed user charges on health services, despite the immediate evidence that it reduced access and service use for the poorest. The standard package of reform which the Bank began systematically promoting with the adoption of its 1987 *Agenda for Reform* includes:

- User fees in government health facilities

- Health insurance schemes to draw in extra resources for health care

- Encouraging the private sector and non-governmental providers including NGOs to develop services for which patients would be prepared to pay

- Decentralisation of planning, budgeting, purchasing and management of government health services.
  (World Bank 1987)

Opposition to the continued use of 'unaffordable' fees for treatment was raised by MPs in the run-up to the 2002 elections (Orlale 2002). The government at that time agreed under heavy public pressure to lift fees and charges for treatment and tests in three highland areas subject to an especially virulent malaria outbreak, but stressed that this was an exceptional measure that was 'too expensive' to apply to other districts (Omanga 2002).

Fees are levied for all treatment: a hernia operation could cost £500-£800 depending on the hospital and the surgeon, while setting a broken leg could cost £50-£120. The state-run National Hospital Insurance Fund (giving partial coverage to at most 25% of the population, all of them people in formal employment, who pay premiums of up to £3.20 per month from their salaries) will reimburse only the bed costs of hospital treatment, paying up to £14 per day for an inpatient – but nothing towards costs of outpatient care (Njeru et al 2005). This would leave the hernia patient receiving a subsidy of £28-£42 towards a total bill of £500-£800 (Stenton 2002).

Even the cheapest reasonable standard of hospital bed costs £15-£20 per night, with additional charges for consultation with doctors, drugs, bandages and other consumables, most of which have to be imported and paid for at world market prices. Government hospitals also operate on a 'cost-sharing' basis, leaving the patient to cover around 70% of the costs of health care: many people have to sell their houses to pay for medical care (Stenton 2002, Gatheru and Shaw 1998).

In outpatient centres, the user fees of US$0.33 for visits brought initial drops in attendances averaging 37%, and as high as 52%. When the fees were suspended, visits rose by 41% (Ugwumba 2000). Fees at Nairobi's clinic for sexually transmitted diseases brought a reduction in attendances of 40% among men and 65% of women in nine months: but here, even after the fees were abolished, attendance levels never fully recovered (Brugha and Zwi 2002).

Moreover – as in many African countries – the fees failed to generate the expected contribution towards the health budget, yielding just 2.1% of Ministry of Health spending by 1993 – well below the 10-20% forecast by the World Bank, even before the cost of administering the charges was taken into account. Kenya has also attempted to 'cascade' charges in such a way as to encourage patients to go first to the lowest appropriate level of care – but by implication imposing financial penalties on those who have more serious illness (Creese and Kutzin 1995).

As Kimalu argues:

> The government policy on cost sharing was aimed at establishing and sustaining high quality health services. Specifically it was aimed to improve effectiveness and efficiency of health programmes, generate more revenue for the health sector, improve the quality of health care, improve equity in the health delivery system and control expenditure in the public sector spending on curative care. [...] But the programme has not performed as expected (Kimalu 2001:16).

This heavy burden of private payment impacts with most severity on the poor. A 1998 survey showed that 9% of the population had chosen not to visit a government health facility because they could not afford the fees: but 76% had decided they could not afford to visit a private medical facility. Just over a third (37%) of Kenyan mothers gave birth in a hospital. 70% of the rural poor and 81% of the urban poor cannot afford private health charges, while 20% of urban and 8% of rural poor people cannot afford the lower costs of government-funded health care (Kimalu 2001:11).

However such problems have not deterred external agencies such as Management Sciences for Health offering their assistance to tighten up and enforce the imposition of charges. A new system of networked cash registers was installed by MSH in the Coast Provincial Hospital in Mombasa, the country's second largest. 'Within four months the cost of the cash registers was recovered', primarily through 'efficiency measures' but also by 'modest increases in patient fees' (MSH 2001). Thus new technology has been employed to remove more money more systematically from the pockets of Kenya's poor to 'increase financial resources for health and family planning services'.

But of course as Arhin-Tenkorang (2000:14) argues, the reality is that systems which hinge on payments only by sick people and their families 'do not equate to additional sources of funds for the health sectors of developing countries': this could only come from sharing risk among both the sick and the healthy. This is why user fee systems have generated negligible – if any – funds for fresh investment in primary care or more local hospital facilities.

More recent studies have shown that the system of user fees, coupled with systematic under-funding of health care facilities by the Ministry of Health generates a degree of dependence on even the small sums of money generated, so that the system of waivers that should exempt the very poorest from payment of all or part of the fees has often not been fully implemented. Fewer than 1% of patients were being granted waivers totalling less than 5% of the amounts collected in fees in the two years 1999-2001: two-thirds of hospital inpatients were apparently unaware that any system of exemptions existed (Korir 2003).

3 Regulating drug costs

Donor funding has focused largely on HIV/AIDS and on health promotion and prevention. But HIV/AIDS has spread rapidly (increasing 150% in the five years 1993-98) along with increased poverty: in 1999, according to UN figures, Kenya was spending just US$0.76 per capita on AIDS. The country cannot afford modern anti-retroviral drugs, and has been among the African countries seeking to import cheaper generic drugs: the cost of the branded products has been as high as $15,000 per patient per year, compared with an average Kenyan annual income of just $270 (Achieng 2001). By September 2004 concerns were growing that even some of the patients being treated in Nairobi with donated anti-retroviral drugs through Medecins Sans Frontieres, and others receiving treatment at Kenyatta National Hospital, were dropping out of treatment because they could not afford the Ksh500 (less than £4) monthly fees for tests and drugs (Okwemba 2004). NGOs and the Global Fund to Fight Aids Tuberculosis and Malaria have pressed the government to ensure that fees are waived where they could prevent the poorest patients accessing the treatment they need. The Fund supplies drugs free to governments, and expects governments to pass them on free of charge to patients: a high drop-out rate from treatment could trigger a halt to Fund support. NGOs have also been critical of the lack of adequate testing of patients at the Kenyatta, which has not been carrying out viral load tests to facilitate more precise treatment regimes.

These problems underline the fact that even when AIDS drugs are donated, there are problems in arranging the effective distribution to those in greatest need. A study by German development agency GTZ found that the value of donated drugs to prevent mother to child transmission of the HIV virus in East Africa would amount to just 1.2% of the total cost of the programme – with the remaining costs falling to local services (Heaton 2001).

Those struggling with the AIDS epidemic in Kenya received a fresh blow in 2005: the Indian government made clear in March that it was bowing to pressure from the World Trade

Organisation and putting through new legislation that would end the production of cheap generic versions of anti-retrovirals, which had brought systematic treatment within the reach of poorer African countries. Indian generic retrovirals cost less than £12 per month, compared with £230 for patented drugs. An angry protest by HIV/AIDS sufferers through the streets of Nairobi to the Indian High Commission reflected the anger at a new law which will protect the profits of the multinational drug companies at the expense of the lives of millions in Africa, Asia and other poor countries (Opinion 2005).

With malaria a major cause of death, killing 750,000 children in Africa each year, affordable treatment and prevention is vital for Kenya. But the more modern drugs such as Larium and Malarone, costing £40 per fortnight, are far too expensive for most Kenyans to afford (Rocco 2003).

Even the donation of a million doses of Malarone by GlaxoSmithKline has brought serious problems, raising questions over the sustainability of any application of the drug, and carrying restrictive 'strings' on its use which meant that by December 2000 only 223 patients had been treated with it, while research indicates that up to 500,000 children would benefit from treatment (Heaton 2001). By contrast quinine hydrochloride, derived from cinchona trees grown in Congo, can be produced for just 50 pence a course (Rocco 2003).

Market-style reforms

1 Decentralisation

Attempts at decentralisation, creating more district level planning, have also failed to deliver many of the expected improvements, especially in the context of limited resources for information systems and appropriate training of staff (Owino et al 2000, Owino et al 2001).

Eighty percent of doctors and dentists still work in urban areas where just 20% of Kenyans live. Attempts at decentralisation of services were hampered by lack of managerial capacity at local level and financial resources nationally (Collins and Green 1994, Stenton 2002). However top health officers have continued to promise decentralisation, most recently Health Permanent Secretary Patrick Khaemba, who told The Nation on March 20 2005 that public hospitals would be given greater local decision making powers – but admitted that no funds had been allocated to finance any such changes.

2 Purchaser/provider contracts

Kenya has not implemented this aspect of market-style reform.

3 Provider autonomy

Kenya's government took the advice of the World Bank and others and in 1987 turned Nairobi's Kenyatta hospital into a 'parastatal', a state corporation with a degree of autonomy from the Ministry of Health (Collins et al 1996, Govindaraj and Chawla 1996).

However the results of this reform have not been an unambiguous success. Impatient at slow progress, the government attempted to contract out the management of the hospital to a European company in 1991, only to retreat in 1992 in the face of opposition. But chronic and unresolved shortages of financial and other resources, compounded by the need to compete for professional staff with private sector hospitals paying higher rates have limited the extent to which the Board has been able to demonstrate improvements.

Collins and colleagues are not convinced that the exercise offers a model that could or should be followed with other (much smaller) hospitals in Kenya (Collins et al 1996:7). Another assessment by researchers from DDM found that hospital autonomy in Kenya had brought no change on quality, accountability or equity, but some improvement in efficiency and resource mobilisation (McEuen 1997:14).

Govindaraj and Chawla, whose study includes the Kenyatta and autonomous hospitals in four other countries, are more categoric in their warnings that corporatisation and autonomy are no panacea for under-resourced public sector hospitals:

> An incontrovertible overall conclusion of the five case studies [India, Zimbabwe, Ghana, Indonesia and Kenya] is that autonomy in public sector hospitals has not yielded many of the hoped-for benefits in terms of efficiency, quality of care and public accountability. [...] It would seem that a flawed conceptual basis for hospital autonomy in the public sector as much as the poor implementation of the autonomy measures is to be held responsible for this failure (Govindaraj and Chawla 1996:3-4).

Among the failures, the authors point to 'an inability to successfully transplant private sector structures and incentives to the public sector hospitals'. And to make matters worse, far from leading towards the World Bank goals of a smaller state and public sector, the result from exercises in corporatisation have 'increased the government expenditures on public hospitals – both in absolute terms and as a share of government health expenditures' (op. cit:25).

In what might seem heresy among some World Bank and USAID researchers, Govindaraj and Chawla conclude that in the context of developing countries:

> It is not implausible that introducing autonomy and private sector measures in the public sector might actually increase inequity without significantly increasing efficiency. [...] Therefore in our opinion what is required in order to ensure that public hospitals discharge their functions effectively [...] is not a blind emulation of the private sector. Instead we would recommend a hybrid institutional system, consisting of participative, decentralised decision-making and goal-setting, performance and outcome based management structures and processes, and appropriate incentive systems (op. cit:26).

4 Provider payment reform

Not implemented in Kenya

5 Purchase from private sector/expand private sector providers

The expansion of the private sector has been hampered by the lack of insurance cover and the inability of most of the population to pay a viable fee for treatment, especially in the rural areas (Wang'ombe 1997). Despite a rapid growth of non-government providers since 1990, Berman and colleagues (1995) found 'very limited' evidence on the quality and efficiency of the services they provide, and that regulation is weak. There is no substantial for-profit private hospital sector in Kenya. But in 2001 only 600 of the country's 5,000 doctors were practising in the public sector. The IFC reports with approval that the:

> Private health sector is vibrant and the government is supportive of it. Half of all the hospitals are private. Recently, quality of public health has been declining. Population is accustomed to user fees at public facilities (IFC 2002:49).

All of the substantial private sector hospitals are run as 'not-for-profit' enterprises, though this still requires them to balance their books and generate a margin within their fees to cover maintenance and investment in stocks and new equipment. There are also many mission hospitals, which receive over 90% of their funds from USAID or international religious organisations, and are thus as dependent on them for survival as the public sector hospitals are on state support (Amrith 2001).

The chronic lack of resources has led to shortages of even the most basic supplies in public sector health facilities, and not surprisingly brought low levels of satisfaction among service users. One survey found that 54% of Kenyans who used private rather than public health care did so because of the non-availability of drugs (Kimalu 2001). This makes it appear as if private services and those provided by NGOs or the private sector rather than the state are necessarily and by definition 'more efficient': and this type of statistical data reinforces the World Bank and USAID's largely ideological preference for working through NGOs rather than lending support to public sector services. By 1994 no less than 95% of USAID's funds for Kenya were paid to NGOs and private companies (Amrith 2001).

There is little doubt that the efficiency of Kenya's public sector hospitals is inadequate, although factors driving this include inadequate numbers of professional staff, shortages of consumables or breakdowns of equipment leading to non-functioning theatres and laboratories, and problems importing or paying for drugs and supplies (Owino and Korir 1997). However, many private facilities are also under-resourced, and offer questionable quality of care: a 1998 survey found that less than a third of Kenya's private clinics offered laboratory services (ICHRSI 1998). A study in 1994 by DDM found that:

> ...there is no clear evidence that the private sector is more efficient than the public sector (Berman et al 1995).

6 Competition and Privatisation
Not implemented in Kenya

7 Expand private medical insurance
One of the reasons why the World Bank and other agencies have insisted on the need for user fees has been to nurture the emergence of insurance schemes even in the poorest countries:

> ...user fees are vital to the introduction of any type of insurance system (McEuen 1997:11).

However it appears that this dogmatic approach represents a triumph of hope over experience. Extensive surveys of developing countries by researchers for the USAID-funded Data for Decision Making found limited evidence of success:

> DDM research... indicated that only small percentages of the populations studied had any kind of health insurance, and that insurance schemes currently do not contribute significant resources to total health financing. Current insurance schemes also tend to cover mainly the more wealthy income groups or the formally employed, limiting the reach of such schemes into the lower income or rural populations (McEuen 1997:16).

In fact the chances of establishing health insurance are undermined by the World Bank/IMF Structural Adjustment Programmes, which in almost all cases result in a reduction in size of the formal employment sector, and cut the incomes of the rural and urban poor along with public employees (Simon et al 1995). Only a small proportion of Kenya's workforce – and less than 10% of the entire African labour force – is employed in the formal sector, and many more are on extremely low rates of pay, limiting the scope for any European-style insurance system (Turshen 1999:61). In fact the IFC makes clear that its target audience for such schemes is not Kenya's poor: rather it is aimed at facilitating the use of private health care by Kenya's (far from numerous) 'middle class' (IFC 2002).

However less than 12% of the population has private health insurance, and the largest private insurer has an annual turnover of just $12.6 million a year, covering 200,000 subscribers. Other schemes are so small that they were threatened with extinction by a provision in the government's Insurance Act which, after years of little or no regulation or supervision of the private insurance sector, would have required them to maintain a capital base of $1.3 million (Kimani 2002).

In the absence of any viable basis for large scale private health insurance schemes, academics working with the World Bank have been keen to promote the notion of community-based health insurance schemes which would target the poor: but in Kenya the only scheme investigated by Partnerships for Health Reform, centred on Chogoria Hospital, had managed to enlist only 1,400 people, just 0.3% of its target population, and by 1998 had only the hospital's staff as members.

Other such schemes surveyed by Musau in Uganda, Tanzania and the Democratic Republic of Congo had either targeted very small communities or failed to achieve any significant wider support (Musau 1999). A prepayment scheme in Rwanda managed to recruit just 4.6% of the target population, while the user fee system reduced attendance at health centres and thus drove up their costs (Schneider et al 2000). There are no serious grounds to believe that such schemes will ever be much more than token exercises to cover over the lack of public health provision for the majority of the country's population.

8 National Social Health Insurance

Plans by the National Rainbow Coalition government to transform the limited National Hospital Insurance Fund into a new universal health care scheme were first drawn up in 2003, and have come under heavy fire from private sector critics, large employers and by trade unions concerned that workplace taxes would be used to subsidise a system that will cover all Kenyans.

The scheme could mean that employers and employee contributions increase by up to 135%, while the NHIF and its assets, until now an institution financed and benefiting the best organised formal sector workers, would be absorbed into the new scheme.

From the beginning there have been doubts and unanswered questions about the costs and viability of the scheme, which had at first proposed monthly contributions of Ksh400-600 (£2.90-4.40) from each worker, and twice as much from employers, who would for the first time be liable to contribute to the health care of all their staff.

Running costs of the scheme have been (optimistically) estimated at around £290 million per year, and government measures to cover the extra costs of covering the 56% of Kenyans who live in absolute poverty include the use of value added tax, levying contributions from those working in the informal sector, a new airport tax on foreigners travelling to Kenya, donations and grants (Munaita 2003).

The opposition has been led by an angry private sector, which has stressed the unrealistically low cost estimates for the scheme, in which a maximum of 1.5 million Kenyans employed in the formal sector will, together with increased taxes on business, effectively support the health care for 30 million. Thakker (2004) estimates the actual costs of 'basic in and outpatient care' at closer to Ksh300 billion (£73 per head per year) than the government's Ksh 40 billion projection, and points out that this is almost the entire Kenyan national budget. He goes on to ask whether the plan is to provide a half, a quarter or even lower proportion of 'basic care'. Other objections focus on the high level of bureaucracy in the new scheme, and

Kenyan governments' poor track record at spending health budgets effectively.

Patel (2004) claims that 93% of the Ministry of Health Budget is currently spent on 'administration, salaries, buildings, maintenance and sundries' – although these salaries will clearly include those of front-line medical and nursing staff and crucial support services. By contrast, she argues, while the government spends just 7% of its budget on drugs and dressings, the private sector typically spends 45-55%. And ministers spent £1.5 million fighting SARS in 2003, despite the absence of even a single case, while spending a mere £116,000 fighting actual epidemics.

And while Patel, as a prominent executive of Avenue Healthcare, may be seen as having a vested interest in questioning the public sector, a survey by Njeru and colleagues (2005) also highlights a series of concerns over the ability of public sector services to deliver the planned NHSIF, and the low level of public confidence in existing public health services, and concludes that there is little option but a much more gradual process of change:

> Kenya lacks the key prerequisites for introducing and sustaining a universal social health scheme. The scheme can hardly be supported by the current status of the economy and health care infrastructure (Njeru et al 2005:3).

By the autumn of 2004 business lobbies stepped up the pressure against the new scheme, proposing instead a merger of the National Hospital Insurance Fund and the existing National Social Security Fund, along lines implemented in Tanzania and Ghana (Akumu 2004). Another alternative plan is to establish separate schemes for different sectors of the population: one for those in formal employment, another for the rural population, and so on. One key objective of these proposals – much of which had already been conceded by the government by September 2004, is a reduction in the share of the Fund to be paid by the employers compared with their workforce, from the original 2:1 to closer to 1:1.

By November the combination of financial problems with the scheme and pressure from opposing interest groups had forced a split in the ruling coalition and a retreat by the government. Finance Minister David Mwirara told MPs that he had been misled on the cost of the scheme by Health Minister Charity Ngilu: the projected annual cost had almost doubled to Ksh72 billion, and the Treasury was apparently expected to find an extra Ksh6 billion (£44 million) towards this total. Mwirara went on to claim that he had never been asked his views on the scheme, which would more than double the Health Ministry's share of government spending (Standard Team 2004).

As this study is completed, it seems that ministers may try once again to push through the National Social Health Insurance Bill, despite its failure to secure presidential assent after passing through Parliament in 2004. The contradictions of a divided coalition seeking a progressive reform in the teeth of such powerful opposition on the basis of such a weak infrastructure remain unresolved (Opiyo 2005).

SOUTH AFRICA

Background: population and pressures on health care services

South Africa is the most prosperous of the SSA countries, classified by the World Bank as an 'upper middle-income' country, with a GNP of $113 billion in 2001 and a population of 43 million. However more than half the population can be classified as poor, in many cases still reflecting the stark racial inequalities inherited from the apartheid regime, with poverty concentrated among black people and the rural areas (McIntyre et al 1998).

Despite high comparative and absolute levels of health spending in South Africa[150], life expectancy has fallen from 62 to just 48 years during the 1990s, largely as a result of the raging HIV/AIDS epidemic, which had infected almost 5 million adults by 2005 (almost 20% of the adult population): 84,000 infants were born with HIV in 2001 (World Bank HNPstats 2003).

Apartheid South Africa's health policies were regressive in every way, with more than 75% of public health spending allocated to hospitals, most of which are in urban areas, with academic and specialist hospitals taking 44%. Just 11% was allocated to primary care. A burgeoning private sector employed the majority of health staff, and controlled 61% of the country's health spending.

The allocation of hospital beds and every other aspect of health care resources was consistently focused on the richest districts (and therefore the white minority of the population) which enjoyed almost double the allocation of hospital beds, almost seven times as many doctors, double the number of nurses and nearly four times the health budget per head compared with the poorest (Gilson et al 1999).

However despite the overwhelming mandate for change secured by the new ANC government after the end of apartheid, there has been no South African equivalent of the dramatic post-independence upturn in health investment and outcomes seen in most SSA countries. Instead the general line of policy had already been established as one of collaboration with the private sector. This is in the very nature of the ANC as a cross-class liberation movement, and Lucy Gilson and colleagues trace the roots of this policy at least as far back as a 1991 speech by Nelson Mandela in the USA, where he declared that:

> The private sector must and will play the central and decisive role in the struggle to achieve many
> of these [ANC] objectives… The rates of economic growth we seek cannot be achieved without
> important flows of foreign capital (cited in Gilson et al 1999:25).

The ANC government has therefore effectively followed a variant of the World Bank model for health sector reform, without being compelled to do so by external pressure.

But on a wider level, the same approach has informed the ANC government's leading role in promoting the 'New Partnership for Africa's Development' – a continent-wide initiative launched in Abuja in 2001, aiming to resolve Africa's chronic problems of under-development and dependency through encouraging additional direct investment from the main centres of capital. NEPAD is at pains to present itself as an African-owned and led initiative, but its objectives are clearly to reform and strengthen African states to encourage and facilitate a major injection of foreign direct investment. As such, it seeks to embrace and repackage essentially the same neoliberal methods that have been urged on African countries by the IMF and World Bank for decades (Calamitsis 1999). Like the IMF, NEPAD sees the solution to Africa's under-development and exclusion from the world's economy as 'private sector-led growth'. The founding document identifies 'an annual resource gap of US$64 billion':

> The bulk of the needed resources will have to be obtained from outside the continent.

---

150 Equivalent to around half the entire health budget for all the SSA countries: see Appendix A.

The task of governments is to ensure that their countries:

> ...become attractive locations for residents to hold their wealth. Therefore there is also an urgent need to create conditions that promote private sector investments by both domestic and foreign investors (NEPAD 2001:36).

As we have seen, in other countries this has meant wholesale privatisation of state-owned corporations, big reductions in the public sector workforce, and a tax regime that leaves profits intact. Partly because of this, the limited goals for health improvement are tied not to any commitment for long-term government investment, but to appeals for a $10 billion per annum increase in external donor assistance, which even if it were forthcoming would leave health services dependent on the charity of the advanced economies into the indefinite future.

South African critics of NEPAD warn that the entire policy amounts to little more than 'globalisation with a human face' (Patel and Pretorius 2002a). There are also signs that the scheme is failing to convince many other African governments. By summer 2003 only 15 of the 53 member countries of the African Union had signed up to join NEPAD's 'peer review' system for checking adherence to the scheme's principles (Bell 2003, Madlana 2003). Thabo Mbeki has complained that some presidents who have endorsed the deal appear not to have told their cabinets (Fabricius 2003).

Ten years after the end of apartheid, leading medical experts point to the disappointing progress, both within South Africa itself and in its contribution to health care in the continent:

> We have provided 80% coverage to prevent mother-to-child transmission of AIDS. South Africa leads the world in this[151]. But I still don't see the political commitment yet to rolling out the programme of treatment with anti-retrovirals. We see the Director General's post is still vacant, and now we have a vacancy for the head of the AIDS programme (Coovadia 2004).

Indeed the planned roll-out of the Anti Retroviral Therapy (ART) programme is running into problems, with just 3,600 patients receiving treatment so far in the 2004 financial year, way short of the target figure of 53,000. Researchers now argue that the £37 million budget for ART drugs would be enough for just 7% of South Africa's AIDS patients (Kamaldien 2004).

National Health Bill

The political and economic policies of the ANC in government have also meant that the much-promised National Health Bill (NHB), which after its first appearance as a draft in 1995, and years of debate and delay, has only passed through Parliament in 2004, and has been held up awaiting the Presidential signature that would make it law.

This process has been further impeded by threats from the private sector and other political opponents of the ANC that they will go to court to challenge central aspects of the legislation, most notably the powers granted to the Minister of Health to grant – or refuse – any health care facility a 'Certificate of Need', without which it will be illegal to continue to practise (Kane-Berman 2004).

Although these same regulations would also apply to public sector hospitals – some of

---

151 ART drugs administered to women in labour in Gauteng have saved an estimated 58,000 babies from contracting AIDS in the last three years, according to researchers – restricting incidence of the virus from 33% of babies to just 8% (Park 2004).

which are predicted not to survive scrutiny – they are widely interpreted as an attack on the private sector, which has continued to show itself reluctant to direct resources to poorer and more rural areas, where less income can be generated (Y Pillay 2004). However the ANC has established itself as a keen proponent of public-private partnerships, and the Bill itself stresses from the very outset its objective of 'establishing a national health system which encompasses the public & private providers of health services' (Y Pillay 2004).

Indeed the NHB does not, as its name might suggest, focus on funding a health care system to allow the elimination of user fees, but on seeking to regulate the private sector and establish a more equitable allocation of resources and more decentralised structure – while retaining full powers at government level in the hands of the minister. Its supporters argue that the Bill does represent a real step forward for some of South Africa's most vulnerable people (K Pillay 2002).

It does, for example, seek to ensure that all South Africans have access to a package of free primary health care – although even where such services are provided free of charge, many people face physical and financial problems travelling to and accessing them (Connolly 2002). There is no specific health insurance system for the whole population, and the main trade union confederation Cosatu, in its initial response to the Bill strongly urged that further measures should be brought forward to establish a system of National Health Insurance, which would ensure universal access to comprehensive health care, and allow all health services to be incorporated into the public sector (Cosatu 2002).

The Health Minister has been quoted describing the public sector provision as 'in a shambles'. Chronic shortages of resources in the more isolated rural areas have contributed to an exodus of doctors, dentists and other trained professionals – to the cities, to the private sector, or often overseas to work in developed countries for higher salaries – creating an atmosphere of growing crisis in public sector health care (Cullinan 2003).

Market-driven reforms

1 Cash limits and spending cuts

Levels of government health spending have been constrained by the controversial economic policy known as Growth, Equity and Redistribution (GEAR), and a programme of privatisation, which have brought conflict with trade unions and other sections of the ANC's own base support, while delivering few of its objectives on poverty or health. (Gilson et al 1999:36, Patel and Pretorius 2002b).

The largest health union, NEHAWU, has complained that 29,000 posts nationally were not being filled because the hospitals and clinics did not have funds to recruit staff (NEHAWU 2002).

2 Rationalisation

Even in the midst of an AIDS epidemic some public sector hospitals are struggling with low levels of bed occupancy, with only two provinces exceeding 75%. Reformers are pressing for a rationalisation, with the closure of surplus beds and hospitals and resources redirected into primary care (Boulle et al 2000). However the more fundamental problem remains – the unequal distribution of hospital and other services, which can only be addressed by the injection of serious new resources as part of a planned reform aimed at equity of access.

Many hospitals still show the scars of neglect during the apartheid years: many are in the wrong places, while other areas lack access. An audit in 1996 found a third (by value) need to be replaced or repaired, with a growing backlog and ongoing deterioration of the building stock, and equipment maintenance requirements of over one billion rand a year – well above current spending (Boulle et al 2000:12). Problems included a third of buildings with unreliable supplies of water or electricity. The most neglected buildings, often again in the poorest rural areas, also have underpaid, neglected and depleted numbers of staff (Mtshali 2003).

3 User fees

The new South African government from 1994 confined itself initially to two substantial changes, bringing in free health care to pregnant women and children under six, and also instituting free primary care for all. These policies appear to have increased the attendances at public sector clinics, but did little to ensure that the required services would be available where required, and left hospital fees for those other than indigent patients intact (Gilson et al 1999).

Estimates of the scale of revenue that would be generated if the government carried out its pledge to introduce Social Health Insurance show that it could raise around double the current amount collected in fees: but as Cosatu has pointed out, in pressing the case for the alternative policy of National Health Insurance, the cover would be only for those in formal sector employment and their families, and leave the larger share of resources in the private sector.

Raising what amounts to a workplace tax would leave the wealthiest minority paying little or nothing into the system, and make the poor pay for the poorest. However in the absence of either this or a national health insurance system, the government share of health spending has actually fallen back, with social sector spending increasing at a lower rate than general public spending since 2000. As a result the largest share of the increases in health spending have come from households (out of pocket payments for fees, drugs and private medical insurance) – the least equitable source (Doherty et al 2002).

Market-style reforms

1 Decentralisation, purchaser/provider contracts, provider autonomy, provider payment reform

Although the National Health Bill proposes what appears to be a level of decentralisation, this appears to be largely a diversion to conceal continued centralised control. As a result, these policies as market-style reforms have not been implemented in South Africa.

2 Purchase services from private sector

A 1996 report suggested moves to establish more cooperation between public and private sectors, including restrictions on the licensing of new private hospitals; competition between the sectors for paying patients; and the use of spare capacity in private hospitals to treat publicly funded patients (Monitor Company, cited by Gilson et al 1999:86). Some of these proposals have now been legislated, though several have not been effectively implemented.

While health spending seems set to continue increasing, the expansion seems likely to be greatest in the private sector, which is still expanding, and larger as a share of GDP than public health services, though less than 20% of the total population makes use of it. One reason for restricted use has been cost escalation which has affected private medicine in South Africa – especially the for-profit sector – just as it does everywhere, making it more difficult for those other than the wealthy and the top-paid workers to afford the premiums and charges: in 1998-9 medical schemes spent almost six times more per head of beneficiaries than national and local health spending per public sector dependent, and the gap is widening (Doherty et al 2002, Connolly 2002).

3 Competition

In a lop-sided competition for patients and fee income with a private sector that currently has the advantage, public sector hospitals are responding by fitting out plush new private wards designed to compete head to head with private hospitals for insurance-funded patients, who will be able to choose which hospital to use under new regulations scheduled to take effect in 2004. The government hopes that this will enable the public hospitals to draw in new funds – and create a competitive pressure to hold down private sector charges (Jacobson 2003).

But while this may lure in a number of paying patients, there are fear that the introduction of SHI could result in thousands more patients, like many who are already in medical schemes, using their new insurance cover to head in the opposite direction, and seek care from private rather than public sector hospitals.

And while the highly visible battle shapes up for the billions in fees that can be made in the hospital sector, the result could well be even less cash left for primary health care for the majority who depend upon it (Hoffman 2003).

4 Privatisation

The dominance of the private health care sector may be one explanation for the government's lack of initiative to further privatise South Africa's hospitals, despite a generalised drive towards privatisation that has seen water, electricity and telecom services among those sold off (Bond 2003).

South African private health care providers are expanding into other countries, including the contract to fly in doctors and nurses from South Africa to Oxfordshire (one of the most prosperous counties in England) to perform elective cataract operations in a new treatment centre (Timmins 2004a, Carvel 2004).

5 Private and social health insurance

Long-promised moves to establish a system of Social Health Insurance (SHI) were not brought forward, while large private hospitals continue to compete with the public sector both for staff and for revenues from paying patients.

More than seven million people – 18% of the population – are members of some 200 'medical schemes', voluntary, non-profit funds (though administered by for-profit companies) which offer a range of benefits packages that can reimburse anything from primary care costs or reimburse costs of hospital care. Schemes allow members to use public or private hospitals: most go private (McIntyre et al 1998).

6 Managed care

An attempt to transplant the US model of 'managed care' (even as it showed itself unable to control costs in the USA) proved an embarrassing disaster for United Health Care, whose 'Southern HealthCare' venture wound up adrift with 'many enemies, few friends, and no market' (Gould 2001).

Shorter country summaries – Africa

ZAMBIA

Zambia is described by Abt Associates Project Director Marty Makinen (1998) as possibly 'the world's most aggressive reformer'. As with many other Sub-Saharan African (SSA) countries, the reforms follow a worsening of health outcomes beginning in the late 1970s, despite initial gains after independence, which had brought the nationalisation of health services (Nwuke and Bekele 1995:11-12).

Among the features of Zambia's reforms is an explicit commitment to work in partnership with the private sector, and in 1994 it brought in the Harvard-based DDM to advise on further measures. A National Conference on Public/Private Partnerships for Health was financed in 1995 by USAID. Despite the 'nascent' stage of development of private medicine in Zambia (most private provision coming from church-affiliated institutions) the agenda was fairly explicit in its direction:

- To provide a forum for the government to express its commitment to forging partnerships with the private sector
- To offer various components of the private sector the opportunity to communicate with government
- To define the contractual relationship between government (as purchaser) and private sector (as sellers) of care
- To identify constraints to the development of the private sector and explore feasible solutions
- To recommend appropriate policy reform for maximising private sector (provider) participation in the public health agenda
- To identify critical next steps in the development of public/private sector partnership. (Nwuke and Bekele 1995:13)

The conference heard not only Zambia's health minister, but also the acting director of USAID, who was much more categoric in stressing the need for 'private provision of health care services'. With total health spending running at just $12 per capita annually, half or more of this coming already from service users and out of pocket payments, it was of course clear from the outset that the scope for private sector expansion would hinge on capturing a growing share of an increasing government health budget.

However the emphasis on the private sector comes in a context of wholesale privatisation of much of the Zambian economy during the 1990s, under the watchful eyes of the IMF. Out of a target list of 282 non-mining public enterprises, 224 had been privatised between 1991 and 1998 with fresh efforts to privatise the mines, the power industry, the National Bank, the State Insurance company and the National Savings and Credit Bank by 2000. The civil service and remaining public sector jobs were to be further scaled down, reducing the share of wages of national wealth, while the IMF urged a widening of pay differentials between management and staff (IMF 1999a).

The Zambian reform package that so impressed Dr Makinen reflected a similar approach: it included a substantial decentralisation of health management to 72 districts, the creation of a professional-led Central Board of Health to allocate funds to districts, excluding government health workers from public service status, contracting out a wide range of non-clinical services to the private sector, restricting public funding to a basic package of 'cost effective' service, introducing user fees, and establishing a voluntary insurance system for residents of two main cities.

The system of user fees, introduced in 1991, involves fees set by each government facility, varying from 10-20% of the cost: children under five and adults over 65 should be exempt, (although it appears that only about two-thirds are able to escape payment) and the poor can apply for 'certificates of indigency' (Makinen 1998, Nwuke and Bekele 1995). The theory is that the user fees 'free up' resources from the hospital sector for the development of lower levels of care.

A 1996 survey by PHR found that utilisation of services was 'equitable across income groups', since around 40% of people in each income group sought health care when ill. It also showed that almost half of the richest 20% choose private health providers, while 70% of the poorest choose a government health centre. But since the poor get no exemptions at private facilities, while the private sector employs more doctors and specialists, this is no great surprise (Makinen 1998, 1999).

The PHR survey also showed that the probability of getting care for a sick child – at just 52%, was better than the general average (43%) – but the elderly face a much lower (36%) probability of care.

Nor is it surprising that the 'risk sharing' insurance scheme has mainly been patronised by the rich, who accounted for over 70% of those in the scheme since they were best able to afford the premium payments. Since there is little else in the way of health insurance available in Zambia, leaving out of pocket payment as the source of a majority of health funding, it makes sense for the rich to cover themselves against possible costs. The PHR survey confirmed the general picture of inequality: the richest 20% spend about 1.3% of their income on health, compared with more than double this percentage among the poorest 40%. Yet the richest also spend five times more money on drugs and three to six times more on other forms of health care, with greater use of outpatient services than the poorest.

In other words the user fees and 'reforms' in Zambia have simply institutionalised and perpetuated the inequalities. Life expectancy in Zambia has fallen since 1990 by about ten years to just 43, while infant mortality has risen by a third (Wynne 2000). By the summer of 2003, *The Times* of Zambia, while welcoming a new promise of cheaper drugs for the poorest in society from a Western pharmaceutical corporation, noted that:

> Ten years down the line of liberalisation, the ordinary citizen had borne the brunt of medical costs (Editorial 2003).

Even top DDM consultants have been forced to the conclusion that the package of reform in Zambia has not delivered what it promised:

> Zambia's local districts are receiving less funding than before the reform, and user fees may be limiting access. In most countries insurance reforms have been associated with shifting of resources from the general 'solidarity pool' to private insurance and private providers who attend wealthier patients... (Berman and Bossert 2000:10)

As in many other low-income countries, the moves towards health system reform came at a time of financial pressure, forcing a reduction in government spending: health spending in Zambia also fell as a share of government spending 1994-97. Nevertheless the same years saw a substantial ('unprecedented') shift of spending from (largely urban) hospitals to local districts (Makinen 1999).

But the drain of resources had an impact on hospitals: the main one, the UTH, has suffered a sustained reduction in budget, from a colossal 25% of the Ministry budget, to 17% in 1994 and 11% in 1997 (Purvis 1997). The IMF noted a deterioration of facilities and equipment, shortages of drugs and a poorly staffed system that was still predominantly publicly owned. Nevertheless it endorsed the government's 'goal' of siphoning even more cash from hospital care to provide by 2001 a range of health services well below the World Bank's 'essential package' that had been costed at $12 per head per year back in 1993:

> ...a package of essential services (costing about US$7 per person) to all Zambians, compared with an allocation of about US$3.20 in 1997. This increase will be financed by the reallocation of resources from lower-priority ministry and hospital expenditures (IMF 1999a).

ZIMBABWE

The economic collapse and political repression in Zimbabwe have received considerable exposure in the world's media in the last few years: but the problems of its health services began at the end of the 1980s, long before the degeneration of the Mugabe regime drew public attention. Like many SSA countries, Zimbabwe's first years after independence (in 1980) were marked by heavy and progressive investment in health care, which after years of institutionalised racism and inequity[152] began to deliver substantial results in the form of expansion of primary health care, and reductions in child mortality rates.

User fees for all earning less than Z$150 per month were scrapped – exempting 70% of the population. Five hundred rural clinics were built and staffed, and child immunisation rates rose from 25 to 80%. Life expectancy rose from 56 to 64 years, and the use of modern contraceptives rose from 14 to 36% – the highest level in SSA (Johnston 1998, Sahn and Bernier 1995).

However after the economy fell back in the global market, and the support of the IMF and World Bank was requested in 1988, health spending was reined sharply back – falling from 6.8% of government spending in 1991 to just 2.7% by 1994. The government also agreed in 1990 to introduce user fees – which eventually rose four-fold over the next five years (Kemkes et al 1997). During the 1990s the HIV/AIDS epidemic has also had an especially brutal impact on Zimbabwe, with up to 20% of the population – 1.4 million people infected with HIV by 1998.

The spending cuts brought shortages of medicines, a lack of functioning equipment and the closure of some rural hospitals: the user fees brought a sharp decline in hospitalisation, but also deterred poor people from seeking treatment for venereal diseases, thus contributing to the transmission of HIV.

By 2001 amid mounting economic and political chaos in the country, Zimbabwe's health care system, moulded by the World Bank, was branded the worst in the world by the WHO's controversial 'league table' (WHR 2000). Among the policies which the Bank had proposed were a few familiar notions:

- Promote private and NGO provision of health services
- Privatising some ancillary services (laundry, catering, ambulances)
- Increased cost sharing with local and municipal governments
- Boosting cost recovery from insured and uninsured patients.

(Hecht at al 1995:54)

---

152 Pre-independence health spending on whites was running at 36 times the level of rural blacks, and infant mortality among blacks more than five times higher than whites (Stout 1998).

Of these the most consistently applied has been cost recovery. Strict guidelines were spelled out in a bid to ensure that all appropriate cash be collected at point of treatment:

> A patient account should be opened immediately upon admission. Charges should be posted daily to allow the accounts personnel to have a current invoice available at all times. [...] This means striving to collect a cash deposit early in the patient's stay, and to settle bills before patients leave the premises (op. cit:60).

Bank advice was that if these measures were consistently enforced (by evidently reluctant staff) it would generate Z$11.8 million in 1990, and if adjusted upwards to cover inflation, the charges could raise over 11% of recurrent hospital spending – though clearly all of this 'extra' money would be paid by sick, poor people and their families. These projections have since been criticised by a Bank analyst as 'excessively optimistic' (Johnston 1998:33).

However while the Bank sought ways to get poor people to fund their own care, the government has been spending steadily more of its scant health budget subsidising private provision, within which the only section clearly enhancing the equity of health care are the not-for-profit (mainly missions) which run services for 70% of the rural population (49% of the total population). In the absence of sufficient information, an informed guess by Mudyarabikwa (2000) puts the level of private sector subsidy at a third of government health spending. Insofar as some of this takes the form of tax breaks for financiers, for-profit providers and wealthier individuals it clearly undermines any other efforts at increased equity.

Zimbabwe has also carried through a far-reaching decentralisation of services to Rural District Councils, with an accompanying increase in autonomy at hospital level (Hongoro 1997). As the public sector provision has come under pressure, there was an expansion of private health care and insurance schemes in the 1990s, with health insurance covering (the more prosperous) 8% of the population by 2000 (Campbell et al 2000). This insurance takes the form of not-for-profit Medical Aid Societies, with no for-profit health insurance available in Zimbabwe. While the poor cannot afford a choice, those opting for private care predictably said they preferred the shorter waiting times, improved chances of seeing a doctor and greater availability of drugs. However the growth of the private sector has increased problems in staffing public health services (Johnston 1998).

The private sector itself has incurred major problems of rapid cost inflation, opening up a debate on the merits of adapting US methods of 'managed care' to constrain provider-driven demand and more than a suspicion of fraud, especially at the level of primary care (Campbell et al 2000). There are fears that if their efforts to contain costs prove unsuccessful, then insured patients may face the prospect of co-payments after years of rising premiums.

The reform package ushered in on the advice of the World Bank has in general failed to yield the promised results, while cost has now become 'a significant barrier to access of services by the poor, especially in urban areas' (Stout 1998:34). The impact of fees is underlined by the example of under-five use of services, which reached its lowest point after a sharp (2.5-fold) increase in fees in 1994, but increased rapidly after the abolition of fees at rural health clinics in 1995 (Johnston 1998:48).

UGANDA

Uganda's health status indicators were seen as the best in SSA following independence in 1962, but years of unrest, repression and instability brought a mass exodus of doctors and pharmacists, and the 16 years to 1986 brought an estimated 90% reduction in real health spending (Bossert et al 2000). With a GDP of around $250 per capita in 2004 it is one of the world's poorest nations, and with 90% of its wealth held by 10% of the population, one of the most unequal. It is also one of those most ravaged by HIV and AIDS, and one that has responded by a comparatively effective containment policy.

Uganda is held up by the World Bank as a prime example of seeking private sector solutions to the provision of health care, resulting in what Okuonzi (2004) describes as the 'abdication' of responsibility by the Ministry of Health. And he argues that the appearance of self-sufficiency and 'sustainability' were always an illusion. As with most other SSA countries, the key to any private expansion is receiving an increased share of government spending, and between half and two-thirds of health spending comes from international donors.

The Bank singles out for special praise:

- The government commitment to increase public spending on health to ensure an 'essential package of health services'

- Uganda's experiment in transforming public health facilities into self-governing trusts

- The plan to contract out services including ancillary services and even blood transfusion and the training of clerical and management staff

- The introduction of 'vouchers, insurance schemes and other cost recovery mechanisms'

- A project for District Health Services that will provide equipment for privately run facilities in under-served areas.

(World Bank Group 2000b)

With around 90% of Ugandans living in rural areas, the decentralisation of health services has been a crucial element, though it has run alongside a substantial (110%) increase in funding to hospitals (which still receive around 50% of government health spending and employ 70% of trained staff) and the imposition of user fees. Spending on primary care has fallen by 8% (Okwii 1997, Bossert et al 2000).

However Okuonzi (2004) pinpoints decentralisation as one of the factors that has further widened disparities in the nature and quality of Uganda's health services:

> For example the availability of emergency obstetric services now varies from 4% to 42%. This is because the richer districts and those with powerful local politicians who have been able to persuade non-governmental organisations to work in their district have done better.

There has been considerable public opposition and resentment against the user fees, which are significantly less popular among service users than health care staff, and which, in the context of the general level of poverty in Uganda are unlikely to generate large sums of money (Konde-Lule and Okello 1998). Deininger and Mpuga (2004) have conclusively demonstrated that the user fees work to the detriment of the poorest and most vulnerable potential service users, while generating less than 5% of the total budget of most hospitals and local services.

Birungi and colleagues (1999) point to the fact that in a health system marked by a high level of 'immoral or illegal survival strategies' through which under-paid health workers supplemented their official salaries, the revenue raised from fees was too small to make much difference to their pay and conditions and regularise their work.

The government's objective of working more closely with the 'private sector' is also complicated by the immensely variable and unregulated quality of work done by 'itinerant providers and home providers who constitute the majority of the private providers in the rural areas' (Birungi et al 1999).

The package of market-style measures imposed under pressure from the World Bank in the 1990s is summed up by Okuonzi (2004) as a total failure. By 2003 the technical efficiency of emergency obstetric units varied from 3.9% to 41%, while health care outputs had risen sharply in price:

> Re-establishment of a functioning healthcare system will require heavy investment in infrastructure, which means more dependence on outsiders, not less. Thus in all aspects of health sector performance, the picture is of failure.

Market economic principles, Okuonzi concludes 'are good for generating wealth but poor at improving health and social welfare':

> In the long run, poor countries such as Uganda should adopt a universal health and welfare framework, which they must increasingly finance from internal sources.

However taxation levels are so low that the government has an annual revenue of just 12% of GDP ($7 billion), leaving little obvious capacity for internally generated investment in health care.

GHANA

Ghana was one of the first countries to introduce user fees for health care which had been 'free' at point of use since independence – and one of the first to witness a sharp decline in the utilisation of services as a result. In 1985 as part of an Economic Recovery Programme prescribed by the IMF and World Bank, it implemented a sharp increase in fees for the first visit to a specialist at government hospitals – to ten times the daily wage, plus the full cost of any drugs prescribed: it brought an increase in revenue, but another drop in service use, especially in the rural areas.

However the aim of recovering 15% of health costs through charges was only briefly achieved, and income tapered off to as little as 1%. Perhaps more worrying for governments looking at such policies, a survey showed that many poor people regarded the user fees as instituting a division between the rich who can afford to pay, and the poor who cannot (Arhin-Tekorang 2000).

The move towards hospital autonomy is largely attributed by Govindaraj and colleagues (1996) to attempts to hold down spending. The major teaching hospitals as in so many SSA countries have been consuming a disproportionate share of government health budgets: but the limited autonomy that has been granted has not delivered the expected benefits in terms of efficiency, quality of care or public accountability.

Asia

While World Bank and other advisors have been urging African countries to institute user fees and create new markets for health care, their colleagues offering advice for many Asian countries are counting the consequences of fees that have become unaffordable, and markets that have brought the collapse of once-successful health care systems, leaving a mounting toll of inequality, ill-health and disease confronting the poorest people.

A World Bank Strategy document for East Asia and the Pacific warns that:

> User fees are already widely used in government health systems in most countries in the region, and evidence indicates that they already restrict access of the poor to services (Saadah and Knowles 2000:22).

The Asian Development Bank echoes World Bank criticisms that governments in the region are spending too little – 'underinvesting' – in health care, devoting a smaller share of budgets to health than anywhere else in the world (ADB 1999:66).

This brief country study of China concentrates only on those market-driven and market-style reforms that have been clearly documented.

CHINA

Background

Revolutionary China once led the world in the eradication of disease, the provision of universal access to basic health care, the training of a million 'barefoot doctors' and the emphasis on prevention of ill health. Using techniques very different from the hospital-based Semashko model that had been introduced by Soviet communists, Mao Zedong's party developed an inherently decentralised and rural-focused health care system which, alongside improvements in general nutrition and living standards, delivered some remarkable improvements. Mortality rates from infectious disease in Chinese cities fell from 128 per 100,000 in 1957 to 4.6 in 1998. Immunisation levels exceeded 95% in the 1990s, helping to eliminate polio by 2000 – smallpox had been eradicated as early as 1961 (Li et al 2001). China's system provided one of the models of primary health care which inspired the WHO's Alma Ata declaration and its Health for All 2000 campaign (Hesketh 1997a).

But by the mid 1990s many of the key progressive policies had been abandoned or reversed: privatisation and the market had replaced socialist provision, the communal agriculture system was dropped and the collective provision for health in the rural areas (embodied in the Co-operative Medical System (CMS)) largely collapsed with it. In 1981 71% of Chinese had access to state health care: by 1993 this had fallen to 21%, and China's health spending ranked 144 out of 199 countries (Lampton 2003).

The ageing of the population has also left many older people with little or no cover, and growing numbers unable to afford the care they need. There were fewer doctors per head and fewer hospital beds in 1999 than in 1980 (Liu et al 2002). The situation is even worse for the large migrant population of 80 million rural workers in the cities, and for the unemployed (Bloom et al 2002).

The spending pattern also tends to widen growing social inequalities: the poorest 25% accounted for just 4% of all health spending in 1993. The unequal spending has run alongside unequal health outcomes: the poorest 25% of Chinese suffered infant mortality levels 2.4 times higher than the wealthiest, and 2.9 times more infectious disease (Bhushan 2001). Central government had virtually ceased funding health services, spending just 0.7% of GDP on health, devolving responsibility to local government, while private sources delivered 76% of spending (Saadah and Knowles 2000:11).

China's People's Daily (2001) (cited by Xing 2002) has admitted that over 37% of rural people cannot afford to see doctors, while two-thirds of sick farmers had no access to hospitals.

The decentralisation of health services has also had negative consequences, cutting off provincial-level funding for the Epidemic Prevention Services, and leaving services including TB control subject to user fees. Preventive care has been supplanted by fee-for-service activities, with prenatal care and hospital births among the services that have declined as a result (Jing and Qiongfen 2001:14).

While tobacco sales are soaring, generating a huge health issue of smoking-related deaths[153], the government has been unwilling to use taxation on cigarettes as a means to fund health care, despite estimates that a tax increase of 6.5% could finance essential health services for the poorest 100 million in China (Saadah and Knowles 2000:9). Plans for a 0.5% increase in tax were defeated twice in parliament (Hammond 1998).

But tobacco is far from the only health hazard facing China: in June 2001 China's then health minister stunned the world when he announced that the real level of HIV/AIDS infection was 600,000, compared with previous reports of fewer than 23,000. Many feel that even this new figure is a serious underestimate. The UN AIDS programme estimated in 2002 that there were certainly a million people infected, possibly up to 3 million – it could reach 10 million by 2010 (Gill et al 2002). The disease has spread not only through the familiar routes of heterosexual and homosexual intercourse and needle sharing by drug abusers, but through the unsafe methods used in the 1990s to harvest blood plasma from rural farm workers for use in biomedical factories (Goodman 2002).

The disease finds China with no organised public health system, and few doctors with the necessary training. Unaffordable fees for treatment are compounded by enormous costs of imported drugs – meaning that only the wealthiest can access the care that might prolong their lives. Confusion remains on whether the minority of Chinese people (87 million) who are covered by health insurance can claim reimbursement for their treatment. It is clear that even if they can, their insurance will not cover any AIDS drugs (People's Daily 2002c).

Market-driven reforms

1 Cash limits and spending cuts

Though health spending as a share of GDP increased from 3.17% to 4.82% between 1980 and 1998, the government share of this spending fell by more than half, from 36.4% to just 15.5% (Liu et al 2002).

Public funding was left to provincial and county governments, which can raise money from taxes – but as a result poorer areas are least likely to have funds for health care. This funding covers only a fraction of the spending needed to pay a living wage to health workers, obliging all local health care providers to raise the remainder through user fees: all hospitals insist on cash payments in advance for inpatient care.

2 User fees

By 1998 an estimated 700 million rural Chinese had no insurance or prepayment system to cover health care costs, and were obliged to pay out of pocket for any treatment or drugs they may require. A mere 10% were covered by remnants of the CMS (Liu et al 2002).

Even in the cities, only 45% of the population was covered by workplace-based health

---

153 The most common cause of death in China: Bhushan (2001) estimates that one in six Chinese alive today can expect to die in this way.

insurance, and that number has been falling: policies offer highly uneven entitlements (Hesketh 1997b, Liu et al 2002, Li et al 2001, Yip and Hsiao 2001). In 1992 20% of urban Chinese referred to hospital declined admission, 40% of them blaming the cost: by 1997 this had risen to 32%, with 65% saying they could not afford treatment.

Services concentrate in the most affluent areas, where the largest numbers are covered by some form of insurance or rich enough to pay for themselves. Big city hospitals are swamped with patients, some seeing as many as a million each year, while smaller local services struggle to meet their costs.

Hospitals are restricted on how much they can charge for basic treatment – and are therefore eager to prescribe more drugs, on which they can make a surplus (Bloom 1998). Hospitals can also make money from the wealthy elite by offering high-tech treatments: neo-natal intensive care in Hangzhou Children's Hospital charges a daily fee equivalent to almost double the local average monthly wage (Hesketh 1997b).

3 Regulating drug costs

The country that sacrificed its universal health care system to embark on the road to globalisation and the free market now finds itself unable to afford the price demanded by the western pharmaceutical companies, but unwilling to jeopardise its relations with the leading global powers by breaking patents and manufacturing its own generic drugs, especially having just joined the WTO (Ewing 2001). Instead the vice minister of public health offered the prospect that Chinese people (who can afford it) will be able to visit an experienced foreign dentist, and that the tariffs on imported medicines and medical equipment would be cut (People's Daily 2002a).

Market-style reforms

1 Decentralisation

The chaotic system appears to have generated a wide consensus that more public spending is required and greater responsibility must be taken by central government, although there are unresolved issues over the form this involvement should take (Bloom 2001, Jing and Qiongfen 2001, Bloom et al 2002, Liu et al 2002, Lampton 2003). Liu and colleagues (2002) point out that for all the local-level schemes that have developed across the country since 1949, there is not one example of a scheme totally initiated and sustainably run by a non-government organisation without government support.

It is clear that in the case of China decentralisation has served primarily to weaken the regulatory power of central government to the extent that the same amount of money delivers less in the way of health care: it could even result in a worsening of township (formerly commune) hospitals. As with poor countries elsewhere, the solution to the health problems of China's 900 million rural poor cannot be solved simply within the poor areas themselves (Jing and Qiongfen 2001).

2 Privatisation

The collapse of the public sector brought a mass defection of doctors and professionals to private practice – by 1994 almost half the village clinics were private. The new private sector that emerged was virtually unregulated in terms of quality and the distribution of services, and was under no obligation to deliver any preventive care (Liu and Liu 1997). Almost 60% of rural households and 40% of urban reported in 1993 that they did not use public health facilities because of the cost (Hossain 1997).

A visit to a village clinic could cost a third of a week's income, with township hospitals charging twice as much. A quarter of the people surveyed who had incurred health bills had had to borrow or sell items to pay them, and the long-term impact of health costs are now seen as a major cause of poverty (Bloom 1998:243, Jing and Qiongfeng 2001, Liu et al 2002). By 1997 individuals were paying a massive 85% of total health spending in most rural areas (Bloom 2001).

There have been some moves to improve the system, but they have been piecemeal and covering relatively small numbers: in December 1998 the government established a new social insurance programme for urban workers – but it was to cover only those employed, and not their dependents (Yip and Hsiao 2001). This followed a decision earlier in the year to 'streamline a health care network' to deliver a basic package of care to 900 million rural workers (People's Daily 2002b). But the new rural system will still pool risks only at a local level, perpetuating the inequalities that have grown during the years of China's marketising reform.

Shorter country summaries – Asia

INDIA

India, the world's second most populous country, remains another prime example of the failure of a largely privatised health care system with chronic low levels of government health spending, static for several years at around 1% of GDP – well below the WHO's recommended minimum of 5%.

About 80% of spending is absorbed by the private sector, while 75% is paid directly by households, and only 10% of Indians have some form of insurance. User fees apply even for poor people treated in public hospitals, with upwards of 15% of those hospitalised falling into poverty as a result of the costs incurred:

> Hospitalised Indians spent 58% of their total annual expenditures on health care. More than 40%
> of hospitalised people borrow money or sell assets to cover expenses (Peters et al 2002:5).

Spending is also highly unequal, with the wealthiest 20% receiving three times more government health spending than the poorest – though the pattern varies in different states (Peters et al 2002).

The central government, with a Central Ministry of Health employing no less than 30,000 administrators, exerts direct and heavy-handed control over its network of under-funded and pressurised public hospitals – but little if any regulatory control over private sector providers, many of which are not formally registered. A priority area of the public sector has been the population control programme, which despite a signal lack of effectiveness in reducing fertility rates or population growth, has as Nandraj (1997) points out, resulted not only in the neglect of other areas of health care, but in many rural health services being seen as little more than a population control service.

Curative care services in the rural areas have been largely left to the private sector, which as World Bank-commissioned research has concluded, is at best of uneven quality (Naylor et al 1999, Peters et al 2002). The neglect of rural services is also reflected in the lack of hospital provision: in 1991 just 32% of hospitals and 20% of beds were in the rural areas where 70% of the population lives – giving just one-twelfth of the beds per head available in urban areas (Nandraj 1997).

Overt and covert government subsidies for the private sector include the training of at least 15,000 doctors every year, two-thirds of whom go to work in the private sector. Public hospitals also offer a 'safety net' for under-insured Indians who cannot obtain private treatment, while the public sector also handles almost all treatment of the poorest citizens, allowing the private hospitals to cream skim those best able to pay.

Most accident victims and more serious cases are also passed on to public hospitals from the private sector: a survey in Karnatka found that just 3% of small private hospitals had a blood bank (Naylor et al 1999). Many of the generic problems of private medical provision are exhibited in the context of the unregulated Indian system: perverse incentives for private practitioners to give superfluous, costly 'tests' and treatment, widely fluctuating levels of fees; payments flowing back to referring doctors when patients are sent for specialist treatment; and private hospitals refusing treatment without a cash payment in advance (Nandraj 1997). Small wonder a household survey in 2002 found that health care is seen as the most corrupt service in India (Kumar 2003).

The combination of lumbering, bureaucratic and under-resourced public services and profit-seeking private hospitals leaves India vulnerable to what Mukhopadhyay (2000) describes as 'two shadows': infectious disease like malaria and tuberculosis on the one hand, and non-infectious chronic diseases such as cancer and coronary diseases on the other:

> The large wide-spread health infrastructure that has been set up throughout the country seems to be non-functional and unresponsive in many parts. Instead of moving forward to meet newer health challenges, it is sliding backward (Mukhopadhyay 2000:342).

Mukhopadhyay might have added HIV/AIDS to the list of hazards to be combated: up to 3.5 million people are thought to be infected, and the total is rising (Peters et al 2002).

However the answers to these challenges are limited by world market pressures. Nandraj (1997) blames the lack of government investment in health care on Structural Adjustment Programmes and in particular India's New Economic Policy, though it is clear that some of the chronic lack of public sector infrastructure, the bureaucratism in the public sector and the unequal distribution of health care services have been inherited from the worst aspects of the British Raj.

But Naylor and colleagues point out that however desirable it may be to increase government spending (if only to 'subsidise enrolment by the poor in private prepayment schemes'), this is precluded by India's 'large fiscal deficit' and the extent to which it is reliant on private finance (Naylor et al 1999:21). India's loans from the World Bank totalled $44 billion in 1999, making it the largest single borrower. Ministers justify the imposition of user fees in public health services by the need to prepare for the time the money runs out (Abbasi 1999e).

However the levels of social inequality have also created very difficult conditions for the profitable operation of fully private insurance multinationals. Cigna has withdrawn from the market after two years, and in 2002 BUPA was reviewing a joint HMO venture (Hall 2003).

Boxed in to an untenable situation by its dependent status and by past failure to act more decisively in the interests of its poorest citizens, India's rulers seem to have established their country as yet another stark example of the inability of privatised medicine and market-based solutions to meet basic social needs.

VIETNAM

Still ravaged by the effects of 50 years of war which ended in 1975, and saddled with the debts run up by the US-sponsored regime in South Vietnam, the Vietnamese government was obliged to seek support from the IMF and World Bank in the mid 1980s. The strings attached to this support involved wide-reaching free market reforms. One of these was the introduction of user fees at the district hospitals and commune level centres, which from liberation until 1989 had distributed health care and pharmaceuticals free of charge (Hong 2000).

The infant mortality rate had been halved between 1979 and 1989, and progress had been made on many preventable health problems. The 1989 reforms changed all that. User fees ran alongside deregulation of pharmaceuticals, the legalisation of private practice and a halt to government funding for local level facilities. A World Bank report a few years later surveys the aftermath of a devastating collapse in what had been an effective and localised system:

- Deaths from malaria had reached the highest ever level in 1991, not least as a result of the under-funding of the National Malaria Control Program

- District hospitals were running out of medical and surgical equipment, while 'a large proportion of commune health facilities have become dilapidated to the point of being unusable'

- Outpatient attendances had halved, along with hospital admissions

- Service users at public health facilities were paying twice as much as the government towards health spending, and even more was being spent by patients buying drugs from private practitioners or as self-medication – in total, the state budget paid just 16% of health spending in 1993

- Steps to revitalise and further extend the public health network were 'essential', since 'without government intervention the commune health centers will turn to fee-for-service arrangements... or wither away'. This would endanger TB control, disease surveillance and other community services.

    (World Bank 1995)

The situation worsened further in the 1990s. By 1998 another World Bank analysis, which regarded Vietnam as 'a not uninteresting case study' noted that 80% of health spending was paid out of pocket. User fees for hospital care had risen 1000% in real terms between 1993 and 1998, while fees for private clinics and doctors had risen 600%. There were also charges for commune health centres 'even though these were still supposed to be free in 1998' (Wagstaff and van Doorslaer 2001). The government budget, accounting for 58% of health spending, increased only marginally from 1995-98, and the health system remained dependent on foreign aid (an 'unsustainable resource') for 13% of its resources. Hospital fees were equivalent to 13% of the health budget, but covered 50% of hospital spending (Trong Hai and Schuftan 2001).

A survey for PHR of health care provider payment reform in Asia and Latin America describes Vietnam – and also China – as:

> ...moving away from a British model of public sector delivery and financing of care toward one based on social insurance. [...] As income grew, people became less satisfied by existing public services. Government funding limitations prevented the large facility improvements that would have satisfied the public, and therefore social insurance was seen as a way to mobilise resources

and offer universal coverage to citizens (Bitran and Yip 1998:3).

As we have already seen, there is little evidence to support this extraordinary interpretation of the changes either in China or Vietnam, where the 'public' is not only starkly divided between urban and rural, rich and poor, but also the last to be consulted on its views in the shaping of health policy. Vietnam's social health insurance scheme, introduced in 1993, covered only 12% of the population, mainly among the higher income groups (op. cit:2), falling to less than 10% by 1998 (Trong Hai and Schuftan 2001). Lonnroth and colleagues note that in 1998 there were no health insurance schemes covering private health care provision, despite the fact that a majority of physicians were practising in private clinics. They also noted the limited facilities and equipment used by private doctors (Lonnroth et al 1998).

The reforms have opened a growing gap between the health care for Vietnam's richest and poorest, with the rich making more use of health services in general and hospital services in particular, and spending more than twice as much each year in money terms, but around a third as much as a percentage of their income (Trong Hai and Schuftan 2001, Bhushan 2001:225). Under-utilisation of services by the poor has created problems in sustaining the network of community health stations.

The government has tried to shift the balance of spending, to allocate greater resources in areas of greatest need, such as the impoverished mountain communities which suffer the greatest burden of disease – and therefore incur the greatest cost. The mountain areas currently receive 1.8 times the per capita budget allocated to the more prosperous areas, but this is still not enough to compensate for the additional spending required. Given the differentials in income, and the lack of insurance coverage, spending in the rural areas has to be predominantly financed from government budgets (Trong Hai and Schuftan 2001).

JAPAN

According to Ii (2005) 'Japan's health care system is facing a financial crisis'. This view is echoed in most detailed studies, despite the general consensus that the health status of the 122 million Japanese population is among the highest in the OECD , and the country's relatively low level of spending on health care (7.6% of GDP in 2000: OECD[154] Health Data 2003).

Western medicine began in Japan in 1867, and the introduction of the first limited Bismarck-style social health insurance came in 1922 (Ii 2005). This was subsequently extended at various points to cover the whole population by 1961 (Jeong and Hurst 2001). The Employees Health Insurance System is now financed through compulsory deductions from the payroll, shared equally between employers and employees. It covers workers and their dependents, while the National Health Insurance System covers the self-employed, pensioners and unemployed. The insurance system pays all providers a flat fee-for-service, with fees being revised centrally every two years. Patients are subject to a co-payment of around 14% up to a maximum of £318 per month, out of average monthly disposable earnings of £2,805. These fees are seen as a means of 'dampening demand' (Imai 2002:5). There have also been attempts to set global budgets that would cap health spending, but these have not proved successful (Bitran and Yip 1998).

---

154 Life expectancy is high at 77 years for men and 84 years for women, while the infant mortality rate, at 3.6, is almost half that of the USA.

In 1973 health services for people aged over 70 were exempted from payment, but ten years later co-payments (10%) were reintroduced for the elderly, and are now a feature of all Japanese health care. Health spending on the over-70s is five times the average spend on those aged under 70. A separate system of insurance to cover nursing care for the elderly was introduced in 2000, although the level of co-payments is still seen as a deterrent by some and one factor in a quarter of the 2.5 million elderly whose needs had been assessed not using care services in 2000. The reliance on private provision of services has also left a gap between rising levels of demand for home care services and the availability of services which the private sector does not see as profitable. Problems in tailoring the system to the needs of older service users have meant that the projected reduction in geriatric beds has not been achieved – and as a result Japanese hospitals buck the global trend by maintaining by far the highest allocation of beds per head of population in the OECD[155] (Imai 2002).

Although most care is publicly funded, the Japanese health care system has remained dominated by private sector providers: 80% of hospitals and 94% of private clinics are privately owned and operated, although investor-owned for-profit hospitals are prohibited, and the role of private health insurance is 'marginal'. The funding system is complex, with around 5,000 insurance funds covering different sections of the workforce and wider population, but with little control over the volume of medical services provided, and playing little proactive role in negotiating with providers or checking on the quality and effectiveness of care (Imai 2002).

Japanese health care also lacks any form of 'gatekeeper' system or any rigid demarcation between specialist roles, so that 'virtually all doctors in private clinics try to deal with all the problems of their patients' (Imai 2002:6). Part of this expansion is explained by the rapid ageing of the Japanese population, and the lack of consistent distinction between acute hospital beds and geriatric beds: Japanese statistics define as a 'hospital' any health care institution with more than 20 beds, giving the country a staggering 9,100 hospitals in 2003 (Ii 2005). An extraordinarily long average length of stay of 30.8 days – far longer than any other OECD country, and four times the OECD average – means that despite a relatively low level of hospitalisation (just over half the OECD average) Japan utilises three times the OECD average of bed days per capita, with many of these accounted for through long-term care of frail older patients, known as 'social hospitalisation' (Imai 2002). People aged over 65, equivalent to 18.5% of the population, accounted for over 51% of health spending in 1997.

The lengthy and often inappropriate use of hospital facilities, coupled with extremely high rates of consultations with doctors (second highest in the OECD), high levels of high-cost outpatient treatment and high levels of prescribing have meant that after years in which expansion could be afforded in a booming economy, Japanese health care has continued to rise in cost since the 1980s despite the stagnation of the economy.

However the soaring cost has not been matched by quality of care, and there are concerns both over the length of waiting times to see a doctor and at the short time patients spend in the eventual consultation. Satisfaction levels appear to be relatively low (Imai 2002, Jeong and Hurst 2001) with some surveys suggesting up to 90% of the public is dissatisfied with the health care system (Kondo 2005).

---

155 Estimated by Ii (2005) at ten beds per 1,000 population in 2002. Numbers of doctors, expanded by the opening of new medical schools in the 1970s increased by almost 150% from 103,000 in 1960 to 256,000 in 2,000, 60% of whom are employed in hospitals.

The Japanese system has attracted critical attention from US management consultants who have noted that 'the productivity of the current Japanese system is at approximately 75% of the current US level,' and that despite the dominance of the private sector:

> ...the Japanese system is characterised by low levels of competition in each of the markets that make up a health care system. Competition among payors [sic] for patients and among providers for payor contracts is banned by law (McKinsey MGI Report 2000).

The large scale of Japan's potential market for medical technology (estimated at $21 billion a year), and the looming financial crisis – with a predicted shortfall of $40 billion and the possible bankruptcy of several major insurance funds over the next two to three years also attracted the attention of the US Congressional Ways and Means Committee (2001). They saw the crisis as a possible crucial factor that could drive the Japanese government to contemplate far-reaching reforms including 'market-opening measures'.

Similar dire warnings of bankruptcy for the medical insurance system by 2003 have come from Japan's own Health and Welfare Ministry (Lamar 2000). The downturn, together with the rapid ageing of the population that is reducing the workforce by 0.6% per year, is serving both to reduce income to the medical insurance funds, and to increase health care spending on a larger number of older people, with the 'over-treatment of geriatrics' (Bitran and Yip 1998). Two-thirds of insurance funds were in the red in 2000, with 90% expected to be in deficit in 2001 (Imai 2002). Yet despite the urgings of various analysts and observers, and growing evidence that the fee-for-service system was generating perverse incentives for physicians to over-prescribe drugs at an estimated annual value of $3.5 billion (Pilling 2003)[156], relatively little radical action has yet been adopted by the Japanese government.

The main attempts to stabilise the system have come in a squeeze on the fees paid to doctors and hospitals, while pharmaceutical companies have been left relatively unscathed, and the government has held back from tax increases which might further jeopardise economic recovery (Burgermeister 2004c). The attempt to limit doctors' fees, and to reduce the additional surpluses they can make through the prescription and dispensing of drugs, reflects a loss of political power and influence by the Japanese Medical Association, which for over 40 years worked closely with the governing party and the bureaucracy of the Ministry of Health Labour and Welfare to form an 'iron triangle' protecting medical incomes and opposing radical reform of the system (Kondo 2005). This same level of professional power has also helped maintain a system with wide variation in clinical practices between medical schools and hospitals, making it difficult to develop alternative systems of provider payment based on diagnostic related groups (Imai 2002).

However Ernst & Young (2003) identify three basic drivers of change in the Japanese health care system: the ageing population; transformation from a system of retrospective fees to a system of prospective payment (forcing providers to share risk); and the deregulation of hospital and insurance markets which have been protected up to now from competition[157]. A

---

156 A Vanderbilt University study found that in 1996 physicians in Japan were earning an average $43,000 each year on the 'mark-up' between wholesale and retail prices of drugs which they prescribe and dispense for patients – a link strongly defended by the doctors' lobby (Pilling 2003).

157 'In the Japanese system neither the consumer's choice of health insurers nor the insurer's choice of service providers is possible' (Imai 2002:8).

wider reform agenda has also been urged in OECD investigations[158] (Imai 2002).

Over and above improved use of information technology, other key reforms proposed include:

- The integration of insurance funds into a larger unit, to establish more effective risk pooling and a stronger role as agents for patients

- A strengthened role of insurers as purchasers of care, increasing the accountability of providers and reviewing the quality of services

- A move from fee-for-service towards more inclusive payments which give hospitals incentives to reduce costs (Imai 2002).

KOREA

Kwon (2004) sums up the curious and contradictory features of the social insurance-based health care system in this country of 47 million people, which launched its system of social insurance in 1977, and only established complete coverage of the population in 1989:

> Health care in Korea can best be described by inefficiency, for-profit domination and fee-for-service system.

Of these three features perhaps the most decisive is the for-profit domination, which thrives on some of the inefficiencies in the system. 90% of all hospitals and all clinics are privately owned, half of them in theory as 'not-for-profit' corporations, although they appear to behave as if they were for-profit (Kwon 2003). Without government funding or philanthropic funds to draw upon, they are all funded largely through fee-for-service payments from National Health Insurance – which is the single fund created in 2000 through the merger of the previous 350 separate insurance funds.

Fee-for-service has given health care providers an in-built incentive to increase the volume and intensity of treatment provided, in order to maximise their income, and has also skewed treatment towards more complex (and profitable) services and those which are outside the National Health Insurance list, and therefore unregulated (and uninsured). Perhaps the clearest example is the extremely high number of babies delivered by caesarean section – 43% of births in 1999, four times the level recommended by the WHO (sharply up from just 6% in 1985). The obvious explanation for this is that the fee for the caesarean procedure is 2.7 times that for a normal delivery (Kwon 2003:86).

The predominance of the private sector has also helped to force up prices for treatment well above those achievable in the public sector, without any discernible difference in quality of care. Children can be vaccinated in public sector health centres for a third of the price charged by private clinics; costs for ambulatory care patients range from one-third to half the cost of private treatment, and those needing treatment for chronic diseases pay as little as a fifth of the fees charged by private hospitals. Public hospitals also treat a tenfold higher proportion of poor patients funded by the Medical Aid Programme. And while the 200 health centres are well distributed, covering every district, the accessibility of privately funded hospitals is uneven, with fewer facilities available to serve the rural population, and greater concentration of doctors and hospitals in the biggest cities (Colombo and Hurst 2003).

Meanwhile the lack of any regulation or capacity planning has meant that private hospitals have expanded in number, bringing a four-fold increase in bed numbers between 1980 and 1999, running at very low levels of occupancy (65.8% in 1998), which in turn pushes up unit costs. Hospitals also operate with a very long average length of stay, which might be accounted for by the use of acute beds for chronic care, or by the fact that with a relatively low level of admission rates (just over half the OECD average), Korean patients who are admitted may in fact prove to be more seriously ill, and require more extended treatment (Colombo and Hurst 2003).

The system of payment also helps explain Korea's high use of prescription drugs (double the OECD average). Before 2000, physicians were able to charge not only a fee for consultation but also to make a surplus on the mark-up price of drugs they dispensed directly to patients: this gave a double incentive to prescribe, and revenue from pharmaceuticals often accounted for more than 40% of physicians' total income. By 2000 Korea was the world's tenth largest pharmaceutical market, worth $8 billion a year, 15% of which was imported.

But new regulations passed in 1994 and implemented in 2000, aimed at squeezing down the soaring drugs bill, insisted on a separation between physicians prescribing and pharmacists dispensing drugs. Angry doctors retaliated with a series of strikes which resulted in a compensating 45% increase in physicians' fees – landing the problem back onto patients. Further efforts to hold down drug spending include new legislation on Economic Evaluation of the cost-effectiveness and availability of new products, and a system of 'reference pricing' which set a top limit on the amount that would be reimbursed by NHI – leaving patients to pay the remainder. This was clearly intended to push doctors and patients in the direction of cheaper, home-produced and generic drugs – and triggered an angry response from the major pharmaceutical manufacturers (Yang 2003, Ward 2002). However with no financial reward on offer for prescribing lower-cost drugs, doctors have resorted to prescribing more expensive, branded drugs: 14 of the top-selling drugs covered by NHI in 2002 were produced by multinational companies (Kwon 2004).

With little infrastructure of primary care, and therefore no 'gatekeeping' function, most patients tend to be seen by specialists who compete with each other rather than cooperating in the interests of better patient care. All of the inflated costs in Korea's health care system have an especially negative impact on the poorest and those with chronic disease, not least because the fees are fixed without reference to the ability to pay, subject to only minimal exemptions, and not limited by any annual 'cap'. The higher costs of private sector provision, thriving in the absence of sufficient lower-cost public sector alternatives, have helped fuel a constant upward pressure in health spending that has brought the insurance system to the brink of bankruptcy (Kwon 2004, Kwon 2003, Yang 2003).

The limited scope of government investment in hospitals and health centres flows from another underlying characteristic of the Korean health care system, which was put in place 'top-down without social consensus among major stakeholders' by an authoritarian regime seeking greater legitimacy and acceptance. The aim was to ensure rapid extension of low-level coverage at low cost (contributions from employees began at 4% of income) rather than the development of a comprehensive public service (Kwon 2004). Korean health care spending thus began very low by OECD standards, and has grown from this small base towards the OECD average: but a much larger than average share of health care spending has always come not from government or insurance funding but from out of pocket payments by individual patients. In Korea less than half of health care spending (46% in 1998) is from public sector funds, compared with an OECD average of 72%. This means that the remaining cost has to be made up of co-payments and fees for services and treatments and not covered by National Health Insurance (Colombo and Hurst 2003). As a result the NHI system has come to be viewed not as a system of full coverage, but one offering 'discounts' on the cost of health care (Kwon 2004).

The financial crisis at the turn of the century can be seen as the product of a number of factors:

- Low levels of contribution to NHI, depressed by the stagnant economy during the Asian economic crisis of 1997-98, and generally rising more slowly than health insurance expenditure
- The addition of new benefits to NHI coverage since 1994 without adequate funding
- A decline in government subsidies to cover benefits for the self-employed and unemployed
- A rapid increase in NHI spending (up tenfold from 1982-1999) driven by a rapidly ageing population, an expanding hospital sector and increased volume of treatment, with claims per capita increasing at over 9% per year, and rising medical costs.

(Colombo and Hurst 2003)

By the end of 2001 the deficit had reached $2.6 billion, equivalent to about 20% of the total NHI budget: steps to resolve the crisis included a temporary cash injection using money from a sharply increased tobacco tax that had been earmarked for a health promotion fund. This subsidy is due to end in 2005 (Kwon 2004). The government's plan of action to tackle the financial crisis also included steps that, rather than confront the powerful provider interest groups (doctors and hospitals), would foist the cost onto service users:

- An increase in co-payments
- Improved income assessment for the self-employed
- A 9% per year increase in contributions until 2006.

But even if these measures can stave off the prospect of a financial melt-down, as Kwon argues, a system so skewed in favour of for-profit hospitals and private doctors requires more fundamental changes, in particular:

> ...a new paradigm of NHI policy in order to empower consumers and to counteract the overwhelming influence of the medical profession... [because] unless there is a government commitment or mechanism to induce health care providers to contain expenditure, more compensation to them is simply a reward for inefficiency (2004).

Kwon argues that early trials of provider payments based on Diagnostic Related Groups in Korea have shown that it is possible to reduce costs, reduce lengths of stay and reduce tests and use of antibiotics without harming patient care: but the introduction of this was interrupted by the doctors' strikes in 2000. Together with Colombo and Hurst (2003) Kwon also floats the notion of Medical Savings Accounts, which have proved such a controversial policy in the US and elsewhere. But the most obvious model for an alternative to the rampant profiteering and high cost private sector would be an expansion of the existing network of publicly owned hospitals and health centres, coupled with a tariff of reference prices based on public sector costs, pressurising the private providers to make health care more affordable to the NHI and to the patients who need it most.

Chapter eight

Country summaries: North America and Australasia

North America

CANADA

Background

Canada has a population of almost 31 million in a huge country of 10 million square kilometres. It is a federation comprising 10 provinces and three territories, each of which has its own Ministry of Health or equivalent, and as a result Canada has been described as having 'not one health care system but 13' (Romanow 2002b). Although showing similar patterns of spending in terms of share of GDP from the early 1960s, Canada has always spent less per head on health than the USA.

In the late 1960s Canada broke from a US-style health system based on private insurance to establish a single-payer publicly funded system, beginning with the 1966 Medical Care Insurance Act. It established its Medicare system in the 1984 Canada Health Act, which offers universal coverage for medically necessary services delivered by a physician or in hospital.

Private for-profit hospitals account for less than 5% of Canadian hospitals (Armstrong et al 2001, PAHO 2002). The system avoided the sky-high overhead costs which continued to escalate in the unreformed US, but in terms of share of GDP spent, Canada's remained one of the most expensive of the health care systems in the OECD countries until the early 1990s. However as Table 8 shows, the gap between the health spending per head in the US and the equivalent in Canada has vastly widened since 1984, from around 50% to the latest estimate of 133% (OECD 2003). It is also important to note that the Canadian figures cover a system delivering universal coverage for the whole population, while the higher spending in the US still leaves an estimated 42 million people (far more than Canada's whole population) completely without health insurance.

Table 8

Total current expenditure on health/capita, US$ exchange rate			Total current expenditure on health as % gross domestic product	
Year	USA	Canada	USA	Canada
1960	138	110	4.8	4.9
1970	328	256	6.6	6.5
1980	1025	735	8.4	6.8
1990	2683	1795	11.6	8.7
2000	4475	2019	13.7	8.8
2001	4819	2070	13.7	9.3

OECD HEALTH DATA 2003

As a single-payer system, Medicare has incurred the anger of neoliberal critics who resent the level of public funding and the resulting restrictions on for-profit private health provision: but it has held down administrative and transaction costs to around a third of those prevailing in the USA[159] (Woolhandler et al 2003). Treatment costs for Ontario cancer patients and Alberta cataract patients sent to private US hospitals are six times as high as the costs of the same treatment in Canada (Deber 2000:42). Despite the damage to public confidence and the extended waiting times that have resulted from the extended squeeze on federal spending during the 1990s[160], the Medicare system remains not only lower in cost, but 'wildly popular' (Deber 2000) and public opinion has repeatedly favoured an increase in federal funding to sustain publicly funded care rather than privatisation or neoliberal reforms (CMA 1998, Lewis et al 2001).

In 1998 74% of Canadians over the age of 12 had supplementary insurance coverage for prescription costs, while 99% of physician services and 70% of total health care spending were financed by the public sector. Medicare coverage has always been strongly linked to services provided by 'hospitals, physicians and dentists', giving little support for new models of care such as home and community-based services (Deber 2000).

This has meant that in some cases policy reforms seeking to downsize the hospital sector and shift care closer to patients' homes have appeared to be advocated most strongly not by

159 Per capita costs of administration were estimated at $1,059 in the USA in 1999 (and 31% of total US health spending), and $307 and 16.7% in Canada. By 1999 more than one in four (27%) of the US health workforce was an admin & clerical worker, compared to 19% in Canada (Woolhandler et al 2003).

160 Health care spending fell as a percentage of Canadian GDP from 10.2% in 1992 to 9.5% in 1996, and was expected to fall to 9.2% in 1997, bringing five successive years in which annual growth in per capita spending was below 1%. Over the same period hospital spending fell as a proportion of total health spending, from 38.9% to 35.5%, resulting in a decline in access to a range of services, lengthening waiting times, and crisis measures in Ontario, British Columbia, Quebec and Alberta to tackle bed shortages (CMA 1998).

progressive campaigners seeking to improve patient care, but by governments seeking to cut public spending and seeing the new model as a means of shifting costs from the public sector on to individuals and their families (Williams et al 2001).

In April 2001 Roy Romanow, a former social democratic prime minister of Saskatchewan, was appointed by the Federal government to chair a Commission on the future of Canada's health care system: this conducted extensive consultations and reported in November 2002. Outlining plans for a £10 billion increase in spending over three years, and a permanent increase of over £4 billion a year (Laghi 2002a,b,c), it noted a widespread consensus in favour of the principles of Medicare as a single-payer tax-funded system, and proposed a modernisation of the Canada Health Act that would expand its coverage to include two 'new essential services': diagnostic services and 'priority home care'.

Romanow calls for improved primary care and prevention services, to establish 'comprehensive primary health care available to Canadians 24 hours a day, 7 days a week'. The new system should aim to reshape health care, by:

> ...taking away the almost overwhelming focus on hospitals and medical treatments, breaking down the barriers that too frequently exist between health care providers, and putting the focus on consistent efforts to prevent illness and injury, and improve health (Romanow 2002:116).

The report also calls for increased resources for mental health ('the "orphan child" of health care') which Romanow notes is now 'largely a home and community-based service': it should be included as medically necessary services under the Canada Health Act, and made available across the country (ibid xxxi).

However the report retreats from a full-scale inclusion of home care (notably avoiding any commitment to include continuing care for older people) in the 'medically necessary' services to be covered by Medicare:

> Because of the significant costs that would be involved in including all home care services under the Canada Health Act, priorities should be placed on the most pressing needs. There is little doubt that effective home care support is vitally important to people with mental illnesses, to people who have just been released from hospital, and to those who are in their last months of life. These three areas – mental health, post-acute care, and palliative care – should be the first three home care services to be included under a revised *Canada Health Act* (Romanow 2002a:172).

Romanow also rejects any tax increases to pay for the new injection of resources into Medicare, which he argues could be funded from the federal budget surplus.

While Romanow's report firmly rejects a further expansion of the private sector, a rather less categoric conclusion was promoted in the findings of a separate, concurrent report from the Senate's standing committee,[161] which favours continued government funding, but argues that care should be purchased from either public or private providers. However despite the fears of some campaigners that it would open the door for an expansion of for-profit care (Barlow 2002), the sixth and final volume of a Senate report, chaired by Michael Kirby, examines – and *rejects* – alternatives including the expansion of for-profit hospital services,

---

161 Which also began work in 2001 (Lewis et al 2001).

diagnostics and outpatients. It declares in favour of maintaining the Medicare model, but does not do so unconditionally:

> The single, public insurer model was in fact the first principle enunciated in Volume Five. As a corollary, private insurance for publicly insured health services should continue to be disallowed, *provided that* such publicly insured services are delivered in a *timely* fashion (Kirby 2002: Chapter 16).

In line with this implicit warning that the alternative could be a move towards a more privatised, two-tier system, the Kirby Report also argues that Canadians would have to spend an additional £2.1 billion a year on Medicare if they want it to survive. The report recommends that this should be raised through a health care premium to be added to the tax bill, ranging from £0.21 per day for the lowest-paid, to £1.68 a day for the highest earners. This should be linked to the introduction of nationwide coverage for 'catastrophic' prescription drug costs (provision of which varies from one province to another), and the fixing of maximum waiting times for major medical procedures – after which patients would be guaranteed funded treatment in other provinces or in the US. Other proposals included an expansion in the numbers of nurses and investment in medical schools (Spurgeon 2002).

While the debates and indecision continue in Canada's 13 health services, it is clear that while there are strong advocates of reform, there has been no equivalent to the 'managed care' policies of the US, or the quasi-markets of the UK. Much of the increased weight of the private sector in Canada has been 'at the margin' of the Medicare system, affecting home care, long-term care and diagnostic services that were not covered by the Canada Health Act.

Market-driven reforms

1 Cash limits and spending cuts

Sustained spending restrictions in the mid 1990s meant that real-terms spending in 1996-7 was lower than in 1991-2 (Romanow 2002b, Deber 2000:17), and the pressure on resources generated continual frustration and debate throughout the 1990s. By 2000, when the federal government finally agreed to increase direct funding in support of provincial health budgets the pressures were making themselves felt in many hospitals across the country:

> Recent problems have included extreme overcrowding of hospital emergency services, severe shortages of medical and nursing staff, long waiting lists for lifesaving surgical operations, and a lack of sufficient equipment and staff, resulting in patients being sent for treatment to the United States at great expense (Spurgeon 2000).

Canada's waiting times for hospital treatment in 2001 were estimated to be 77% higher than they had been in 1993: spending reductions had meant capacity could not match demand (Esmail & Walker 2002).

Yet there has been consistent pressure not only to sustain services, but also to expand the range of services covered by Medicare. In 1997 after 30 months of research and deliberation the prime minister's National Forum on Health called for Medicare to be expanded to cover home care and prescription costs, and for the share of public spending to be expanded (Lewis et al 2001).

The tax-funded system has avoided the unrestrained costs of multi-payer insurance schemes in France and Germany, but at a cost: it has struggled for resources during much of the 1990s, leaving specialists in some high-profile services – notably cancer treatment – demanding urgent action to rectify falling standards of care (Cancer Care Advocacy Coalition 2003, Hryniuk 2003).

2 Rationalisation
However while market-style reforms have generally been held at bay by the weight of popular opposition, there have been market-driven (cost-cutting) moves to rationalise hospital services in Ontario, Canada's most populous province[162] (Deber and Baranek 1998), and to adjust funding formulae to achieve greater equity (Pink and Leatt 2003).

3 User fees, regulate drug costs
Medicare has managed to maintain the principle of free care at point of use, while Canadian pharmaceuticals already retail at much lower costs than the same drugs in the USA.

Market-style reforms

1 Decentralisation
Decentralisation in Canada arises not so much from market reforms as the federal character of the country. Almost 92% of public spending on health care originated from provincial and territorial governments, with just 5.2% coming from direct federal spending, and the remainder from social security and municipal spending (PAHO 2002), although these figures conceal the amount raised and retained by the province from federal taxes through 'tax points' (Deber 2000). This imbalance in funding creates tensions between provincial governments and the centre: while the federal government sets the over-riding principles of health care, it leaves the responsibility for much of the funding to more local level.

2 Purchaser/provider split, contracts and provider autonomy
Health care under Medicare has always been funded through taxation at federal and provincial level, but delivered largely by private practitioners and non-profit hospitals run by community boards of trustees, voluntary organisations or local municipalities.

3 Purchasing care from private sector
In Alberta some clinical services such as hip operations are contracted out to private hospitals, though under strict conditions to prevent extra billing and queue jumping. A report from the province's former deputy premier[163] advocated an increased role for private health care, the imposition of user fees and a possible restriction on the range of essential services to be delivered by the public sector (Lewis et al 2001, Council of Canadians 2002, Spurgeon 2002a). However health ministry figures showed that waiting lists for hip operations in Alberta were just half those of a private clinic in Calgary, and figures also showed that private for-profit MRI scans for Medicare patients in Calgary cost 21% more than public sector provision (McNulty 2002).

In British Columbia, the Vancouver Coastal Health Authority in the summer of 2003

---

162 While Pink and Leatt (2003) argue that the rationalisation is purely to improve efficiency and equity, Deber and Baranek (1998) point to the Ontario government's objective of cutting Can$1.3 billion from hospital spending. The resulting reduction in hospital capacity inevitably contributes to the pressures on an under-resourced system.

163 Don Mazankowski was also previously a Canadian minister for privatisation, and now sits on the board of Great West Lifeco Inc, a private health insurance company (Council of Canadians 2002).

incurred the anger of health unions and opposition leaders when it invited bids from private sector clinics to take on upwards of 3,000 day surgery operations currently performed in the public sector (Lavoie 2003). Alberta and three other provinces have private for-profit MRI and CT scanner services: Ontario decided in June 2002 that it would allow 20 for-profit MRI clinics and five CT scan clinics to open. In 2001 Ontario had allocated Can$60 million of federal funds to help for-profit companies buy beds, bathtubs and diagnostic equipment (Sutherland 2002).

4 Privatisation/private insurance

Canadian legislation prevents private sector insurance covering services already provided by government programmes, though insurers can offer to 'top up' benefits which do not fully cover areas of care such as dental, ophthalmological and complementary medicine services, and prescription costs. In the case of diagnostic services Romanow (xxv) noted that the growing reliance on the private sector for advanced services was 'eroding the equal access principle at the heart of medicare' – a finding echoed by Sutherland's detailed investigation into the effects of an expansion of for-profit MRI and CT clinics[164] (Sutherland 2002).

5 PFI

Campaigners and health unions have also voiced strong opposition to the extension of the Private Finance Initiative to Canada, notably the plans to build and run two new hospitals in Ontario under a Can$500 million Public Private Partnership (P3s) arrangement that would provide all but medical services on both sites.

Critics argue that this arrangement would be more costly in the long term, and offer less accountability than public funding. Any apparent reduction in running costs would – as in the first wave of PFI hospitals in Britain – be explained by the fact that the buildings would be new, and would be both smaller and have fewer beds than the hospitals they are replacing (Auerbach 2002, Barlow 2002).

UNITED STATES OF AMERICA

Background

US academic institutions and US-based agencies may tour the word advising poor countries how to restructure health services, but few of them have added the influence to those pressing for reform of the costly and shambolic health system on their doorstep. The American system is by far the most costly in the world, and plagued by 'soaring costs, low value for money relative to population status and unsatisfactory coverage and access to health services'. Its costs are projected to reach 17.7% of GDP ($3.1 trillion) by 2012 and a third of GDP in the longer term, but it delivers only 'mediocre' outcomes in terms of the population's general health (Docteur et al 2003, Heffler et al 2003).

Indeed the US system has in most cases pioneered and exposed the limitations of all the

---

164 Sutherland points to evidence that opening for-profit clinics could result in longer waits in the public sector; allow people to queue jump without respect to medical need; risk poorer quality but more expensive services; give doctors a financial incentive to increase numbers of inappropriate referrals; and draw skilled staff away from public sector services (Sutherland 2002).

stock proposals made by academics for the 'reform' of health services along market lines in developing countries:

- The entire system is dominated by private provision, and structured around user fees and co-payments for all but the most basic emergency care
- A 'market' of sorts has been created, in which multiple payers and providers compete to offer insurance cover and high-tech treatment
- The predominant role of the private sector leaves a relatively small influence for Federal government, with a large number of functions 'decentralised' to states and local level
- Hospital 'autonomy' has in most cases been developed to the highest level, with both for-profit, non-profit and publicly funded hospitals being obliged to generate income, and balance their own books.

The US experience is that a system based on these principles can fail some of the poorest and those with greatest health needs. However despite the efforts of a gallant few progressive professionals and campaigners (notably the campaign for a single payer system of national health insurance promoted by Physicians for a National Health Program (PNHP)) fundamental reform has been off the mainstream agenda since 1994. Today's situation has long roots in repeated failures to build a sufficiently broad coalition for change, coupled with the political dominance of forces wedded to the prevailing status quo.

History

During the period of radicalism in the early years of the 20th century, in which working class organisations (trade unions and political parties) in many parts of Europe forced the pace towards health insurance and sickness funds, the American labour movement did not unite around this demand. A campaign for health insurance launched by the American Association of Labor Legislation which in 1914 won the support of the American Medical Association was denounced by the American Federation of Labor (as unnecessary and paternalistic) and by the insurance industry. After 1917 proposals for such collective protection were attacked as 'bolshevism' in the Red Scare. In the 1930s concern over health insurance was crowded off the political agenda by mass unemployment and the demand for social security, while attempts to promote legislation in the 1940s were rebuffed for 14 successive years. The post-war US government again brushed aside health insurance as 'socialised medicine', and embarked on the McCarthyite witch-hunts. And by the later 1950s the major trade unions had secured health care benefits to cover their members, and showed little interest in campaigning for wider coverage (Palmer 1999).

In the mid 1960s plans were devised for Medicare and Medicaid programs to finance health care for most of the elderly and provide a form of safety net for the poor, while preserving the private insurance sector and the vested interests of commercial medicine, and were signed into law by President Johnson in 1965. However it has become increasingly clear since that point, as revealed with Bill Clinton's failure to win backing for his health care reforms (Marmor 1998), that the $1.4 trillion US health care sector has taken on the scale and political power of the 'military-industrial complex' of which President Eisenhower once warned Americans: indeed health spending is now four times the level of the military budget, and the pharmaceutical lobby alone spends millions each year promoting its interests. Top congressional representatives from both major parties – including Republican Senate majority leader Bill Frist, whose family founded the giant HCA (Hospital Corporation of America, the country's largest for-profit hospital chain) – have major shareholdings or business links to the health care and pharmaceutical industries (Morgan 2003, Ireland 2003).

Resources without results

A 2002 OECD report on the US health system summed up some of the dimensions of the problem: in 2000, health spending in the US represented 13.2% of the country's enormous GDP, compared with an OECD average of around 8%. This was equivalent to $4,631 per person – 2.5 times the OECD average, and more than ten times the worldwide average[165].

The average annual administrative cost per American enrolled in health insurance schemes was $270 in 2000 (Williams and Treloar 2002:73) – higher than the total spend on health in all but 35 countries (see Appendix A). The total administrative costs of the US system in 2003 was estimated to exceed $399 billion – more than the entire Japanese health spending, and 20 times Canada's health spending (Woolhandler et al 2003): yet it still left 14% of the US population, 38-40 million people, uninsured against potentially catastrophic costs of care in largely private hospitals (Docteur et al 2003:7).

Some US health statistics show services falling short of those in the poorest developing countries. The overall US immunisation level of just 73% in 2001-2 is well below the WHO's Health For All target of 90%, and the targets fixed in the World Bank's 'essential package' of primary care: but 19 US states fall below even this figure, with immunisation levels in Louisiana, Idaho and New Mexico at or below those achieved in Kenya ten years ago[166] (Leatherman and McCarthy 2002, Kaiser Family Foundation 2003).

The levels of social inequality in the US are part of the reason for its relatively high levels of infant mortality (sixth highest in the OECD, with only Turkey, Mexico, Hungary, Slovak Republic and Poland showing higher figures), and one of the lowest levels of improvement since 1990 of any industrialised country.

The US-wide average infant mortality rate of 6.9 conceals state-level variations, with 15 states showing a figure in excess of 8.0, and a top level of 10.7 in Mississippi and 12.0 in District of Columbia (DC) (Kaiser Family Foundation 2003) – worse than any OECD country other than Turkey and Mexico.

More than nine million American families spend over 20% of their income on medical costs, and many poorer Medicare beneficiaries spend half their income: unpaid medical bills result in 200,000 bankruptcies a year (Connolly 2002, Docteur et al 2002:13). It is clear that many of the inequalities that US academics readily point out as grounds for reform in other countries also apply in the US: while the poor can find themselves excluded from all but the most basic emergency care, the wealthiest minority enjoy superior insurance cover, and can also afford to access 'first class' private beds even in non-profit hospitals – such as the Pavilion

---

165   By 2004 it had reached $6,200 per capita (Woolhandler & Himmelstein 2004a).

166   Louisiana achieved 66%, Idaho 65% and New Mexico 61% in 2001-2. Kenya's rate of immunisation fell to 65% in 1993, under the impact of Structural Adjustment Programmes and the imposition of user fees. The US average level of immunisation is well below that currently achieved in many poorer and developing countries including Jamaica, Dominican Republic, China, Vietnam, Mongolia, Nepal, Sri Lanka, Kenya, Tanzania, Malawi, Rwanda, Zimbabwe, and Mozambique.

Table 9

OECD infant mortality rates 1990-2000			
Deaths per 1,000 live births			
Countries	1990	2000	Change
Australia	8.2	5.2	-37%
Austria	7.8	4.8	-38%
Belgium	8	4.8	-40%
Canada	6.8	5.3	-22%
Czech Republic	10.8	4.1	-62%
Denmark	7.5	5.3	-29%
Finland	5.6	3.8	-32%
France	7.3	4.6	-37%
Germany	7	4.4	-37%
Greece	9.7	6.1	-37%
Hungary	14.8	9.2	-38%
Iceland	5.9	3	-49%
Ireland	8.2	6.2	-24%
Italy	8.2	4.5	-45%
Japan	4.6	3.2	-30%
Luxembourg	7.3	5.1	-30%
Mexico	36.1	23.3	-35%
Netherlands	7.1	5.1	-28%
Norway	7	3.8	-46%
Poland	19.4	8.1	-58%
Portugal	11	5.5	-50%
Slovak Republic	12	8.6	-28%
Spain	7.6	3.9	-49%
Sweden	6	3.4	-43%
Switzerland	6.8	4.9	-28%
Turkey	57.6	39.7	-31%
United Kingdom	7.9	5.6	-29%
United States	9.2	6.9	-25%

OECD HEALTH DATA 2003

Suite in the Washington Hospital Centre, where the 35 rooms with chandeliers, carpets and creature comforts including chef and waiter service, cost an extra £220 per night (Morris 2000).

Meanwhile research has underlined the health impact of inequality in the US, with one report estimating that the lives of 900,000 black Americans could have been saved in the decade from 1991 if black patients had enjoyed equal access to timely treatment of new technology (Woolf et al 2004).

The extra spending does buy state of the art technology and a responsive service, delivering almost instant treatment with few if any waiting lists for care – for those who are insured. But as a whole US residents use roughly the same volume of services as other OECD countries, and are hospitalised less often and for shorter stays.

Market-driven reforms:

1 Cash limits/rationalisation

History confirms that the US system has been unable to contain spending at purchaser or provider level: and while this has meant relatively stable employment for staff in the country's hospitals[167], it has driven up the costs of contributions to HMOs – with a predicted increase of 14% in 2004, down 3% from 2003[168] (Milliman 2003). The rationalisation therefore comes not from the health care system but from the patient making cutbacks: there are claims that as the insurance industry tries to keep down premium rates by imposing higher co-payments and deductibles, individual patients fearing the cost are making fewer visits to the doctor and cutting back on care, even when they need it (Flanagan 2003).

2 Regulating drug costs

Heffler and colleagues (2001) have shown that the biggest single component in the price increases has been drug spending, fuelled by an extension of insurance coverage which shields both consumers and physicians from the costs of prescriptions, and has reduced out-of-pocket spending on prescription drug purchases from 59% to 32% since 1990, while average numbers of prescriptions per person have risen by 25% in five years (Heffler et al 2001:198, Berndt 2001, Docteur et al 2002:18). US drug prices are well above the global average: Americans obtained 27% fewer prescriptions per head than the OECD average, but pharmaceutical spending was 41% higher.

3 Market-style reforms

If there was anywhere in the world where market-style solutions should be able to show their effectiveness in delivering high quality, accessible health care to meet the needs of the whole population, it would surely be in the US, the world's wealthiest nation.

Yet despite the ever spiralling levels of public and private spending; the world's most favourable ideological and political climate for market-style solutions; the most advanced medical technology; the large, highly skilled workforce with proliferation of specialists; the vast pharmaceutical enterprises leading much medical research; the competition of providers and insurers; the decentralisation of control; and the long-established corporatisation of its main

---

167 Hospitals, with a combined workforce of five million, now directly and indirectly account for one in every nine US jobs (AHA 2004).

168 Health insurance premiums rose 11% in 2001 and 13% in 2002 (Docteur et al 2002).

hospitals, the American health care system has not only failed to deliver: it stands as the most spectacular example of how market-style policies can go terribly wrong – and have the most devastating impact on the poor.

Even the guru of managed care, Alain Enthoven recently concluded that one of the pillars of the system is crumbling:

> Employment-based health insurance is failing. Costs are once again rising out of control. This will drive up the number of uninsured people (Enthoven 2003).

4 Decentralisation (weak government)

The apparent predominance of private sector providers and payers, and the devolution of many powers and responsibilities to the states means that the Federal government has relatively little power to plan or regulate health care – and that the distribution of services and facilities is necessarily unequal.

While the US average provision of acute hospital beds is 2.9 per 1,000 population, the distribution by state varies from a high of 5.9 in DC and South Dakota, to as low as 1.9 in Oregon, Utah and Washington. Patterns of hospital admissions also vary either side of an average of 119, from a maximum of 230 admissions per thousand population in DC to just 77 in Alaska (Kaiser Family Foundation 2003). Similar inequalities in distribution can be found within particular states.

5 Purchaser/provider split, provider autonomy

The US system has the most world's most developed division between purchasers (insurers, but also Medicare, Medicaid and the apparatus funding county hospitals) and providers. However it has not brought either efficiency or economy in the use of costly assets.

Equally, the large hospitals have been (and have acted as) corporations for a long period, without generating the often-promised responsiveness to the health needs of local populations.

6 Provider payment reform

Despite the eagerness of some advocates of health system reforms to focus on provider payment methods (Bitran and Yip 1998, 1999, Maceira 1998), few seem to have paid detailed attention to the continued predominance in the US of systems of hospital reimbursement – per diem, and fee-for-service – which are generally recognised to give a perverse incentive to provider-led demand (Ranade 1998:6).

Indeed Williams and Treloar draw attention to the dramatic increase in use of these payment methods since 1997, despite years of HMOs and managed care. Per diem rates were used by 90% of HMO plans in 2000, compared with just 53% in 1997: fee-for-service payments increased in prevalence from 16% in 1997 to 78% in 2000. During this period of renewed health price inflation HMOs achieved a relatively small increase in the more cost-effective system of capitation funding (Williams and Treloar 2002:69).

And the impact of the for-profit sector, and the surpluses retained even by the non-profit hospitals, inevitably also contribute to the costs of delivering care. In 2001 Kaiser Permanente retained a 16% profit on revenue of $17.7 billion – largely explained by an average 10% increase in premiums and additional co-payments by patients for treatment. In HCA, the largest for-profit hospital chain, it has been revealed that individual hospital managers were systematically pressurised by corporate executives in Nashville to produce a 20% return – or lose their jobs (Palast 1999).

Berliner (2000) sums up the stock ways in which US for-profit providers hold down their costs, opening up scope for bigger profits:

> They could produce a day of inpatient care at a lower rate than their not-for-profit and publicly
> funded competition, and yet they sold that day of care at the same or a higher rate. [...] They
> were able to produce care less expensively because they neither provided charity care nor
> unprofitable services such as emergency care... used fewer staff per bed, did not have unionised
> workers, did not engage in teaching or research, and were able to secure better prices through
> volume purchasing of supplies and equipment.

But as Ginsburg (2004) argues, the political consensus uniting the two main contenders for the Presidential elections in 2004 was on delivering cost containment for the individual employee covered by a workplace insurance scheme, rather than forcing any actual reduction in costs: both George Bush and John Kerry offered government subsidies or tax credits to relieve the burden of payments – at public expense, and therefore at the expense of low-paid workers without health insurance.

Rejecting Kerry's timid line, and pointing out a Washington Post/ABC News poll showing 62% of Americans in favour of a 'universal health insurance program in which everyone is covered under a program like Medicare that's run by the government and financed by taxpayers', Woolhandler and Himmelstein (2004b) argue that Bush's $534 billion Medicare Drug Bill hands $46 billion in profits to private sector HMOs that had been 'ripping off Medicare for years', and includes a clause prohibiting Medicare from negotiating with drug companies to lower their prices. The Bill had already triggered a fresh round of drug price inflation which will wipe out the promised benefits to US seniors.

During the election campaign drug companies had been alarmed that a Kerry victory might bring fresh, if limited, pressure to limit prices, and afterwards Pfizer promptly issued a statement welcoming Bush's re-election (Roberts and Alden 2004).

Despite the political sensitivity of any restriction on services, however, some HMOs are seeking to rein in costs by bringing back tighter regulation on health care providers which they previously relaxed (Mays et al 2004). And once the election was complete, moves began within the Senate to slow the growth in Medicaid entitlements, with plans for spending reductions totalling $14 billion over five years (AHA 2005).

7 Purchase services from private sector

Just 24% of acute hospitals are publicly funded, by states and local government, including the county hospitals and other safety-net services for the indigent. Numbers of public hospitals have been declining throughout the 1990s as a result of 'facility consolidation, mergers and privatisation' (Williams and Treloar 2002:77). The remainder are privately run, 61% as non-profit and 15% for-profit (Kaiser Family Foundation 2003). Here too the distribution is very uneven: the national average of 15% for-profits conceals concentrations as high as 47% in Florida, 42% in Nevada, and a third of hospitals in Texas and Arizona. At the other end of the scale no fewer than 27 states have less than 10% for-profit hospitals, six of these[169] having none at all (Kaiser Family Foundation 2003).

In 1998, 85% of dialysis programmes, 70% of home care and nursing homes and 64% of

---

169 Connecticut, Delaware, Minnesota, Montana, Rhode Island and Vermont

HMOs were owned by for-profit corporations (Geyman 2002). Devers (2003) and others have drawn attention to the systematic efforts of specialist hospitals – many of them owned by for-profit corporations – to maximise their income by focusing on specific high-paying procedures (notably cardiovascular and orthopaedic surgery), and leaving the other hospitals in the area to cover the more costly and complex treatment of emergencies, the poor and chronic sick.

As in other countries the US also faces a division between urban and country dwellers, with hospitals and health care facilities tending to be concentrated in the wealthier areas of the cities. This unequal distribution of services also applies to managed care plans, which are simply not available in many rural areas (Families USA 2003b).

One overhead cost of the private sector is the profits that are drawn from the system and paid out to shareholders and top executives. US Health Maintenance Organisations (HMOs) reported profits totalling $6.7 billion for the first nine months of 2003, up 52% on the comparable period of 2002 (anon 2004): this profit for the medical industry comes from the contributions of other companies and individuals – per capita spending for health services covered by private insurance rose by 39% between 1999 and 2003, compared with a 14% increase in hourly wages (Ginsburg 2004)[170]. Many of the insurance companies, which in most cases pay the bills for treatment, are also for-profit, with surpluses running into billions. Private health plans typically carry administrative costs averaging 9.5% of turnover[171], attributable to advertising, marketing, and profits. The top executives running private plans averaged a salary of more than $15 million in 2002, plus stock option (Families USA 2003b).

8 Competition

Although competition is generally perceived as a downward pressure on prices, the high overhead costs of a complex multi-payer, multi-provider system in the US have been a constant factor in inflating costs.

A survey of operating room costs in 4,500 hospitals by the California Nurses Association and the Institute for Health and Socio-Economic Policy to identify the country's 100 most expensive, found that hospitals throughout the US were marking up their prices to charge more than 220% above cost.

Among those charging the highest mark-ups were for-profit hospitals (61 of the top 100, nine of the top ten), 44 of them owned by just two companies, Tenet Healthcare and HCA. The highest mark-up above cost price was 1,000% in Arizona; two California hospitals (both Tenet-run) and one in Florida marked up by more then 900%, while six more charged at over 800% above cost. Average mark-ups in Florida were the highest at 334%, with California close behind at 325% over cost (Idelson 2003).

9 Steps to control medical professionals

HMOs seek to constrain the clinical freedom of family doctors by offering bonuses to those who restrict use of emergency room services by their patients: up to 80% of a physician's annual income may be at risk if they fail to restrict service use (Waitzkin 2001:83-84, Kleinke 2001).

Some managed care organisations also operate 'gag rules' that prevent physicians from

---

170 HMO profits increased by a further 32% ($1.4 billion) in the first half of 2004 (Weiss Ratings 2005).

171 Compared with admin costs in Medicare of just 2%, and chief executive remuneration of $130,000 in 2002.

telling patients of diagnostic and treatment options that are excluded by the organisation: this can create a major ethical issue for the doctor concerned, making them effectively 'double agents' serving both the patient and the managed care corporation (Waitzkin 2001:89).

Insurers like Aetna have set out to push up their profits by squeezing their payments to health care providers, including primary care. While most hospitals have managed to retain and increase their levels of fee-for-service payments, growing numbers of family doctors have been pressurised by insurers to agree to capitation-based contracts, which pay a flat annual fee regardless of the level of treatment required by individual patients.

Aetna pays GPs no extra for treating toddlers with severe asthma: and it pays just $19 for administering a meningitis vaccine that costs $58 (Connolly 2002, Geyman 2002).

10 Patient choice

i. Managed care: less choice for lower costs

With health spending rising consistently higher than general price inflation for the last 20 years (Williams and Treloar 2002:8), different measures have been taken to try to bring costs under control. Attempts to contain hospital costs have included the introduction of 'managed care', most notably in the form of health maintenance organisations (HMOs), which – together with the 'threat of health reform' (Altman and Levitt 2002) succeeded in holding down price rises in the mid 1990s by restricting patient choice of provider and treatment, and by hard bargaining to establish fixed price contracts with physicians and hospitals.

Surveys showed that HMOs and other 'managed care' plans served to slow down the growth in hospital spending (Heffler et al 1999, op. cit:9, Docteur et al 2003). However the spread of HMOs, like every other aspect of health policy and health care has been uneven across the US states, with a market penetration ranging from aero in Alaska to highs of 45% in Massachusetts and 54% in California: in 12 states HMOs had less than 10% of the market in 2000 (Williams and Treloar 2002).

Many HMOs also aim to generate a return for shareholders: there has been a five-fold increase since 1981 in the proportion of enrollees in HMOs in for-profit plans, which by 1999 had over two-thirds of HMO enrolment, though HMOs have been unprofitable, with many generating annual losses, since 1996 (Williams and Treloar 2002).

Researchers critical of commercial medicine have published comparisons which show patients get better care from non-profit HMOs than those seeking profits (Marini 1999). Part of the decline in HMO profits is also part of the reason for the enormous administrative costs of US health care: extra investment in sophisticated information technology to keep closer control on spending and the introduction of new technology and drugs. Again for-profit hospitals spend more on this type of administration than public and charitable hospitals (Berliner 1999, Palast 1999).

HMOs also came under increased pressure from state regulators, seeking to uphold the rights of beneficiaries, and a new patients' bill of rights. Some HMOs have passed these problems on, in the form of intensified pressure on hospitals and on primary care physicians to agree to contracts which cut their prices to the bone, even below the price of drugs supplied (Berliner 1999, Williams and Treloar 2002:71).

While HMOs proved especially popular with large employers seeking to hold down their insurance plan payments (which fell sharply to below wage increases and general inflation between 1989 and 1996), they have been more controversial with some general practitioners

(Kleinke 2001), with some hospitals which find their margins, budgets and clinical freedoms squeezed by HMOs, and with significant numbers of HMO subscribers requiring more complex and costly treatment, who have run into delays and obstructions in accessing the care they need (Court and Smith 1999).

An annual survey has identified an increase since 1997 in the numbers of patients who report that HMOs and managed care plans have reduced the time their doctor spends with them, decreased the quality of care for the sick and made no difference to their health care costs (Williams and Treloar 2002:80).

More recently employers have begun to move insurance policies from HMOs to Preferred Provider Organisations (PPOs) which offer patients more choice of doctor and hospital: PPO coverage of employment-based insured workers increased from 28% in 1996 to 48% in 2001, while the HMO share fell back from 31% to 23% (Heffler et al 1999, Williams and Treloar 2002:80).

ii. The uninsured

Limitations on the choices open to Americans covered by HMOs are a minor issue compared with the difficulties faced by the country's army of uninsured and under-insured. A survey of Emergency Room doctors by the American College of Emergency Physicians showed 81% believed that people without insurance were more likely to die prematurely than those who have it: and 71% thought that uninsured patients in the ER tended to be sicker, often having delayed getting help at an earlier stage in their illness. Federal law requires hospital emergency departments to assess and stabilise any patient presented, irrespective of their ability to pay, and this is why uninsured people are crowding into ERs across the country: at one ER in Washington state, 53% of attendances in 2002 were uninsured or Medicaid patients – up 10% on the previous year (Smith C 2003).

Hadley and Holahan (2003) estimate the value of care for uninsured patients at $98.9 billion in 2001, of which about a third is 'uncompensated care' not covered by out of pocket payments or by public or private insurance: they argue that the funds from government, state and other sources which currently cover this would be better spent on establishing an insurance scheme to cover the uninsured.

However proposals by the Bush administration to introduce $1,000 tax credits to allow the poor to buy themselves health insurance have been strongly opposed by Families USA, which points out (among many other issues) that in only three states were policies costing as little as $1,000 available for a healthy non-smoking 55-year old woman: in 19 states even a healthy, non-smoking 25-year old woman could not get a policy for $1,000. Even those policies that were available were inadequate, leaving the policy-holder liable for as much as the first $5,000 of any claim (Families USA 2003a).

Each year since 1996, 70-80% of Americans have reported themselves to be 'very' or 'somewhat' concerned about being unable to afford necessary health care when a family member gets sick: in 2000 18% reported having put off seeking health care because of the cost, while 15% had skipped a recommended test or treatment (Kaiser Health Poll 2003). Estimates by the Congressional Budget Office suggest that as many as 58-60 million people – 'about a quarter of the non-elderly population' – may be without medical insurance at some point in the year: 80% of them are in work, but low-paid and possibly employed by smaller companies that do not offer health cover (Marwick 2002, Pear 2003).

iii. Medicaid

Numerically 76% of uninsured are white, with Hispanics the next biggest group (Docteur et al 2003). However minority Americans are at least twice as likely to be uninsured as whites, and to be among the 50 million dependent upon Medicaid coverage (Kaiser Family Foundation 1999). As a result minorities and poor whites are likely to be the main victims of planned cutbacks in Medicaid entitlements as state legislatures and the federal government attempt to cut back on spending: Bush is seeking to cut federal support for Medicaid by $45 billion over the next ten years (Swann 2005).

Medicaid spending – shared between states and the Federal budget – has risen more than 50% since 1997, with enrolment rising at the fastest pace since the early 1990s. Now as states try to balance their budgets up to 1.7 million could lose their coverage completely, while California, Florida and Ohio are cutting entitlements to dental care and ophthalmic services; Mississippi and Oklahoma cut prescription benefits. Kentucky and Massachusetts cut back on long-term care – for which Medicaid is the single biggest payer (Toner and Pear 2003, Despeignes 2003, Wachino 2002, Docteur et al 2002:12).

A fifth of all children in the US depend for their health care cover on Medicaid. Lack of health insurance can also cause problems in the access of children to primary care services, and mean that children go without medical, dental or other health care they need (Newacheck et al 1998).

11 Debate on solutions

More recently there have been warnings that the combination of soaring costs of health insurance and ever-growing costs of hospital and health treatment could coincide with a new economic downturn and unemployment to create a 'tidal wave' of uninsured, and 'A Perfect Storm' that would push the system into even greater chaos. The answer proposed is to move to an inclusive system of National Health Insurance (Miller 2001).

A California study comparing nine different models of health care reform found that while six 'incremental' models fell short of reform goals, leaving many flawed policies intact, the three which proposed comprehensive reform (two single payer insurance schemes and one a health service model) would provide coverage for all citizens – and save California $8 billion dollars a year in health care costs (McCanne 2003).

It would be a mistake to see the problem lying in a lack of public funding: recent analysis shows that, if tax concessions and other hidden subsidies are taken into account as well as formal spending, the government at national or state level already funds 60% of US health care costs[172]. The issue is the way in which taxpayers' money is used. While most health services are delivered through private sector providers, research for the Robert Wood Johnson Foundation has shown that the tax subsidies that apply to private health insurance benefit the wealthy rather than those on lower incomes (Williams 2003).

Arguing that 'We pay for National Health Insurance, but don't get it,' Himmelstein and Woolhandler (2003) claim that the US system has 'privatised the profits and socialised the risks' of health care.

---

172 Tax concessions on private health insurance introduced during the Second World War was the key to its rapid expansion from just one million pre-war subscribers to 60 million ten years later (Geyman 2002:410).

Businesses complain bitterly of rising health costs, insure the most wealthy and healthy, and reap large tax-breaks (subtracting tax-breaks reduced employers' share of health spending to just 11%).

Reversing the process, argue Himmelstein and Woolhandler, along with others in support of the general propositions of the Physicians for a National Health Program (PNHP) is the only way to get to grips with all of the perverse incentives which keep the US health care system so dysfunctional. They were signatories as long ago as 1989 to a 'Physicians' Proposal' for a 'National Health Program for the United States' (Himmelstein et al 1989).

A single payer system of national health insurance could eliminate the costs complexities and profit-margins arising from over 1,200 separate insurers: the private insurance industry would be replaced by a blend of federal and state government roles, at an estimated saving of $150 billion a year:

> Although likely to be attacked by some as socialised medicine, the single payer system would really be socialised insurance. The private practice of medicine would continue, with a sharp reduction in administrative and regulatory burdens as well as costs (Geyman 2002).

There is some pressure for an alternative. Early in 2003 the prestigious Presidential Lecture of the American Association for the Advancement of Science (AAAS) was used by neuroscientist Dr Floyd Bloom as a platform for a call for a national commission to be established to 'restore the American health system' (Bloom 2003).

A new, updated version of the Physicians' Proposal has been published as a platform to attract popular support among the medical profession. It would, as with Geyman's proposal, leave the provision of health care largely in private hands, though there would be tough restrictions on the ways hospitals could spend their monthly global budget allocation from the National Health Insurance fund. Physicians would be offered a choice of three payments options: fee-for-service; a salaried post in an institution receiving a global budget; or a salaried position in a group practice or HMO. For-profit HMOs would be converted to non-profits.

What seems clear is that the system is so dysfunctional that there is little prospect of success through piecemeal or 'incremental' reform, while as the OECD report, avoiding any potentially controversial points, rather lamely concludes:

> The discussion has demonstrated there are no easy solutions. Fundamental reform lacks sufficient political support (Docteur et el 2003).

Australasia

AUSTRALIA

Background

Medicare, Australia's universal tax-funded health insurance system was introduced in 1984, and maintained by Labour governments up to 1996, but has been subject to substantial reform by the right wing Liberal government that has held power since (Hilless and Healy 2002). The publicly funded system had contributed to a substantial decline in private health insurance (PHI) coverage, from a peak of 70% of the population in the 1950s to just 30% at the end of 1998.

Measures to buttress the private health insurance sector have included substantial (30%) government-funded rebates for more affluent Australians who sign up for private policies, coupled with a 1% penalty tax imposed since 1997 on medium and high-earners who fail to take out private cover (Zinn 2000).

This summary will focus on just three aspects of market-style reform which dominate the Australian situation: the promotion of private medical insurance, the impact of privatisation, and the unusual attempt to control medical professionals.

Promote private health insurance

The government in 2000 lined up with the private health insurers in a combined attempt to frighten more affluent Australians into signing up quickly for health insurance by introducing a system that would levy a surcharge of an extra 2% on PHI premiums for every year a new subscriber is aged above 30 if they failed to join before a July 1st deadline. This could mean a maximum additional cost of up to 70% on health policies for somebody aged 65 or over (Zinn 2000).

The government intervention to rebuild the flagging private sector has been summed up by the European Health Management Association:

> In essence, the Medicare system was proving too good for the private sector, so the government subsidised the private sector to allow it to compete better with the public sector! (EHMA 2000:59)

As a result of such generous treatment, the private sector has become increasingly dominant in key areas of health care: a majority of physicians are in the private sector; private hospitals provide 30% of Australia's beds and carried out 53% of surgical procedures in 2000-01 – up from 35-40% in less than ten years (Hilless & Healy 2002, Zinn 2003). Most therapy services, home nursing, dental services, visual and hearing aids have always been excluded from Medicare cover (Healy 2002). Almost 45% of the population are now covered by private health insurance. However 70% of health spending still comes from state and federal governments (Hilless & Healy 2002).

The increased role of the private sector has come at a cost. The decline in public sector investment has left severe and entrenched inequalities in health status and access to care among rural areas and Aboriginal communities. And while the government has provided lavish subsidies for the private sector (rising to an estimated £1 billion each year in rebates of premiums to many more prosperous taxpayers (Zinn 2000, Mitchell 2002, Hall and Maynard 2005)) the public sector hospitals have been under pressure, with rising admission rates and waiting lists (Hilless & Healy 2002) and reduced income from private insurers (Richardson et al 1999). The situation could worsen, since the Australian Health Care Agreements provide a trigger which would begin to reduce funding for public hospitals once the private sector exceeds a certain level of coverage (RACP 1999).

Richardson and colleagues, in a detailed examination of official data, conclude that under the impact of budgetary pressures, public hospitals increased their efficiency substantially over the 15 years prior to 1997, reducing their share of the national health budget from 34.7% to 28.8%.

But at the same time the private hospitals secured a *larger* share of health spending, rising from 12.6% to 21.5% of the total – an 'increase in market share of 70.6%'. However the team find evidence that private hospitals are both more expensive and more likely to make use of high-cost procedures than public hospitals, raising questions over whether this increased spending is delivering the best value for money.

> If the $1,500 million subsidy to private health insurance in 1996-7 had been allocated to public hospitals, their capacity would have increased at least 14% which significantly exceeds the likely effect of the subsidy – at least in the short run – upon PHI and the indirect effect upon public hospitalisation (Richardson et al 1999:8).

And they refute the claim that without the government steps to rescue the collapsing private sector, public hospitals would have been unable to cope:

> The decline in the percentage of the population with PHI has not been associated with an increase in the proportion of services offered in public hospitals. [...]
> It is unequivocally untrue that private health insurance or private hospitalisation at their present levels are necessary for the viability of public hospitals (op. cit:21).

A more recent study notes that most of the $2.6 billion annual cost of the government subsidy to private health insurance 'goes to the 30% of the population who already hold private insurance – that is the affluent and the elderly' (Hall and Maynard 2005).

The mechanism forcing the subsidy upwards is clear enough to see: the cost of private health premium payments, which had been expected to fall, have continued to rise by 7% each year for the last three years, and each time the premium goes up, so does the subsidy. And since doctors face no constraints on the fees they are allowed to charge, they have been rapidly increasing their share of the health budget: in just 12 months to the end of 2004 payments to hospitals roles by 9%, while payments to doctors rose by 33%.

Hall and Maynard conclude that while the ideological slant of the reforms will endear them to those seeking to maximise private health care:

> Such policies create increased fiscal burdens for government, increase inequality in funding care, and have no observable effects on efficiency. Worldwide the private health insurance industry shows an inability to control costs and micro-manage its workforce.

Privatisation

The expanding private sector has also had a major impact on hospital care, effectively luring many surgeons away from public sector hospitals with the offer of much higher salaries – and leaving only a residual role for public sector hospitals delivering care for the elderly, poor and chronic sick (Zinn 2003a):

> The public hospitals are returning to their status of a century ago, when their role was largely charitable, their clientele were the poor and the more affluent were excluded by the means test (Birrell et al 2003:15).

Official statistics show that while hospital discharges ('separations') increased overall by 33.2% in the years 1993-2001, the vast majority of this increase took place in private hospitals, where discharges increased 73%, compared with a 17% increase in public acute hospitals (AIHW 2002:9). Thirty-seven percent of all hospital admissions were in private hospitals in 2000-01 (Howard 2003).

As with the private sector in other countries, private hospitals in Australia favour minor elective surgery, with almost 50% of their total caseload being day cases. The increased proportion of surgery carried out privately widens the equity gap between rural and metropolitan areas, where the private hospitals are concentrated. But Birrell and colleagues also warn of the danger that the new system will result in a serious shortage of surgeons in Australia, with many of them spending most of their time in private sector work, and few prepared to work in rural and regional areas.

The Royal Australasian College of Physicians has also expressed concern that the switch of subsidies to private health insurance has left a 'run down' infrastructure of public hospitals 'without sufficient incentives for hospitals to be well maintained' (RACP 1999). In a submission to a Senate inquiry, the College also goes on to criticise any move towards 'cost-shifting' policies that 'would add to the already significant out of pocket contribution Australian consumers already pay for their health care, in contrast to most developed nations.'

Steps to control medical professionals

Primary care services are in some disarray. In theory the system offers GPs a choice between 'bulk billing' Medicare for patient visits, which should result in no charge being levied at point of consultation, or charging a scheduled fee, 75% of which would be reimbursed to the patient. But fewer doctors have been implementing on the basis of bulk billing, while increasing numbers have been charging a 'gap fee' over and above the scheduled fee, meaning that some of the poorest are having to pay for every time they visit a doctor.

The Australian Medical Association has been demanding a doubling of the scheduled fee to draw more GPs back into the bulk billing system – while the government has been pressing for a new two-tier system in which seven million pensioners and welfare claimants would be entitled to free consultations, but millions more Australians would see an end to the 'bulk billing' and the imposition of charges to see a GP (Zinn 2003b).

Richardson and colleagues conclude that:

> There is probably no other country in the world where private practitioners face such congenial regulation. In exchange for the underwriting of medical incomes by public and by private insurance there is no requirement that doctors either individually or collectively limit their fees or undertake to adopt best practice guidelines (however broadly defined). The over-billing by some private practitioners (in the order of 100% of the rebate) is consistent with the hypothesis that the entire benefit of public and private insurance has been captured by the practitioner...
> (Richardson et al 1999:21)

NEW ZEALAND

Background

New Zealanders are proud of their claim to have set up the world's first universal health care system, in 1938, as part of an early welfare state (Hornblow 1997). But more recently its health care system has been reorganised five times in 15 years, going from elected hospital boards, to 14 elected area boards, to four regional purchasers with 23 Crown Health Enterprises (CHEs) providing hospital services, to one purchaser and 22 CHEs, and then back to one Ministry of Health and 21 district health boards (DHBs) (Scott et al 2003).

The pace of change, all taking place under the sceptical eyes of an unconvinced electorate – who were especially unimpressed by the sharp increases in user fees which came alongside the reforms – and oppositional health workers, has meant that many of the changes had little time to take shape and develop before being swept away by the next reform (Scott et al 2003:321-2). Little systematic evaluation took place, and the benchmarks for any evaluation would need to include the preceding problems which were alleged by the reformers to include inefficiency, poor management, budget overruns and badly neglected public hospitals, along with rising waiting lists and increased use of private medical insurance (Devlin et al 2001, French et al 2001).

Market-driven reforms

1 Cash limits and spending cuts

Resource constraints have led to the development of criteria for prioritising patients on the waiting list for non-urgent operations. Each patient is scored on the basis of clinical and social criteria designed to identify relative need and ability to benefit from treatment. If the patient scores insufficient points they will be referred back to their GP, and must wait for a deterioration in their condition to make them eligible for treatment.

However there are grounds to believe that this potentially highly controversial measure is merely a device to divert attention from the real criterion, which is the availability of funds and resources to carry out only a certain number of procedures: it appears that the thresholds are set according to financial rather than clinical needs (Howden-Chapman & Ashton 2000:30, French et al 2001:57). Birrell and colleagues quote the example of Canterbury Hospital, where more than a third of the 30,000 patients waiting for surgery or specialist assessments were referred back to their GPs, and the chief executive of the local District Health Board commented:

> It is impossible for us to meet all the demands of elective surgery or assessment with the resources and financial constraints we have (Birrell and colleagues 2003:12).

Partly as a result of this substantial public sector shortfall in capacity, it is estimated that two-thirds (64%) of elective surgery in New Zealand is privately funded. Substantial increases in government health care spending announced in December 2001, giving increases of 7% in 2002-3 and 21% by 2004-5 have yet to register in the statistics (Birrell and colleagues 2003:12).

2 User fees

One of the reforms dropped most swiftly was the highly unpopular imposition of charges for each day of inpatient treatment in hospital – which were abandoned after a few months, after being found to cost as much to administer as they raised (Ovretveit 1996, Hornblow 1997): another unpopular charge, £12 per visit to see a GP, has remained in place and constitutes a significant obstacle to access by the poor (Hornblow 1997).

Most patients other than expectant mothers, children and the poor pay relatively high out of pocket fees for primary care. Forty percent of the population have concession cards, but it is estimated that as many as a quarter of those who should be eligible do not have a card, while another 5-10% of the population who earn just above the threshold for eligibility can find the charges prohibitive (French et al 2001:57). With public spending covering just 77.5% of health care costs, New Zealand is closer to the insurance-funded health care systems of Europe than the UK's tax-funded system (op. cit:60).

Market-style reforms

1 Decentralisation, purchaser/provider split and contracts

The market-style reforms which came into force in July 1993 were implemented by the National government of 1990-96, but flowed out of a generalised market-style reform that was driven through other parts of the New Zealand economy by a Labour government in the 1980s. Even before the full effect of the reforms had been felt, the government suffered a setback in the general election of 1993, but held on, implementing the reforms in a more cautious way (French et al 2001:19-22).

The reforms instituted a purchaser/provider split, and sought to create competition between the public sector providers, and between public and private hospitals. The 23 new CHEs were at first required to run on commercial lines and deliver a profit, despite widespread public unease with the notion of for-profit hospitals (Bale & Dale 1998:121).

They were to derive most of their funding through contracts to be negotiated with the four new Regional health authorities, each covering a population of around 800,000. The regional boards were directly appointed by ministers, drawing heavily on people from outside the health sector in order to strengthen the commitment to commercial practise (Hornblow 1997).

The new government elected in 1999 changed course and abolished the purchaser/provider split within the public sector, by scrapping the Health Funding Authority and transferring its functions to 21 new District Health Boards, which were to allocate budgets calculated on weighted catchment population, and be run by a mix of appointed and elected members, with guaranteed representation for Maori people (Devlin et al 2001). Many of these were soon facing deficits (Healy 2002b:88).

Like the Thatcher health reforms in Britain, the New Zealand reforms had been drawn up in secret without consultation or debate with professionals or the public: they were informed by the ideology of the new right (Hornblow 1997) in the absence of good information or evidence (Wells et al 1998).

The 1996 election saw health care emerge as the top issue among voters' concerns, and the party that had opposed the reforms won a place in the new coalition that was formed. The result was a health policy which stated that 'principles of public service replace commercial profit objectives' and called for cooperation and collaboration rather than competition. CHEs were renamed 'Hospital and Health Services', and the appointed Regional health authorities were replaced by a single purchasing body, the Health Funding Authority (Devlin et al 2001).

While the overt market-style elements of the New Zealand reforms have come and gone and been replaced with a more democratic decentralisation, the underlying problems arising from under-funding continue to have an impact on the public sector. The European Health Management Association concludes that:

> The quasi-market in new Zealand had similar results to its less intellectually 'pure' British counterpart in that neither critics nor proponents have been vindicated. Generally the impact on productivity, crude measures of efficiency, cost containment and service quality have been hard to discern (EHMA 2002:61).

2 Provider autonomy

The CHEs had the appearance of considerable local autonomy in running their own affairs: like NHS Trusts in Britain, CHEs were told they could fix their own local pay agreements for staff – and unlike British NHS Trusts they were permitted to borrow money from private lenders. CHEs were even denied access to cheaper government-backed capital, and charged above-market rates of interest in a deliberate attempt to force them into borrowing from the private sector (Scott et al 2003:313-322).

Their boards' lack of elected representatives was seen as a way of insulating CHEs from hostile public opinion, and thus encouraging them to withdraw from unprofitable areas of care though – with the exception of continuing care of the elderly and mental health care, which many were already preparing to hive off prior to 1993 – few CHEs pressed ahead with such plans [173]. In some cases those that attempted to do so were pressurised not to by ministers (Scott et al 2003:320, 328).

3 Competition

The prospect of competition never seriously developed. The private sector was insufficient in scale (health insurance contributed just 6% of health spending), and private hospitals generally offered prices as high or higher than the CHEs themselves. There were also fears at government level that if CHEs lost too much of their surgical caseload it would undermine the clinical viability of their services. CHEs were also discouraged by ministers from competing in the catchment area of other CHEs (Scott et al 2003:315).

The claims of 20-30% savings as a result of competition were especially unrealistic, and costs of running the Regional health authorities increased 40% over two years. Contract negotiations dragged on months into each new financial year, consuming expensive management time. Other indicators also showed that the system was going badly wrong. Some regions noted an increase in hospitalisation of children which could have been avoided had parents sought primary care at an earlier stage; hospital waiting lists rose, some by as much as 50%; CHEs, far from making a profit ran up losses and large-scale borrowing[174], and required government cash handouts (Hornblow 1997).

By the end of 1996, the Ministry of Health concluded that there was little evidence of success from the implementation of the reforms:

> Health sector performance over the last three years has been disappointing in a number of areas: costs have not been constrained in line with planned funding growth; both CHEs and RHAs have experienced deficits; although total output has increased, access to some services appears to have reduced; and only 35% of public health targets are expected to be achieved (cited in Howden-Chapman & Ashton 2000:29).

4 Steps to control medical professionals

In the case of primary care, the reforms encouraged GPs (most of whom are private practitioners, funded through a combination of government subsidies and patient fees) to form

---

173 The pressure to restructure (or 'exit from') services outside of the 'care business' continued after CHEs were replaced by HHSs. An example cited by French et al is Health Care Otago, which sold off nursing homes, rural hospitals and cut its psychiatric services to reduce its deficits (French et al 2001:30).

174 Private sector borrowings increased from 16% of total hospital debt in 1993 to 69% in 1998: 'the financial claims of banks and other lenders over the public hospital system have grown from a negligible level to around one third of the total capital' (Howden-Chapman & Ashton 2000:35).

larger organisations, often called Independent Practitioner Associations which would take control of a budget for the purchase of a range of primary and ambulatory care – similar in some respects (though more limited) to fundholding GPs in Britain, not least in the prospect that practices could retain any unspent surpluses. By 1999 80% of GPs had joined IPAs: ironically, since it arises from a package of pro-competitive reforms, the result was to eliminate one area where there had been a degree of competition between providers, and establish instead monopoly providers in a stronger position to drive up their own fees (Howden-Chapman & Ashton 2000:34).

Chapter nine

Country summaries: Latin America and the Caribbean

Overview

Unlike sub-Saharan Africa, in which the vast majority of countries are classified by the World Bank as 'low income'[175], only Haiti and Nicaragua are ranked 'low income' in the Bank's 'Latin America and Caribbean' (LAC) region ('World Development Indicators' 2003). However the general label of 'middle-income' spans a range of per capita annual gross national income from just $736 ($2 per day) to $9,075[176]. These average figures inevitably conceal vast inequalities – 'the worst income distribution in the world' (Fleury 2001:4). The Inter-American Development Bank's figures for 1999 show the top 5% of the population receiving 25% of the national income, while the poorest 30% received just 7.5% (ibid). Large pools of poverty and ill-health persist, even in some of the most developed countries. Another factor is the instability of some of the larger economies, exemplified by the recent crisis in Argentina – one of the world's ten richest countries in the early 1990s (Arie 2002).

LAC countries have a total population of 475 million, of whom 25% lack permanent access even to basic health services. Although the proportion living in poverty was lower in 1995 than in 1970, it has risen sharply since the early 1980s, and numbers of poor people have risen rapidly over the same period to more than 150 million. An estimated 218 million people in the LAC region were without social security coverage in 1999: 107 million were thought to lack geographical access to health services, 267 million were affected by a shortage of hospital beds, and almost 16 million had difficulties accessing services from a physician (ILO/PAHO 1999).

While rural poverty has remained largely unchanged, numbers of urban poor have risen more than three-fold since 1970. Average per capita spending on health is just $240 per annum, of which $102 is public spending (Lopez-Acuna 2000b). This level of spending is

---

175 Only South Africa, Namibia, Swaziland and Botswana are classified as 'middle-income'.

176 'Lower middle-income' is between $736-$2,935 per annum: upper middle-income is from $2,936 to $9,075. The definition of as little as $2 per day as 'middle-income' raises serious questions over the usefulness of this criterion, and on the standpoint of the Bank's statisticians, many of whom will spend more than this each day on potato chips, chocolate or cigarettes. The most recent ILO figures (December 2004) show that half of the world's 2.8 billion workers live on less than $2 per day, with 550 million living on less than $1 per day.

facing the added pressure of the 'epidemiological transition' with an ageing population and the coexistence of communicable diseases, chronic disease, the reappearance of old problems such as cholera, malaria, TB and dengue, and the appearance of the new problem of AIDS (Arias and Yepes 1997).

Many Latin American countries have had welfare systems for much of the 20th century, although these were not universal, but based upon insurance schemes for certain key groups of workers. This has meant that in many cases where informal employment has expanded, workers are excluded from social security benefits: 85% of the new jobs in the LAC region have been created in the informal sector (ILO/PAHO 1999). In the post-war period some countries extended social security systems to provide health cover for much of the urban population (Barrientos & Lloyd Sherlock 2000). The health systems in Latin America and the Caribbean would mostly be characterised as 'mixed national health systems' under the framework applied by the OECD and WHO, which focuses on the predominant method of financing. However Suarez-Berenguela (2000:7) argues that any similarities with health systems in the developed countries are more apparent than substantial:

> None of the systems provides the universal and comprehensive coverage of health care services achieved by European national health systems.

Despite the proliferation of poverty, the 'middle-income' status of Latin American countries, and their geographical proximity to the USA makes them much more of a target than Africa for the attentions of US-based corporations seeking expanding markets for health insurance and for-profit health care services. A landmark 1996 conference of US health insurers, significantly held not in the US but in Mexico City, spelled out the need to find new markets and new subscribers in order to sustain a flagging industry (Hart 2003, ref). Evidence of the penetration of the health insurance market in Argentina by US HMOs is noted by Barrientos and Lloyd Sherlock (2000), and by Iriart and colleagues (2000, 2001):

> Our findings demonstrate the entrance of the main multinational corporations of finance capital into the private sector of insurance and health services, and these corporations' intention to assume administrative responsibilities for state institutions and to secure access to medical social security funds (Iriart et al 2001).

Waitzkin (1997) had earlier noted the rapid diffusion of 'managed care' schemes into Latin America:

> In countries like Chile and Argentina, reforms of public systems put emphasis on competition among large private companies under the US model. In other countries such as Ecuador and Brazil, similar proposals are starting to appear, although their development is incipient (1997:2).

A report to PAHO's Executive Committee as early as 1996 listed the ten most widely used health system reforms in the Americas, among which were six market-style measures: managerial decentralisation, financial decentralisation, cost recovery, new contractings forms, hospital autonomy and selective privatisation. The policies were also being introduced in the absence of any developing programme of research to show their effects or compare health systems (Arias and Yepes 1997:3-4). Waitzkin (1997:3) notes that the reforms were being promoted in Latin America before any evidence had been produced to show that they had proved effective in the US or in Europe. Nevertheless, by 1995, 34 of the 38 LAC countries had embarked on health care reform projects (Cardelle 2000).

In a sobering report to PAHO managers, Lopez-Acuna (2000a) argues that the various reform packages had largely failed to deliver progress on any of the key objectives of equity, effectiveness and quality, or efficiency. Progress on sustainability had been largely confined to inflicting cuts in spending to match available budgets, which offered little scope for expansion to meet health needs, while various plans for wider 'social participation' had yet to show any tangible results (Lopez-Acuna 2000a:13). Indeed this evaluation raises serious questions over the motivation and focus of the entire menu of health sector reforms, which:

> ...have focused mainly on financial, structural, and institutional changes in health systems and on modifying the organization and administration of health care. Much less attention has been given to improving the performance of the system and to reducing inequities in health conditions and in access to health care and its financing; to reducing social vulnerability in health; to increasing the effectiveness of health interventions; to improving the quality of care; to strengthening the steering role of health authorities; and to improving public health practice (2000a:13).

One example of this approach was the 'Country Assistance Strategy' for Ecuador endorsed by the World Bank in 2000, a structural adjustment package which involved slashing health spending to *half* the 1995 level[177]; the motivation in this case could only be financial, with health concerns coming at best a poor second (ICFTU Sept 2000; PHR July 2000).

Lopez-Acuna's scepticism over the driving forces for reform is echoed by Fleury who argues that:

> Thus far the reforms' overall result in the region seems to be a private health insurance market covering less than 30% of the population, and a resource-poor public health sector with the responsibility to provide comprehensive health care coverage to the lower-income sectors of the population (Fleury 2001:34).

Despite this evidence of the failure of reform, a marked contrast between Latin America and Africa has been that while the WHO as a whole has retained its opposition to the imposition of user fees for health care, and stood aside from the World Bank's drive towards privatisation of services, PAHO, possibly as a result of more direct US influence, has committed itself to promote the Health Sector Reform (HSR) agenda. This may be due to the commonly argued (if disputable) view that unlike the USA and Europe, where reforms are seen as driven by desire to cut health care costs:

> ...reform of the health sector in most LAC countries has grown out of an attempt to expand coverage and establish equity in the provision of health care services (Langer et al 2000).

Langer and colleagues note an overall increase in public spending on health care, and improved coverage for some sections of the population. Nevertheless it is hard to avoid the fact that the standard menu of reforms in LAC countries is very similar to that elsewhere. Chacon Sosa (1997) reported that PAHO had been providing direct support for 26 national HSR processes in the region, the most frequently adopted policies of which included:

---

177 Ecuador spent just $71 per head per year on health care in 1995, against an OECD average of $1,827.

- Adoption of cost-recovery schemes in the public sector
- New forms of contracting health service providers
- Hospital autonomy
- Selective privatisation of public health services.

PAHO had gone even further, seeking to create the 'political environment necessary to support the HSR processes, and arranging seminars and 'forums of consensus building'. It even served as the Secretariat of an 'Interagency Committee on Health Sector Reform' comprising the World Bank, the Inter-American Development Bank (IADB), the Organisation of American States, the United Nations Children's Fund, The United Nations Population Fund and USAID (Chacon Sosa 1997).

Many of the policies on the HSR agenda have proved controversial with some Latin American health policy academics: indeed PAHO – again unlike the WHO – has reflected some of this unease in its publications (Bambas et al 2000). Yet PAHO's active promotion of the HSR agenda is reinforced by the support it receives from the IADB, whose operational policies on public health spell out as a general principle that in projects supported by Bank loans, wherever 'services are rendered to income groups capable of payment, 'user' fees should be established (IADB 1994).

However, the World Bank's Latin America and Caribbean equity project has been warned that among the regressive aspects of the financing of a number of Latin American health care systems, user fees serve further to increase inequality:

> Cost recovery or fee-for-service schemes may aggravate inequalities in access to quality health care services, as measured by differences in the level of consumption expenditures by income group (Suarez-Berenguela 2000:3).

Suarez-Berenguela argues that there is 'ample room to improve what governments can do' by increasing the level of resources, switching to less regressive tax systems, and 'more intensive use of direct taxes' (ibid). This has not been the general line of approach of ongoing reforms in Latin America.

The sample country summaries focus only on those market-driven and market-style reforms that have been documented.

ARGENTINA

Background

In 1999 the public sector covered 46% of the population, owned 37% of health facilities and 54% of hospital beds, but accounted for just 23% of total health spending, while the private sector covered just 7% of the population, owned 61% of health facilities and 43% of hospital beds, and accounted for 42% of spending (Burki et al 1999).

The other substantial player in the system is 'social security' (the trade union-run 'Obras Sociales', OSs) which covered 47% of the population and accounted for a third of health spending (Barrientos & Lloyd Sherlock 2000). By the 1990s there were over 300 of these funds, many of which were too small to provide services directly, but purchased services from the private sector.

Argentina also has a separate insurance fund for older people, offering services for insured people over 60, and uninsured people aged over 70 (ibid). However PAHO (2002) reports that many of those covered by the public sector (31% of the population, but almost 46% of those on the lowest incomes) are in fact 'not covered by any formal system' (2002:26).

Major inequalities have persisted even in one of Latin America's most prosperous countries. Casas and colleagues (2000) note that numbers living in poverty in metropolitan Buenos Aires had increased since 1994, and that levels of infant mortality in some provinces in 1995 were over 30 per 1,000 live births, more than double the rate in Buenos Aires.

Although the reforms have delivered questionable results, the biggest challenge to Argentina's health care system has come from the instability of the capitalist economy, which brought what was tantamount to a collapse of the Obras Sociales as a source of funding for treatment.

Market-driven reforms

1 Cash limits and spending cuts

Under orders from the IMF and the World Bank government subsidies to the Obras were cut back, leaving many people without cover seeking care from the public health sector, and creating a financial squeeze which Ernst and Young (2003) warn could result in 'widespread provider withdrawal'. Numbers of people defined as 'poor' increased by 20% in 2002, while the numbers in extreme poverty doubled.

2 User fees

The value of coverage by the Obras Sociales was called into question by the combination of new co-payments designed to tackle financial pressures on the schemes on the one hand, and new fees unilaterally imposed by doctors and other professionals, who decided that they were not being sufficiently rewarded by the OS payments. Some low-income OS subscribers found they could no longer afford the additional charges to access the care to which they were entitled, and were forced to seek treatment from public hospitals. Five percent of OS members hospitalised in 1994 reported that they had used public hospitals in this way (Belmartino 2000:5).

Market-style reforms

1 Decentralisation

Argentina's health care underwent two waves of decentralisation, in 1978 and again in the early 1990s – the first to shift some of the fiscal burden of health services from the central government to provincial level, and the second to switch some provincial responsibilities to municipal level. Management of what had been a number of national public hospitals was transferred to the provinces.

2 Provider autonomy

The reforms also brought in the concept of the 'autonomous public hospital', free to decide how to spend any fees raised from patients with OS or other insurance cover, and to create local-level incentives for staff efficiency and productivity (Burki et al 1999:78, Abrantes 1999, Belmartino 2000:10).

3 Competition

Reforms first proposed in 1993 began not from equity issues, but the introduction of more market-style competition not only between providers for contracts from the OSs, but between

CHAPTER NINE

the funds themselves, offering affiliates a free choice of which fund to subscribe to – a choice they have enjoyed since January 1997 (Barrientos & Lloyd Sherlock 2000:418, Belmartino 2000:12). However this immediately triggered a loss of higher-paid workers from the largest plans to smaller schemes offering more attractive terms. This left the OSs with reduced income, but with a continued commitment to cover the lower-paid members (Bertranou 1999:29).

OSs have responded to the new situation in various ways: some smaller ones have merged into federations or larger funds in order to widen the pool of risk; some have opted to seek support and subsidies under a scheme backed by the World Bank; and some have begun to group with local or foreign companies to establish new managed care agencies for their members (Belmartino 2000:14).

The consequence has been to reduce but by no means eliminate the fragmentation of the health care system. The new arrangement leaves high transaction costs and a multiplicity of relatively small funds in which the private for-profit sector appears to be gaining ground in the area of managed care, and competition and market forces have been placed at the centre of the system, in preference to any considerations of equity (Belmartino 2000:16).

4 Health Insurance

A World Bank loan of $400 million was proposed in 2003 to launch a new system of maternal and child insurance to plug some of the gaps opening up in the health care system as a result of the recession and the uneven extent of insurance coverage. The Bank notes that:

> Two out of four Argentines – mostly poor – do not have health insurance coverage and rely exclusively on the services provided principally by provincial public health facilities. However installed public sector capacity is unequally distributed, with a relatively high concentration in richer jurisdictions. [...] Among the insured, co-payments tend to be high. There are significant differences in the package of services (and co-payments) between different insurers, which result in high out of pocket expenses (World Bank 2003c).

The proposal would establish a new insurance scheme 'though a new system for payment to the providers of the basic package of services for eligible mothers and infants on a per capita basis', thus leaving the basic structures of the Argentine system intact.

CHILE

Background

Chile's health care system was 'reformed' by the Pinochet dictatorship in the early 1980s, with the primary objective of expanding the role of the private sector in both provision and financing, as well as improving resources allocation and promoting decentralisation (Barrientos & Lloyd Sherlock 2000:418).

The old Bismarck-style social security system that had been in place for the best organised workers since the 1920s (de la Jara and Bossert 1995, Fleury 2001:7) was replaced by a new one that gave priority to the best paid workers, who were encouraged to 'opt out' of the publicly funded FONASA health fund, and pay instead for private insurance (ISAPREs). Substantial resources were also transferred from the budgets of state-run clinics and hospitals to the ISAPREs (Vergara 1997).

Per capita spending on health fell from $29 annually in 1973 to $11 in 1988 (Petras and Vieux 1992). By 1989 44% of Chileans were living in poverty (Vergara 1997). In 1990 the elected government of President Patricio Aylwin pronounced a new policy of 'growth with equity' – in sharp contrast to the neoliberal policies and widening inequality of the previous 17 years. Taxes were increased to help fund increased social spending, which by 1993 had risen to 15% of GDP – although still below 1970 levels in per capita terms (Vergara 1997:209).

Market-style reforms

Privatisation

Up until 1981 the government health system had provided 90% of all hospital beds: by 1992 as a result of private sector expansion almost a quarter of beds were in private hospitals (Bitran et al 2000:173). The trend to privatisation continued after the dictatorship had ended: by 1999 the private sector ran more than one bed in three (PAHO 2002:163). The system brought new inequalities: the right to health care was still limited by the purchasing power of the individual.

In 1991 private insurance covered only 19% of Chile's population, but spent 50% of total health expenditure. Subsequent investments by democratic governments have reduced the public:private sector differential to 2:3 (Fleury 2001).

However the significance of the additional spending by the private system is enhanced by the fact that it covers largely higher-income groups and the young – those at least risk of serious illness – while the poor and elderly are reliant on the publicly funded scheme. Bertranou (1999:24) notes that more than 70% of ISAPRE subscribers were less than 40-years old, with less than 2% over 65.

> The ISAPREs focus on providing insurance cover for high frequency, low cost services for high income, low health risk groups (Barrientos & Lloyd Sherlock 2000:421).

As a result the publicly funded scheme carries the majority of the most costly cases. While it offers a 'safety net' for older people and others excluded from ISAPREs, this could also be seen as subsidising the profits of the private sector through an institutional system of cream-skimming.

Nor is there any evidence that the private sector offers enhanced efficiency: administrative costs consumed 18% of ISAPRE budgets in 1997, compared with just 1.8% in the public sector (Fleury 2001:17). Even an ardent proponent of the Chilean system as 'one of the most progressive health systems in the world' admits that the ISAPREs collect premiums 'far in excess of the costs of needed medical care. This leads to wastefulness' (Savedoff 2000:2,6).

NICARAGUA

Background

One of the poorest countries in the sub-continent, Nicaragua was been wracked by a US-sponsored counter-revolutionary war during the early 1980s, in which health workers and health facilities were among the chosen target of the US-backed 'contra' terrorist attacks. The war brought 40,000 deaths, the destruction of health care infrastructure worth an estimated $1.4 billion, hyper-inflation of the economy, the suspension of normal lending by the World Bank and Inter-American Bank, and the emigration of around 20% of the population (Birn et al 2000).

The Sandinista government which came to power in 1979 had been committed to the provision of universal and free health care, and conducted massive immunisation and health education campaigns. There was a four-fold increase in staffed health units delivering primary care, extending access to care from 30% to 70% of the population.

Polio was eradicated (1982) and diphtheria (last case 1987) and health indicators improved: infant mortality was reduced from 80 to 50 deaths per 1,000 live births. The increased availability of care to the majority ran alongside the abolition of the separate health care system, which offered privileged access to services for just 8.4% of the population covered by the Nicaraguan Social Security Institute (INSS) (Birn et al 2000).

More recent problems have been compounded by the impact of Hurricane Mitch, which in 1998 destroyed more than a third of the country's primary health network (PAHO 2002).

Market-driven reforms

1 Cash limits and spending cuts

Health care in Nicaragua has been subjected to 'reforms' dictated by the World Bank and IMF as a requirement for assistance under the Heavily Indebted Poor Countries initiative (HIPC). Real terms spending on health care declined by over 12% in Nicaragua in the four years to 1996.

By 1996, Nicaragua was dependent upon international agencies for almost half the country's annual health budget ($60 million a year). One of the conditions attached to this assistance was severe reductions in public spending, especially in the social sector (Birn et al 2000, Zuniga 2000:297, PAHO 2002).

The 1990s brought a reversal of the Sandinistas' emphasis on primary care services: by 1993 just 30% of health spending was allocated to primary care, compared with 50% under the Sandinistas, and by 1995 primary care was receiving just 26% of the health budget, while secondary care spending increased to 56%. This shift took place in spite of the World Bank's formal commitment to improved primary health care in developing countries (Birn et al 2000).

This was followed from 1996 by an even more extreme right wing government headed by a follower of the ousted dictator Somoza: its minister of health began by demanding the resignations of departmental directors and senior hospital managers, and closing down the National Health Council which had attempted to involve wide sections of civil society in the development of health policy.

2 User fees

From 1997 the privatisation of services accelerated, and fees for services and medicines increased (Zuniga 2000:298-300). Although the Sandinistas had imposed a standard $1 fee for X-rays and prescriptions in an attempt to contain demand for health care in the growing economic crisis, they had exempted all of primary care services, and the poorest areas: the new fees, imposed in a country in which according to government figures 65% of the population are living in poverty or 'extreme poverty' (PAHO 2002:410), have been applied across the board, exempting only pregnant women, children under five and some suffering from 'chronic, vector-borne or sexually transmitted diseases'.

Private ward fees are intended to generate up to 12% of hospital budgets, though in practice they yield far less than the World Bank's projections (Birn et al 2000:118-9).

One outcome of the new system has been a sharp increase in the incidence of malaria which by 1995-97 had reached three times the average incidence achieved in 1980-1990, when a system incorporating a large force of volunteers had helped in early detection of treatment of the disease. Now some malaria services charge for diagnostic services.

Market-style reforms

1 Decentralisation

However the right-wing government that was elected in 1990 was committed to neoliberal policies – interpreted as 'budget cuts, defunding of primary care, promotion of user fees and privatisation,' as a result of which:

> Though the 1990s Nicaraguan health services decentralization has generated small efficiency improvements in budget allocation at subnational levels, its main outcome has been a dismantling of the principles and structures of universality, accessibility and primary care that were developed under the Sandinistas (Birn et al 2000:112).

Indeed any theoretical benefits of decentralisation in Nicaragua are limited by the lack of any legal authority or democratic structures at provincial level, or any revenue-raising powers to supplement funds from central government and those generated through user fees. Instead it has enabled central government to distance itself from any direct responsibility for a failing system.

2 Provider autonomy

Other market-style reforms urged on by the World Bank have included the corporatisation of hospitals to 'incorporate business values', and the restoration of the privileged coverage to the elite of formal-sector workers with social security coverage, based on the Chilean model of ISAPREs.

3 Privatisation/extension of private insurance

The private sector (which also includes NGOs) is now the largest element in health spending (45%), with the public sector contributing 41.5% and external agencies the remainder. However, almost 80% of the country's $55 million spending on pharmaceuticals in 1998 was by the private sector, and only 45.3% of the population has access to medicinal drugs, which are almost never available at Ministry of Health-run facilities (PAHO 2002).

Twenty-six such funds (EMPs) have been established (21 of them private for-profit, two non-profit and just three public), into which high-paid workers contribute monthly subscriptions for benefits similar to an HMO – although the plans exclude high-priced care such as cancer treatment, and support for chronic diseases (PAHO 2002). The EMPs, which now cover 15% of the economically active population (but only 6% of the population as a whole), offer no reduction for retired contributors, few of whom can afford to keep up the same level of payments, and who therefore lose their entitlements to care – ensuring that the EMPs carry little risk of covering large numbers of older and potentially sicker people (PAHO 2002, Birn et al 2000).

CUBA

Background

The Cuban Revolution of 1959 opened the way for a substantial progressive reform of the country's health care services. Despite the country's dependence upon military and economic support from the Soviet Union, the Cuban leadership maintained a distinct and independent style of politics, ensuring that the model of health care was very different from the Semashko system introduced in post-war Eastern Europe[178].

The influence of Che Guevara, himself a trained doctor gave added impetus to the progressive aspirations of the new government, which has kept loyal to its commitment to provide health services free to all (Bernal 2001).

Guevara's early emphasis on training doctors and professional staff[179] combined with the establishment of a network of polyclinics to expand access to medical care across the country, and the initiation of community-level action involving nurses as well as doctors in Health Areas of 3,000-5,000 inhabitants. By the end of the 1980s all Cubans had full access to free health care, numbers of doctors had almost trebled, numbers of dentists had increased 30-fold, and qualified nurses 22-fold (Sanso Soberats 2003:189).

Cuba, which saw half its trained doctors (3,000) leave the country after the Revolution in 1959-60, now has over 51,000 trained doctors, and has sent thousands[180] to work with health services overseas, almost three-quarters of them in six Latin American countries: Cuba's medical schools also provide training for over 3,000 medical students from 23 developing countries in Latin America and sub-Saharan Africa (PAHO 2002:210). And Cuba, with its free training packages, appears to have no shortages of qualified nursing staff to sustain services (Moran 2004, Canter 2001).

The strong focus on public health measures brought very substantial gains: the rate of mortality from infectious diseases fell from 62.7 per 100,000 inhabitants to 9.3; life expectancy increased from around 50 for Cubans born in the early 50s to 75 by the early 1980s; and infant mortality fell over the same period from 60 per 1,000 births to 16.

The system and the gains managed to survive the collapse in the 1990s of the Soviet Union, which for almost 30 years had been Cuba's most powerful trading partner and military protector. A visit by six fellows of the Kaiser Media Fellowship programme to Cuba concluded:

---

178 The author of this study has elsewhere outlined a detailed critique of the politics and regime established by Fidel Castro and his July 26 Movement (Lister 1985). However, the available evidence from the WHO (1998), US academics, and other sources not noted for political sympathy to Castro's regime has now been supplemented by a substantive endorsement of Cuba's health policies by none other than the World Bank (2003). It seems that there is a growing recognition that this country's unique example of ignoring the Bank's neoliberal and market-style proposals has delivered real health gains to the Cuban people.

179 In 1961 the government converted a large convent into a teaching hospital linked to the University of Havana (Bernal 2001).

180 'Currently about 6,114 Cuban doctors and paramedical personnel work in other countries' (Sanso Soberats 2003:197).

> Cuba is quite proud of its health care system and seems to have every right to be. [...] Cuba is a
> shining example of the power of public health to transform the health of an entire country...
> (Essif 2001)

PAHO (2002) reports:

> Despite the economic constraints and socio-economic adjustments that followed the crisis of the
> 1990s... Cuba's development strategy has remained focused on achieving the essential objective
> of social equity by ensuring universal availability of free social services, such as education, health
> care, and social assistance (PAHO 2002:198).

From a low point in 1994 the Cuban economy has gradually recovered and grown, while health spending grew by 59% from 1994 to 2000, when it accounted for 11% of the state budget (PAHO 2002:210).

Unlike Vietnam and China, Cuba's leadership has not responded to economic pressures by reversing previously progressive health care policies, by wholesale privatisation and market-style measures, or by cutbacks and closures in public provision (Sanso Soberats 2003:191). As a result the country has been able to sustain the early progress which began after the Revolution. Infant mortality has continued its downward trend in the late 1990s, falling from 7.9 per 1,000 births in 1997 to 7.2 in 2000 – the lowest of any developing country (ibid). In 1996 Cuba's infant mortality rate was half that of the city of Washington DC (AAWH 1997).

Since 1995 a new set of strategies and priorities have been adopted which have tilted the focus further towards decentralisation and primary care services. In 2000 this resulted in a reduction in numbers admitted to hospital.

However there are problems: 40 years of economic blockade by the US, and the more recent economic problems have had an impact on the Cuban health care system, which faces shortages of supplies and crumbling buildings. A detailed year-long study by the American Association for World Health[181] found that the embargo had:

> ...dramatically harmed the health and nutrition of large numbers of ordinary Cuban citizens. ...it
> is our expert medical opinion that the US embargo has caused a significant rise in suffering – and
> even deaths – in Cuba (AAWH 1997).

Medications such as insulin, aspirin, drugs to treat asthma, and penicillin, all of which have to be imported, are in short supply. Specialist drugs, equipment and isotopes for treating cancer have become harder to obtain in Cuba since American multinationals have taken over the companies that formerly offered supplies: of 1,297 medicines available in 1991, only 889 were available, some intermittently, in 1996 (AAWH 1997).

The economy has also slumped backwards since 2000, making it harder to sustain the level of resources for the health care system. In the quest for hard currency, Cuba has begun to market its expertise, selling packages of private treatment to wealthy patients from Latin America, the Caribbean, Europe, and Russia. Some 25,000 patients were treated in this way

---

181 Based in Washington, the AAWH was founded in 1953 as a private, non-profit organisation serving the US Committee for the WHO and PAHO. It set up a multi-disciplinary team to conduct a 12-month investigation into the implications of the embargo, which visited 46 treatment centres in Cuba, interviewed 160 medical professionals and others, and published a 300-page report in 1997.

in 1995-6 raising some $25 million in revenue, but inevitably at the expense of reducing capacity to treat Cuban patients (Chanda 2002).

The blockade has forced Cuba towards a large degree of self-sufficiency: its national manufacturers produce 86% of the drugs consumed in Cuba, and this includes more than 1,000 generic drugs. Cuban laboratories have developed innovative drugs and treatments, including vaccines for hepatitis B, meningococcus and leptospirosis (PAHO 2002:209). More than 30 million doses of the meningitis vaccine have been used in Brazil, Colombia, Argentina and other countries. The country now has 40 biotech institutions, employing 12,000 staff, and exports vaccines and medical products to over 50 countries. Cuba also holds the patent on over 20 advanced anti-cancer drugs which could prove highly profitable if they are shown effective in clinical trials (Sample 2004).

Cuban-produced anti-retroviral drugs have been reported to be effective in combating opportunistic infections among Cuba's HIV-AIDS patients. Even though Cuba has a prevalence of HIV 17 times lower than the Latin American average (Reed 2001), Cuban scientists have been working on AIDS vaccines.

But it is the combination of high-tech, hospital and primary care that has laid a firm foundation for health improvement. This was why Cuban President Fidel Castro was awarded the WHO's Health for All Gold Medal in 1998 for his 'strong commitment to the health sector in his country'. The citation explains that:

> The country's national health system, with its emphasis on primary care managed by a 'health team' is widely considered to be exemplary. Few developing countries have adopted such a comprehensive range of health policies... Clearly the spirit of Alma-Ata and of health for all is alive and well in Cuba (WHO 1998).

This finding is echoed by academics and public health professionals in north America: an enthusiastic article in the Harvard Public Health review proclaims Cuba's national health system as 'an international success story', although there are problems in reading across to the very different situation in the USA:

> Cuba's commendable health care system is a product of a socialist revolution – so whether its methods can be feasibly applied to the United States remains an open question (Merz 2002).

While many US socialists envy and admire the achievements of the Cuban Revolution, it is not clear if any would advocate trying to transplant Cuban health care to the very different context and culture of the USA. Cuba's methods have however been effective in a developing country facing the disease burden and problems of the Caribbean climate, and it is quite remarkable to note how little attention is paid to these successes by those global organisations which profess to offer advice on health care policies and reforms to other developing countries.

The most deafening silence has come from the World Bank, whose vast Health Nutrition and Population publications database has a mere handful of superficial references to Cuba. A major new 467-page World Bank study *Inequality in Latin America and the Caribbean* also managed to avoid more than a few passing references to Cuba and the progress it has made in health and education. Only in one section is there a grudging admission of what has been achieved by a country that has ignored all of the Bank's policy advice and endured the destructive attentions of the US:

> With regard to decentralisation, Cuba has the best education system in the region by many measures, and remains highly centralised... (De Ferranti et al 2003:314)

The silence over Cuba's achievements on health care has run alongside the failure to evaluate the effectiveness and costs of the market-style reforms and expansion of private sector provision which the Bank, USAID and other global advisors urge as the way forward for developing countries. It helps to confirm that the driving force behind these reforms is not meeting health needs or confronting inequality, but promoting an ideological approach shaped to the needs and aspirations of capital.

It was a particular surprise for many, therefore, to find included in the World Bank's 2004 *World Development Report* a two-page 'spotlight' feature on Cuba (157-8), which makes it quite clear that the foundations of its success have been the 1961 nationalisation of health services that left the government as sole provider, along with centralised control, tight monitoring and evaluation, and the motivation of doctors and medical staff. This open expression of division in the 'Washington consensus' came at the same time as mounting belligerent threats against the Castro regime from George W Bush's administration in the White House (Frank 2004).

The example of Cuba is a timely reminder that not only do the market-style reforms hawked by the World Bank and its sponsored academics often themselves carry reactionary conclusions, but they suffer from an even more fundamental problem: *they don't work*, and they set health care systems in poor countries facing in the wrong direction to tackle the very real problems that confront them.

Shorter country summaries – Latin America

BOLIVIA

30% of Bolivians are covered by public sector health coverage, another 30% by the private sector. Social security covers another 14%, leaving 26% with no access to health care or reliant upon traditional medicine (Burki et al 1999, Odegbile 2001:28). It is difficult to equate these estimates with those put forward by PHR (1998), which show that 39% of health spending in 1995 was from employer contributions from private companies and institutions (almost all of it through a system of health funds), while households contributed another 31% (1998:01): yet the PHR report breaks down health spending, while Burki and colleagues are investigating the proportion of the population covered.

PHR figures show that government spending covered almost 20% of health spending, with almost 10% more coming from foreign sources and NGOs, while insurance companies contributed less than 1%. However private for-profit services accounted for 11% of spending, even though their charges were so high as to deter middle- and low-income populations (PHR 1998:01.2). The private sector may be small and expensive, but it siphons off demand which leaves public sector facilities under-used and forces up their unit costs.

By contrast, the public sector takes the lead in the implementation of special prevention and health promotion programmes, work which is national and provided without charges. PHR (1998:3) admits:

> It would be difficult for another sector of the economy to carry it out as it is not a profit-making activity.

The reforms in the mid 1990s led to a reduction in state budgets and a decentralisation of government functions to the municipalities, which Berman and Bossert (2000:5) argue was not intended primarily as a health sector reform. It nevertheless brought a reduction in spending on health care until the municipalities were specifically instructed to earmark funds for health. The reform was carried through with little debate and no pilot schemes (Caballero and Lopez 1997).

Although the reforms have aimed to improve equity in access to care, the contrast between rich and poor is still substantial: in 1998 women from the wealthiest 20% were on average three times more likely to receive more than two pre-natal visits than those in the poorest 20% – while even among the poorest there was a difference between the 47% receiving visits in urban areas and the 31% in rural areas (Odegbile 2001:31). The contrast is even greater between the proportion of deliveries attended by trained personnel: fewer than 20% were attended for the poorest quintile, while 98% of the richest quintile had professionals present at time of birth (op. cit:36). There is a five-fold difference between the highest and lowest allocations of nurses per head in Bolivia's nine Departments (op. cit:34).

BRAZIL

In the 1970s Brazil's authoritarian military government attempted to secure a degree of legitimacy in the wider population by extending social security coverage to workers previously excluded, and by offering a new entitlement to emergency health care to the whole population, regardless of social security status. The Institute of Medical Care and Social Security (INAMPS) contracted with the private sector to buy in the expanded volume of services required: by 1976, 73% of all hospital beds were in the private sector. The government further encouraged this development by offering subsidies for the building of new hospitals, with guarantees of future contracts to provide care. Existing private hospitals were encouraged to provide services to INAMPS on a fee-for-service basis, which resulted in widespread fraud. Companies were offered generous subsidies if they took responsibility for the health care of employees (Lobato and Burlandy 2000).

As the power of the military government began to unravel in the 1980s, a powerful lobby group, the Health Movement, including Communists inspired by the health reforms being carried out by their comrades in Italy in the 1970s, began to press for a democratisation and decentralisation of health care, funded and provided by the state – clashing as they did so with the power of the medical profession and the private sector providers, and with the existing health and social security bureaucracies.

In the event the campaigners won most of their demands, the centralised power of INAMPS was abolished, and in the early 1990s responsibility for planning and providing health care was decentralised to states and municipalities, enabling a number of progressive reforms including the introduction of family doctors and investment in primary care and health centres (Lobato and Burlandy 2000:8-14).

Serious problems remain, not least in the fight for sufficient resources to run local services, and in the fee-for-service model for agreements, which gives providers the incentive to provide (or bill for) maximum services rather than support prevention and health promotion measures (op. cit:16). There is a serious shortage of nurses, the overall funding level is inadequate, and there are conflicts of interest between public and private sectors and between some sections of health professionals.

However, the Brazilian reforms appear unlike many others to have delivered a more accessible and democratic structure, and positive rights to the population, sections of which had previously been cynically appeased and annexed by populist and authoritarian governments.

The sub-continent's largest country spends 7.4% of GDP on health, of which almost two-thirds (4.7%) is private (involving workplace health insurance schemes for workers in the formal sector, plus private insurance for the wealthy and fee-for-service care). The Unified Health System (SUS) derives the bulk of its funding from taxation (9.8% of tax revenue at federal level, plus a share of state and municipal level taxes). The SUS is decentralised, with separate administration at federal state and municipal level, and provides 95% of the country's primary care services, funds outpatient services and reimburses the costs of inpatient care, though it also levies some fees on service users, through co-payments and deductibles.

Most of Brazil's health care providers are still in the private sector (Burki et al 1999): the public sector owns fewer than 30% of hospital beds, most of those in small units (Fleury 2000). The private sector owns 66% of hospitals, 87% specialised hospitals, and 95% of diagnostic support and therapy facilities. The public sector runs 73% of ambulatory care units (PAHO 2002:110). Some private hospitals are chiefly dependent for core funding on delivery services to the SUS, but also offer more luxurious care for the wealthy, while others are linked to separate insurance plans and local networks.

With signs of discontent over the poor quality of public health services, the middle and upper classes have opted for private health care, which now covers an estimated 30% of the population (Ernst & Young 2003). Almost 80% of Brazilians with private insurance cover live in the prosperous and populous south eastern region: 95% of them live in urban areas (Odegbile 2001:10).

The private sector has been able to 'cream skim', since people who could afford to pay for health insurance have been able to use public hospitals for emergencies and for treatment not available under health plans: while covering only 70% of the population for secondary care, the SUS provides complex and tertiary care for 90% (Odegbile 2001:9). More than half the 2,874 private hospitals are for-profit institutions, and direct out-of-pocket payments accounted for 40% of Brazil's national health expenditure, along with 26% coming through contributions to private prepaid health insurance (Suarez-Bereguela 2000:8).

Problems of equity in access to services persist, with a marked increase in use of prenatal care and attendance of trained personnel at delivery among women from the higher income groups and in urban areas compared to poor rural dwellers (Odegbile 2001:17). The prosperous south east region had more than three times the doctors per head of the north, more than double the coverage in the north east, and more than 50% more doctors per head than the south and central west regions (op. cit:18).

Almeida and colleagues (1997, 2000) are critical, warning that the reforms have not brought a more equitable distribution of resources. They argue that even though the regulations set out to pursue equity objectives, this was not matched by a corresponding allocation of resources to the various regions.

COLOMBIA

Several waves of health sector reforms since the 1960s have driven Colombia in the direction of decentralisation and privatisation, with the most substantial changes taking place in the 1990s. The decentralisation process was furthered by new legislation in 1993, which transferred budgets for health and other services to municipalities. More legislation at the end of 1993 set out to promote competition between insurance suppliers and between service providers, while extending a new subsidy to enable the poor to pay for a basic package of health care services. Hospitals were to be converted into 'autonomous social enterprises', drawing their funding from services provided, with discretion on how to spend revenue from user fees – through the process of autonomisation was held up by disputes over liabilities for health workers' pension entitlements (Beeharry 1999:33).

The objective of the reforms was to 'take advantage of market forces and regulated competition to make social spending on health more efficient' (PAHO 2002:173). However Beeharry's survey of decentralisation processes in six Latin American countries concludes that they tend to have an upward pressure on government spending, while the positive results are not always forthcoming. The implication is that such policies on their own are not sufficiently driven by the disciplines of the market:

> To the extent that autonomous hospitals do not face credible budget constraints, it is sometimes argued that corporatization or privatization might be preferable to improve the efficiency of service delivery. The experiences of Colombia and Argentina will need to be closely monitored to see whether hospital autonomy indeed improves efficiency (Beeharry 1999:27).

PAHO's analysis of subsequent developments shows some of the pitfalls of applying the 'menu' of market-style reforms in the context of a poor 'middle-income' country like Colombia: it points to a six-fold crisis for the General Health and Social Security System:

- A 'major hospital crisis', primarily in the public institutions which remain as the safety net provision for the poorest
- 'Paralysis' in the extension of health coverage because of the spread of unemployment and falling government revenues
- Deterioration of public health programmes
- 'Lack of commitment' to public health services among professionals and health workers who have been alienated by downsizing and the imposition of 'flexible working'
- Problems with quality control
- Administrative problems caused by a range of factors including 'mistakes made by the health authority, fragmentation and anarchy in the organisational structure'. (PAHO 2002:174)

GUATEMALA

Guatemala has suffered many years of authoritarian military rule, and never enjoyed any genuine welfare state or social security programme. Social security coverage has never extended beyond 15% of the population and no more than 35% have ever been covered by public sector health services (Verdugo 2000:282).

Neoliberal health policies were introduced into Guatemala from 1991, under the guidance of the Inter American Development Bank, and then in accordance with World Bank proposals:

> In 1993 the country committed itself to health reform through an IDB loan that follows guidelines laid out by the World Bank in its *World Development Report* 1993… and the different administrations between 1991-98 have had to assume the commitment to fulfil the credit

conditions agreed upon with the IDB in order to receive the progressive loan disbursements (Verdugo 2000:281).

The policies introduced included:

- A reduction in health spending, with resources targeted at the poorest
- Decentralisation
- Privatisation
- Subsidies to encourage expanded private sector provision
- Redefining the role of the Ministry of Health to emphasise its 'steering and regulatory role while leaving the provision/management of health care services to the private sector'.
  (Verdugo 2000:282)

Private sector provision includes a very large number of NGOs (over 300), governed through contracts almost identical to those for any commercial provider (Cardelle 2000:223).

Verdugo argues that the transformations under way – inspired as they are by the World Bank – 'are laying the foundations for a highly inequitable health system' (2000:284). The government has continued to declare its commitment to increasing public health spending while in fact leaving the system dependent upon funds from donors and international agencies, user fees, and social funds which are in decline and which cover only a small part of the population.

The system has also been fragmented by the moves to decentralisation, under which 'each hospital, health centre or health post administered by the State or a private organisation would autonomously manage its personnel' (Verdugo 286-7).

HONDURAS

A review of the decentralised user fee system brought in by the Ministry of Health in 1989 found that it created inequalities and that administration costs consumed 67% of the revenues collected.

Eliminating the charges in all but the national and regional hospitals would actually save money, and offer relief to the poorest 20% of households who were the most likely to have to pay fees for their care (Fiedler and Suazo 2002). The authors conclude that decentralised fee systems are not necessarily equitable and that any gains that they may offer are far from automatic.

MEXICO

Health and education were the two social programmes most affected by the massive cut in public expenditure as a share of Mexico's GNP in the prolonged financial crisis that struck during the 1980s[182]. Health spending was halved as a share of GNP in the six years to 1988. Meanwhile the population grew by 20% in the decade (Laurell 1991).

---

182 Public spending decreased from 10.1% to just 4.3% of GNP between 1980 and 1989 (Tamez and Molina 2000).

Three large schemes dominate the provision of health care in Mexico, where the health care system took its modern shape back in the 1950s, as a result of government moves to tie the most powerful groups of workers (the military, civil and public service workers and some sectors of the working class) to the state and the ruling party (Tamez and Molina 2000).

- The Social Security Institute provides comprehensive health insurance to 41 million people, with two-thirds of its budget coming from payroll taxes and the remainder from inflation
- The Ministry of Health covers 42 million uninsured people
- And a third scheme covers another 11 million mainly rural workers.

Just two million Mexicans have private health insurance (Burki et al 1999) despite the entry to the health care market of a number of managed care organisations. More than a third of Mexico's hospitals are private, many of them offering relatively high-tech services, and their largest customer is the social security system. The weakness of the insurance market means private sector care is funded almost entirely through out-of-pocket expenditure. Government spending on health in 1997 was just 5.3% of GDP, US$223 per capita (Ernst &Young 2003).

In the hospital sector, half the funding for the public sector hospitals comes from payroll taxes on employers, while the federal government contributes 39%, leaving workers to contribute the remaining 9%. The three sectors of the health care system work separately from each other, and each remains bureaucratic and centralised. The system thus generates duplication and inefficiencies at the same time as inequality:

> In short, the health care system features incomplete coverage, stratification by population group, and excessive centralisation, as well as serious problems of duplication, poor quality and inefficiency (Tamez and Molina 2000:4).

The reform package brought forward by the government in 1995 set out to extend a minimum package of health care protection to some ten million Mexicans who were excluded from the previous schemes. Under the new proposal the population would be divided into three groups: employed workers with social security; those with private insurance; and those dependent upon state-level public health schemes. However the potentially progressive element of the reform has been undermined by the inclusion of another ostensibly positive move – the introduction of user choice in the social security system, which opens the way for low-risk, relatively high-paying workers, who earn more than three times the minimum wage and therefore pay an additional contribution, to transfer to private insurance plans, while the high-risk, low-paying section will inevitably gravitate to the protection of publicly funded services: this could lead to a reduction of up to 50% in the income to the social security system, while leaving over 70% of the existing contributors on its books. The new scheme also reduced the levels of social security contribution from both workers and employers, requiring a seven-fold increase in government funding (Tamez and Molina 2000:10-13).

For the poor, a package of basic services was agreed by the government to be affordable through a combination of federal and World Bank resources as well as contributions at state level: it was intended that the whole responsibility for funding the package would be devolved to the state governments. The package included 12 interventions in the area of primary care and public health:

- Basic household sanitation
- Family planning

- Prenatal, delivery and postpartum care
- Nutrition and growth monitoring
- Immunisations
- Oral rehydration therapy for diarrhoea
- Anti-parasite treatment
- Treatment of acute respirator infections
- TB prevention and control
- Prevention and control of hypertension
- Accident prevention and first aid
- Community participation for self-care.

(Gonzalez Block and Frenk 1997:14)

The Ministry of Health reported that the package covered six million people by 1996, and had led to an expansion in numbers of physicians and nurses delivering these basic services (op. cit:15). However it is clear that this limited list of treatments will leave many sections of Mexico's poor at risk of catastrophic expenses in the event of serious illness or accident.

Barranza-Llorens and colleagues (2002) stress the minimal extent of the coverage for the poorest, arguing that half of the country's 100 million citizens are effectively 'uninsured', and more than half of the country's annual health spending is out-of-pocket (more than three times the level in the US and 16 times the level in the UK). They point to continued inequalities that give a tenfold difference between infant mortality rates in the poorest areas compared with the richest:

> For persons at the top of the socio-economic spectrum, Mexico's multiple, parallel health care subsystems provide excellent care as assessed by any standard. But for those at the bottom of the distribution, the system provides little more than vaccination (Barranza-Llorens et al 2002:48).

Meanwhile the private sector since 2002 has offered comprehensive health insurance to those able to afford it, and this is expected to 'make private medical practice function more as a corporation'. The private sector remains largely unregulated, offering variable quality of care at varying prices, often in small hospitals: 48% of private beds were in facilities with fewer than 15 beds (PAHO 2002:ii, 6).

PERU

The Peruvian health care system was thrown into crisis by the 'shock treatment' administered in 1990-91 by President Fujimori as part of a structural adjustment programme: the cost of care rose in that year by 8,400%, while numbers of Peruvians officially classed as poor rose from 7 million to 12 million. By 1992 many health centres had closed down, while those still open had no supplies and little to offer in the way of services (Kim et al 2000, Cotlear 2000).

Urged on by the World Bank and IMF, Peru also began a large-scale programme of privatisation of utilities and industries: many newly privatised companies refused to pay for the health benefits which employees had previously enjoyed. The ongoing neoliberal reforms led to the Health Law of 1997, which aimed at reducing 'unnecessary spending on health', removing the government from any role in administering or providing health services, and required individuals to buy their own health insurance from competing providers. The state would assist only in the financing of a 'basic package' for those too poor to afford insurance (Kim et al 2000:133-135).

Kim and colleagues point out that the Peruvian 'reform' was a clear case of ideology prevailing over any evidence or concern for the health of the population:

> The most influential consultants in international health settled on privatisation as their policy instrument of choice, despite lacking any real evidence that its health benefits or fiscal advantages would accrue to the entire population. Their leap of faith, it seems, drew upon a deep cultural cache, a powerful investment in free-market prescriptions (Kim et al 2000:136).

The collapse of the early 1990s was followed by a rapid expansion of health spending in the years 1994-7: the Ministry of Health budget doubled in this period, and the number of clinics expanded by 51% in four years – only to face a new round of cutbacks (Cotlear 2000).

One new factor in the expansion was the emergence of over 500 local health committees (CLAS) which acted as private, non-profit providers of ambulatory care services. Legislation allows these to receive public funds to deliver services on three-year contracts. They hire staff on short-term contracts under private sector legislation, circumventing public sector trade unions and staff entitlements. They charge fees for treatment, which they use to pay staff and update facilities. Publicly run clinics also charge user fees, including the full cost of drugs plus a mark-up. A normal birth delivery can cost $100, a caesarean or hernia operation can cost $400. Less than 20% of the poor are exempt from outpatient fees, and only a quarter of the poor are exempt from fees for inpatient care. There is no risk-pooling or cross-subsidy – each establishment has to balance its own books (Cotlear 2000:7, 8,9).

URUGUAY

Uruguay has been trumpeted by the World Bank as a glowing example of downsizing the state and public provision and maximizing the role of the private sector in health care[183].

> To capitalise on private providers' comparative advantage and avoid developing a two-tier health care system that can offer only sub-par services to the poor, government is getting out of the provision business while at the same time developing its powers as watch-dog over the quality of care. The World Bank's Health Sector development Project supports these efforts (World Bank website 2000).

This policy switch, embracing the full scale of the neoliberal agenda, flies in the face of findings by Slack and Savedoff (2001) that private sector providers are substantially more expensive in delivering high-tech treatments than the public sector. The Bank argues that 'public providers trail their private counterparts in quality and efficiency' (ibid).

The plan so strongly endorsed by the Bank aims to reduce still further the public provision of services currently used by 40% of the population (28% remain uninsured). While the for-profit private sector is still small, the Bank points out that 'most middle class Uruguayans (more than half the population) get health care through the country's 53 private medical non-profit cooperatives' which are financed through transfers from the social security system. Co-payments are levied by these co-operatives for everything except hospitalisation.

----

183 'Uruguay seeks more private, less public health provision'
(www.worldbank.org/html/extdr/hnp/health/ppi/contents.htm accessed 8/7/02).

Appendix A

World's major countries by population, GDP and health spending, most recent available figures

Country	Population 2001 (thousands)	Total GDP 2001 millions $	1990-98 Health spend as % GDP	Health spend millions $	1990-98 Health spend per head $
China	1,271,850	1159031	4.5	52156	33
India	1,032,355	477342	5.4	25776	20
United States	285,318	10065265	13	1308484	4306
Indonesia	208,981	145306	1.6	2325	8
Brazil	172,386	502509	6.6	33166	309
Russian Federation	144,752	309951	4.6	14258	133
Pakistan	141,450	58668	4	2347	18
Bangladesh	133,345	46706	3.6	1681	12
Nigeria	129,875	41373	2.8	1158	30
Japan	127,035	4141431	7.6	314749	2284
Mexico	99,420	617820	4.7	29038	202
Germany	82,333	1846069	10.6	195683	2697
Vietnam	79,526	32723	4.8	1571	18
Philippines	78,317	71438	3.7	2643	33
Turkey	66,229	147683	5.8	8566	177
Ethiopia	65,816	6233	4.1	256	4
Egypt, Arab Rep.	65,177	98476	3.8	3742	48
Iran, Islamic Rep.	64,530	114052	4.2	4790	128
Thailand	61,184	114681	6	6881	112
France	59,191	1309807	9.6	125741	2377
United Kingdom	58,800	1424094	6.7	95414	1686
Italy	57,948	1099754	8.2	90180	1676
Ukraine	49,093	37588	5.1	1917	42
Korea, Rep.	47,343	422167	5.1	21531	349
South Africa	43,240	113274	7.1	8042	230
Colombia	43,035	82411	9.3	7664	227
Spain	41,117	581823	7.1	41309	1043
Poland	38,641	176256	6.4	11280	264
Argentina	37,488	268638	10.3	27670	852
Tanzania	34,450	9341	3	280	8

	Population 2001 (thousands)	Total GDP 2001 millions $	1990-98 Health spend as % GDP	Health spend millions $	1990-98 Health spend per head $
Country					
Sudan	31,695	12525	3.4	**426**	126
Canada	31,082	694475	9.2	**63892**	1899
Algeria	30,835	54680	3.6	**1968**	68
Kenya	30,736	11396	7.8	**889**	31
Morocco	29,170	34219	4.4	**1506**	49
Peru	26,347	54047	6.1	**3297**	141
Uzbekistan	25,068	11270	4.1	**462**	87
Venezuela, RB	24,632	129948	4.2	**5458**	171
Malaysia	23,802	88041	2.5	**2201**	81
Nepal	23,585	5562	5.4	**300**	11
Uganda	22,788	5675	5.9	**335**	18
Romania	22,408	38718	4.1	**1587**	63
Saudi Arabia	21,408	186489	8	**14919**	611
Ghana	19,708	5301	4.7	**249**	19
Australia	19,387	368726	8.5	**31342**	1692
Sri Lanka	18,732	15911	3.1	**493**	26
Mozambique	18,071	3607	3.5	**126**	8
Yemen, Rep.	18,046	9276	5.6	**519**	18
Syrian Arab Republic	16,593	19945	2.4	**479**	116
Cote d'Ivoire	16,410	10411	3.8	**396**	29
Netherlands	16,039	380137	8.6	**32692**	2139
Madagascar	15,976	4604	2.1	**97**	5
Chile	15,402	66450	5.9	**3921**	289
Cameroon	15,197	8501	5	**425**	31
Kazakhstan	14,895	22389	5.9	**1321**	86
Ecuador	12,879	17982	3.6	**647**	59
Zimbabwe	12,821	9057	6.6	**598**	49
Cambodia	12,265	3404	6.9	**235**	17
Guatemala	11,683	20496	4.4	**902**	78
Burkina Faso	11,553	2486	3.9	**97**	9
Niger	11,184	1954	2.6	**51**	5
Mali	11,094	2647	4.2	**111**	11
Greece	10,591	117169	8.3	**9725**	957
Malawi	10,526	1749	6.3	**110**	10
Belgium	10,286	229610	8.9	**20435**	2184

	Population 2001 (thousands)	Total GDP 2001 millions $	1990-98 Health spend as % GDP	Health spend millions $	1990-98 Health spend per head $
Country					
Zambia	10,283	3639	6.9	251	23
Czech Republic	10,224	56784	7.2	4088	392
Hungary	10,187	51926	6.4	3323	290
Portugal	10,024	109803	7.5	8235	803
Belarus	9,970	12219	6	733	387
Senegal	9,768	4645	4.5	209	23
Tunisia	9,674	19990	5.1	1019	108
Sweden	8,894	209814	8	16785	2145
Rwanda	8,691	1703	4.1	70	10
Bolivia	8,515	7969	6.4	510	69
Dominican Republic	8,505	21211	4.8	1018	93
Austria	8,132	188546	8.3	15649	2153
Haiti	8,132	3737	4.2	157	21
Azerbaijan	8,116	5585	1.8	101	9
Bulgaria	8,020	13553	4.7	637	69
Chad	7,916	1600	2.9	46	7
Guinea	7,580	2989	3.6	108	19
Switzerland	7,231	247091	10.4	25697	3835
Burundi	6,938	689	3.7	25	5
Honduras	6,585	6386	8.6	549	74
Benin	6,437	2372	3.2	76	12
El Salvador	6,400	13739	7.2	989	143
Israel	6,363	108325	9.5	10291	1607
Tajikistan	6,245	1056	6	63	13
Paraguay	5,636	7206	5.2	375	86
Turkmenistan	5,435	5962	5.1	304	31
Slovak Republic	5,404	20459	7.2	1473	284
Lao PDR	5,403	1761	2.6	46	6
Denmark	5,359	161543	8.3	13408	2707
Georgia	5,279	3138	2.2	69	14
Papua New Guinea	5,253	2959	3.2	95	27
Finland	5,188	120855	6.9	8339	1722
Sierra Leone	5,133	749	5.5	41	8
Jordan	5,031	8829	9.1	803	123
Kyrgyz Republic	4,955	1525	4.5	69	15

Country	Population 2001 (thousands)	Total GDP 2001 millions $	1990-98 Health spend as % GDP	Health spend millions $	1990-98 Health spend per head $
Togo	4,653	1259	2.6	33	8
Norway	4,513	166145	8.9	14787	2952
Lebanon	4,385	16709	9.8	1637	361
Croatia	4,381	20260	9.6	1945	428
Moldova	4,270	1479	8.4	124	33
Eritrea	4,203	688	2	14	14
Singapore	4,131	85648	3.2	2741	841
Costa Rica	3,873	16108	6.8	1095	266
New Zealand	3,849	50425	8.1	4084	1128
Ireland	3,839	103298	6.1	6301	1446
Armenia	3,809	2118	7.8	165	27
Central African Republic	3,771	967	3	29	9
Lithuania	3,482	11992	6.3	755	183
Uruguay	3,361	18666	9.1	1699	621
Albania	3,164	4114	4	165	36
West Bank and Gaza	3,090	3972	8.6	342	81
Panama	2,897	10171	7.3	742	246
Mauritania	2,749	1007	4.8	48	19
Jamaica	2,590	7784	5.7	444	157
Latvia	2,359	7549	6.7	506	167
Kuwait	2,044	32806	3.3	1083	551
Macedonia, FYR	2,044	3426	6.5	223	113
Slovenia	1,992	18810	7.6	1430	746
Namibia	1,792	3100	7.8	242	143
Botswana	1,695	5196	4.1	213	127
Estonia	1,364	5525	6.9	381	219
Gambia, The	1,341	390	3.7	14	13
Trinidad and Tobago	1,310	8842	4.3	380	204
Gabon	1,261	4334	3.1	134	121
Mauritius	1,200	4500	3.4	153	120

Source: World Bank website, accessed 15 June 2003

Appendix B

Mental health – a case study of the inappropriateness of the main health reform agenda

The contradiction between the scale of the unmet need and the level and development of policy debate is especially stark in the case of mental health – quite possibly because of the close correlation between mental health and poverty on the one hand, and the social stigma widely attached to mental health patients on the other (Knapp et al 2002, Sturm and Gresenz 2002, Patel 2001, Weich and Lewis 1998, WHO 1996, WHO 1999, Brundtland 1999). As a result, while mental health problems blight the lives of tens of millions of people around the world, policies for the development of mental health services appear to rate low on the list of priorities of health care reformers, even where they are included on the list at all.

Nor is the failure to address issues of mental health care restricted to the poorest countries. The contrast in attitude among the world's wealthier nations to the issues of mental health and those relating to ageing was summed up in the launch in 2001 of a three-year Health Project by the OECD. This announced the intention to confront the growing challenges facing health policy and health care systems, and set out to measure and analyse the performance of health care systems in member countries. But while the project designated long-term care for frail elderly persons as a specific area of study, it made no reference at all to mental health, despite the fact that it is a substantial health issue among older people (OECD 2001 b, c).

Mental health care in wealthy countries

The problems and contradictions faced by capitalist societies in dealing with mental health reflect the fact that the inverse relationship between level of illness and ability to pay for treatment is as wide if not wider in mental health than any other area of care. The link between mental illness and poverty is well established, while it has been estimated in various contexts that between 10-30% of psychiatric service users with severe needs utilise as much as 80% of the services available (Torrey 1997; Lien 2003). These are also the people least likely to have well-paid formal sector jobs or the means to be covered by insurance, or to be able to pay fees to cover the sometimes extremely high costs of their care, which may be required for many years.

This means that the greater their level of health need, the less attractive a mental illness sufferer is as a client to a for-profit private sector provider, and the less easily such needs can be met within a market-style health care system or through 'managed care' (Chisholm and Stewart 1998). There are also indications that poverty and unemployment can serve to prolong the duration of mental illness, resulting in even higher costs of care (Weich and Lewis 1998).

The focus for policy makers and service providers therefore tends to switch away from those with the greatest needs to those with the least, or most manageable problems, and those already within the system. As one senior executive of a for-profit mental health service provider in the US summed up:

You don't go looking for people who are going to be the highest risk unless you want to go
bankrupt (Quoted in Torrey 1997:125).

In 1990 Lave and Goldman noted that less than 3% of Medicare spending in the USA was
on mental health, and that:

> ...policies regarding mental disorders differ from those for physical disorders. Coverage of mental
> disorders is more limited, and payment rules sometimes differ for specialty mental health
> providers (Lave and Goldman 1990:20).

More recent studies confirm the ongoing pattern of unequal US health spending:

> ...mental health benefits in private health insurance plans are typically much less generous than
> benefits for physical health care services, with separate deductibles, higher coinsurance
> requirements, and lower annual and lifetime maxima (Zuvekas et al 1998).

This approach appears to have largely continued among most of the key makers of health
policy during the 1990s. In the more prosperous countries, where the use of improved but
more expensive drugs as part of a new system of community-based care could be financially
feasible, there has been a reluctance to channel the necessary resources into mental health:
attention and investment has tended to remain more focused on acute surgical and medical
treatment.

Modern psychiatry, which developed in the post-war period with the growing use of new
drugs, notably Chlorpromazine, in the 1950s, has been one of the first to embrace the notion
of 'evidence-based' practice, running randomised controlled trials which established the
effectiveness of anti-depressants and anti-psychotic drugs in the 1960s (Rivett 1998, Geddes
et al 1997). The growing effectiveness of the drugs, especially the more modern anti-psychotic
drugs with fewer harmful side-effects, made it possible to devise new, community-based
services to replace much of the institutionalised care in large psychiatric hospitals[184] (WHO
1999). The new generation of anti-depressants are substantially more costly – but also more
efficacious than the previous type of drugs they replace: control of costs needs to be seen in a
wider rather than a narrower sense if patients are to benefit and long-term costs are to be
contained (Stewart 1998).

However the driving force in mental health care reforms is not technique and innovation,
but the quest to minimise spending: no matter how eager the pharmaceutical corporations may
be to capitalise on their investment, new drugs that cost more will only be used when it is
shown they can generate savings for those holding the purse strings. Even within the relatively
neglected area of mental health, the care of older people is even less of a priority in the
allocation of resources. In the UK, research into Alzheimer's disease receives just £11 per
Alzheimer's patient, compared with the £289 per cancer patient (Salari 2003).

In Britain, government policy since 1959 has looked to develop 'community care' as the
model for mental health – a policy reinforced by the then Health Minister Enoch Powell in a
landmark speech in 1961, in which he proclaimed the old-style Victorian 'asylums' to be the

---

184 Torrey (1997) argues that the biggest impact on deinstitutionalisation of care in the USA came
not from new drugs but from changes in federal funding of mental health and the opportunity for
widespread 'cost shifting' by states.

'defences we have to storm' if a new model of care was to emerge (Ham 1999, Caldwell et al 1998). In practice the lead in closing down the large mental hospitals was given by the Italian government, beginning in the 1970s (Knapp et al 2002). More than 40 years later, however, it is not only the British government that has lagged behind in implementing its own self-proclaimed policies.

A 'backwater' specialty

Over the same period psychiatric medicine has failed to attain the public prestige and professional predominance that has been accorded to other medical specialties, despite the high hopes expressed in a *Lancet* editorial back in 1963, which proclaimed that:

> From being a backwater, ignored as much by the rest of medicine as by the public at large, psychiatry is becoming one of the major specialties (cited in Rivett 1998:159).

There is little doubt that one of the reasons for the almost universally low status of psychiatry and mental health compared with other sectors of health care (notably the prestigious specialties such as cardiac surgery, orthopaedics and other acute hospital treatment) is linked to the generally low economic status and often the low social status or social exclusion of mental illness sufferers.

There are very few wealthy patients who can realistically be expected to pay the full costs for their own mental health care: any expansion or enhancement of service provision therefore requires either an increase in overall premium payments by those in private insurance schemes, or increased state spending, whether funded from social insurance or general taxation.

Even in the US, which has the most private of health care systems, public spending covered 53% of all mental health treatment costs in 1996, while private insurance covered only around a quarter (Hogan 1999). Torrey (1997) estimates that the public share of US mental health spending is even higher.

In Britain, the closure of the asylums was also urged on by mental health campaigners concerned at growing evidence that long-term incarceration in a large-scale institution could deprive patients of any chance of regaining a normal life (Caldwell et al 1998, Lister 1999). But while the closures appeared to unite the Thatcher government with the liberal and libertarian campaigners, the vital issue of resources for new community-based services was overlooked. During the 1980s, when the programme of 'downsizing' and closure of the large mental hospitals began in earnest (40% of psychiatric beds closed 1982-92) it was at first assumed that a community-based service could be as cheap as or even cheaper than hospital beds.

This approach was harshly criticised in 1985 by an all-party committee of MPs, who insisted that:

> A decent community-based service for mentally ill …people cannot be provided at the same overall cost as the present services. […] Community care on the cheap would prove worse in many respects than the pattern of services to date (Commons Social Services Committee 1985, xiv).

Any change in the configuration of mental health services required investment – in new drugs, in the training of staff to work in new community-based services, and in housing and alternative accommodation for people who would otherwise have been long-stay hospital inpatients.

The US shrinks its mental health services

A very similar set of problems seem to have also arisen in the USA, where the market and its associated ideology have reigned supreme. Torrey (1997:8-9) shows the extraordinary and rapid 'deinstitutionalisation' which reduced the number of inpatients in psychiatric beds from 558,239 in 1955 to just 71,619 in 1994 – over a period in which the total US population increased by 50%.

Not only were the psychiatric institutions emptied, they were also closed down, leaving no services for later patients who would previously have been admitted. Even allowing for 10,000 inpatients in Community Mental Health Centres, and another 40,000 in psychiatric beds in general hospitals, Torrey argues that more than three quarters of a million severely mentally ill people – 'more than the population of San Francisco' – are now living in the community who would have been hospitalised 40 years ago (Torrey 1997:9).

Perhaps equally concerning is the fact that in the world's largest and leading developed economy, according to the US National Advisory Mental Health Council, only around 60% of severely mentally ill adults – suffering from conditions including schizophrenia – received treatment in any given year.

This means around 2.2 million people with severe mental illness receiving no treatment (cited by Torrey 1997:6). The problem is also compounded by the fact that as Ustun (2000) argues, nearly half of those who need mental health treatment do not seek it, while many of those who do suffer from the side-effects of the cheapest available medicines, social stigma, poor continuity of care, and inadequate follow-up from under-resourced community teams.

One conspicuous area of underinvestment, the impact of wide-scale drug abuse, and its knock-on effects on law and order in the USA, has frequently been discussed in the mass media. Cartwright estimates the total cost of this to US society at $110 billion in 1995. However spending on drug abuse treatment amounted to just 1% of health insurance costs (Cartwright 1999).

Far from addressing or resolving the gaps and problems in mental health services, government policy and the emergence of 'managed care' and for-profit medicine have simply made things worse in the USA. The introduction of Medicaid in 1965 with a provision to fund mental health care was seized upon by states as a way to shift cost burdens onto the federal government.

Whereas in 1963 98% of mental illness treatment was funded by state and local governments, Torrey argues that by 1994 the federal government was underwriting 62% of the total costs, largely through Medicare and Medicaid. This served to speed up the inappropriate discharge of tens of thousands of patients from hospital care; fuelled the expansion of low quality and institutional nursing home care; encouraged the expansion of psychiatric beds in general hospitals – which can be substantially more expensive than publicly-run psychiatric hospitals; and led to a disjointed system:

> The result is the most expensive, yet least coordinated system of psychiatric services in the Western world (Torrey 1997:105).

By 1995, the US mental health managed care industry was described by the Wall Street Journal as a $2 billion industry with potential for additional growth, 'boasting margins of 15% and more'. In part this profitability has been created by 'skimming' to take in only the least ill patients, and 'dumping' those seen as higher risks (Torrey 1997).

Markets and mental health

The market-style reforms in Britain and in many countries during the 1990s have raised a different, though related series of questions: can such a system result in a progressive reform of mental health services? Hadley and Goldman (1995) appear to answer this in the negative. These Pennsylvania University researchers were among the first to question the impact of market-style reforms on mental health care in Britain, finding that the situation of perverse incentives and multiple payers had created a 'difficult and complex' system from a relatively simple one, and left clinicians struggling to provide services:

> The situation is therefore reminiscent of the mental health system in the United States, where funding and responsibilities have been fragmented and the relation between specialist services and primary health care has become poorly defined and in many cases non-existent (Hadley and Goldman 1995).

More recently Lien (2003) has explored the effects of market-style policies on mental health services in Norway. He notes that these reforms have a strong focus on increasing the productivity of the acute hospital sector. However mental health was specifically exempted from Norway's new payment-by-results funding system, making it less likely that – in merged health care trusts spanning both general medicine and mental health – any expansion of mental health services would be seen as a financially attractive prospect by providers.

Lien argues that mental health, as an area of health care in which the level of risk is especially hard to predict, is in general especially unsuited to conventional market forces. It was excluded from the system of prospective payment based on Diagnostic Related Groups when this was introduced in the USA. In New Zealand and Australia there is evidence that payment by Diagnostic Related Group tends to lead to misclassification of patients, to make it seem as if their condition is more serious and complex – and thus qualify for higher payments.

Lien also notes that the introduction of new funding mechanisms in the USA through Medicare in the 1980s served to reduce average length of stay in psychiatric hospitals, but also led to a rising rate of readmission.

The transition to outpatient and day case treatment of patients who would previously have been admitted to hospital can cause problems for others: while it may be cheaper as far as service providers are concerned, some of these savings come at the expense of unpaid carers who support patients between episodes of treatment. Only in the longer term – if at all – do these carers see the benefit of their increased effort (Creed et al 1997).

However Trieman and colleagues have shown properly planned and resourced care in the community can be beneficial for most patients and has few detrimental effects on their new neighbours (Trieman et al 1999). Murray and colleagues, assessing a community team's work warn that many of those most needing treatment do not seek it, even from community teams in England:

> Our single most important shortcoming has been the failure systematically to reassess patients who may not seek help (Murray et al 1996).

Mental health care is perhaps the most extreme example of the need to invert the traditional hierarchy of professional-led services, to empower the service users, and enlist their active participation and cooperation, both to sustain their own treatment and to help shape the services they require (Gureje and Alem 2000). Yet this runs so far counter to the existing power relations within the health care systems that progress on these issues has at best been slow and uneven (Simpson and House 2002, Lund and Flisher 2001, WHR 2001). Health reformers have in general not even begun to address this issue.

Mental health in developing countries

If discussed at all in the context of developing countries, mental health care has been largely dealt with as an adjunct to the more central issue of establishing a minimum package of primary health care services, and setting up new structures of user fees as a device to establish various forms of health insurance.

Perhaps because it doesn't easily fit into any market-style reform package, mental health has also remained largely neglected as a subject for policy research by the otherwise active global agencies and consultancies. A search of the World Bank's 14,000 online publications for the term 'mental health' early in 2003 drew just 19 references, none dealing in any depth with policy issues.

The extensive final collected works of the USAID-funded Partnerships for Health Reform also contain only a few scant references to mental health or psychiatric services. PHR publications in general make only occasional and passing references to mental health care: a report of a Social Health Insurance Working Group, meeting in Zimbabwe in 1998, for example, examines the possible outlines of a benefits package to be secured through SHI, but asks (without attempting to answer the question):

> Should mental health services be included? (Kress et al 1998:32)

Another PHR study notes without further comment that private sector health insurance policies 'generally exclude dental and mental health coverage…' The same authors point out that private policies also exclude treatment for other conditions which are commonly assigned to the care of mental health services – alcoholism, Alzheimer's and bulimia (Hollander and Rauch 1998:15).

A similar picture of exclusion also emerges from the privatised insurance system which the post-Sandinista government in Nicaragua introduced in 1994, to cover just 6% of the population (Bitran et al 2000). Cohen contrasts the radical and progressive changes that were ushered in to Nicaragua's mental health care under the Sandinista government, which achieved a drastic reduction in the 'custodial' treatment of psychiatric patients, with the subsequent reversal of policy after the right wing regained power in 1990:

> Mental health services were eliminated from primary care. Psychiatric patients cannot be admitted to general hospitals, and conditions in the national mental health hospital have deteriorated because of severe budget cuts (Cohen 2001:19).

Mental health on the periphery

The peripheral importance of mental health to pro-market reformers of health services is again underlined in a PHR-funded study on Rwanda. This mentions in passing that the country has three public referral hospitals and 'one mental health care hospital': its subsequent policy analysis does not discuss the integration of that hospital or mental health care into the prepayment system that is the main focus of the study (Schneider et al 2000).

Another PHR report on Rwanda details the imposition of a $15 fee for each electroencephalogram, and a sliding scale of fees (ranging from $1.50 to $9) for consultations at the country's first mental health outpatient centre. The report fails to make any comparison between these charges and the average income of Rwandans in greatest need of mental health care – but nevertheless concludes by asserting that:

> Patients are willing to pay a fee for services they perceive as valuable (PHR 2000c).

The fact that psychotropic drugs are available at a subsidised price from the clinic, whereas they are far more expensive if purchased through private pharmacies, is not recognised by the authors as the decisive factor in this 'willingness to pay'.

The exception that underlines the general rule of the marginalisation of mental health care within the debates on health sector reform is a PHR study of Jamaica. It makes the point that the authors deliberately set out to include mental health services in their survey of the impact of policies on the 'indigent' because:

> There is a dearth of data on this chronic illness in Jamaica. Mental illness is also proving to be very costly to the Jamaican government since it incurs the longest average hospitalisation for chronic illness (Henry-Lee and Yearwood 1999:xiii).

The authors report that schizophrenia and delusional disorders accounted for over 9% of inpatient care, with an average length of stay of almost 92 days. They note that France singles out mental health for exemption from relatively high co-payments which apply to other sectors of health care, and point out that a number of countries in practice also recognise the difficulty in charging mental health patients the high costs of continuing care and of inpatient treatment. And they quote Glaser (1991), who argues that for as long as mental health consisted largely of 'custodial' inpatient treatment it had no place in health insurance.

Warning that the Jamaican government's National Health Insurance Plan is seriously under-funded to deal with the numbers of people suffering chronic conditions, the authors also warn of the detrimental effects that are likely to arise from government plans to halve the number of inpatients in the country's main psychiatric hospital, unless adequate services are put in place to support those who would be sent home (Henry-Lee and Yearwood 1999:35).

It is hard to avoid the conclusion from the approach in each of the above studies that mental health is in general seen as a side-issue or an optional extra by governments and by many of the key global players in health policy reform.

A worldwide problem

In the late 1990s the WHO, the one global agency that has given a high profile to mental health issues, began to draw attention to the size of the gap that was opening up in provision for this area of health care, especially in the developing countries. The WHO summed up the situation in 2001:

> Globally, the mental health resources in countries present a dismal picture of severe shortage and neglect. Often the services and resources are one tenth to one hundredth of what is needed (WHO 2001d:4).

The most recent available WHO figures show that mental health disorders account for 12% of all disability-adjusted life years and almost a third of the years lived with a disability. They account for six of the top 20 causes of disease burden among the world's population aged 15-44 (Knapp et al 2003) and for five of the ten leading causes of disability worldwide (manic depression, schizophrenia, bipolar disorders, alcohol use, obsessive compulsive disorders) (WHO 1999d).

At any one time as many as 1.5 billion people world-wide are suffering from mental or neurological disorders, or from problems related to alcohol and drug abuse. It is estimated that as many as one in four people on the globe will suffer such a disorder at some point in their lives (WHO 1996b). There is also a link to ageing, with the WHO warning that the increase in life-expectancy brings with it greater risk of age-related mental illnesses (WHO 1996g).

Numbers suffering from senile dementia in Africa, Asia and Latin America are projected to increase from 20 million in 1990 to at least 80 million by 2025. Urbanisation intensifies rates of abuse of alcohol and illicit drugs and leaves tens of millions of adults and children homeless in sprawling 'megacities'. It also erodes traditional forms of family and social support for elderly people and those with mental illness (WHO 1996c).

Again the inverse care law

Once again the available information – in this case much of it painstakingly collated by the WHO, which has compiled a comparative study covering 185 of its 191 member states – underlines the prevalence of the 'inverse care law', both at national level and internationally. At the root of much mental illness is the constant pressure of grinding poverty: as Brundtland (1999) argues 'For the WHO, mental well being is an integral part of mental health,' and poverty is a major obstacle to such well-being.

Worse: the chances of having to pay 'out of pocket' for any mental health services are the greatest for people living in the poorest countries. Cash payment without the benefit of any insurance or public funding was the most common means of financing care in 40% of low income countries, compared with 12% in lower-middle income, zero in higher-middle and just 2.9% of high-income countries.

The problem is worst in Africa and South-East Asia (WHO Atlas 2001). While the median number of psychiatrists available in all countries is one per 100,000 population, the high-income countries actually have NINE per 100,000, while the poorest African Region countries average just one psychiatrist per two million people. Forty-four percent of the world's population has access to less than one psychiatric nurse per 100,000 people[185] (WHO 2001d).

All of the 18 countries which reported in excess of ten psychiatric hospital beds per 10,000 population were either OECD countries or in Europe. By far the highest use of inpatient beds was recorded by Japan (28.4 beds per 10,000 population) and Belgium (25), while the next heaviest user of hospital care was Canada on 19.3. By contrast the average bed availability for the whole of Africa was 0.78 per 10,000 population, and even this is distorted by the atypical and relatively high bed numbers in Mauritius (8) and South Africa (4.5).

South Africa topped the African provision for psychiatric nursing staff, with 7.5 nurses per 100,000 population, but many African countries had fewer than one per 100,000. Twenty-four wealthier countries reported coverage three times or more higher than Africa's best, with a highest level in Finland (176) followed by the UK (104), Netherlands (99) and Ireland (96.5).

The inequality reaches beyond the issue of beds and staff: a third of the world's population has no access to essential drugs for treating mental health problems, including psychotropic drugs. The problem is even worse in the rural areas of the poorest countries.

In India only 20% of people suffering from schizophrenia and epilepsy received treatment,

---

185 The WHO's 2001 survey of mental health care provision around the world underlines the stark inequalities that prevail between the poorest and richest countries.

compared with an average of 80% in the established market economies. But mental health remains the poor relation of health services: only an estimated 35% of patients suffering from depression receive treatment, even in countries with well-developed health care systems (WHO 1999b).

WHO researchers found that 40% of countries had no explicit mental health policy at all, and a third had no mental health programme. Thirty-eight percent provided no community-based mental health care, while 33% did not report having a specific mental health budget, and a similar percentage allocate less than 1% of health spending to mental health: most devoted less than 5% (WHO *World Health Report* 2001).

The user fees which are being promoted as the solution to funding problems in other parts of the health care system are central to the continued exclusion of millions of mental illness sufferers from the care they require. Even more than the frail elderly, it is those with mental illness who find themselves outside the health care framework, looking in, while the attention of reformers is firmly focused elsewhere, on issues affecting acute hospitals, insurance systems and the role of private sector providers.

Appendix C

(Not) caring for an ageing population – a case study of the inappropriateness of the main health reform agenda

The dramatic growth that is taking place in the numbers of older people within the world's populations in the industrialised and developing countries around the world is described by the Second World Assembly on Ageing as a 'demographic triumph' (UN 2002). However it is clear that the celebrations will not be joined by many of those governments and agencies that are calculating the likely costs of health and social care provision.

There are of course obvious economic and political reasons why the interests of older people should be seen as so unimportant to those driving the health policy agenda at national and international level. From the standpoint of government finance ministers, big business and policy-makers, most older people are seen as a net cost and a 'burden', possessing neither the money to pay for treatment, nor the potential labour-power that might generate future profits for capital.

The illnesses of ageing in wealthier countries

Within the health care systems of the advanced economies care of the elderly has generally been regarded as a low-priority 'Cinderella' specialty, very much subordinated to the glamour, headlines and blue lights of front-line emergency care, and lacking the emotive pull of heroic surgery and breakthrough science. In Britain, where large numbers of hospital doctors come from overseas, there have been complaints that many black and Asian doctors and nursing staff have effectively been 'sidelined' into the less popular and lower status geriatrics and mental health services, while their white colleagues land lucrative posts in orthopaedics, paediatrics and cancer treatment (Lister 1988, Esmail and Everington 1997, Ahmed 2001, Coker 2001, Laurance 2004).

Hospital managers, too, implementing market-style reforms and techniques based on the New Public Management, and seeking improved 'throughput', are aware that older people tend to stay longer in hospital and be harder to discharge than the young or adults of working age.

Experience in some high- and middle-income countries suggests that older people can also be the victims of 'cream-skimming' by private health insurers, who may seek to exclude them (either overtly or by inflating the premium payments for clients above a certain age) on the assumption that they represent a high risk of making extremely high claims. In Chile for example the private ISAPRES HMOs, which cover only 12% of the population, include just 3% of over-60s in their coverage, while the much larger public sector includes 12% (Lloyd Sherlock 2002, Vergara 1997).

Tens of thousands of NHS elderly care beds closed in Britain in the market-style reforms and rationalisation of the 1990s. The desire to remove older patients who are seen as 'blocking' front-line acute beds has now led the government to copy a Swedish system, and levy fines on local social services departments which fail to provide a nursing home place or supporting services to allow them to be discharged promptly.

The level of provision that has been established for the support and care of older people (pension systems in most countries and Medicare in the USA) was generally the outcome of the post-war settlement, and pressure on political leaders from well-organised trade unions. In the case of Medicare, a large network of private providers and pharmaceutical corporations now have a vested interest in sustaining a costly system.

OECD calls for reforms

However, the growing pressure of global competition, coupled with the rising numbers of pensioners, has meant that many governments have been seeking to revise and scale down some of these very costly provisions. Pensions have been a target for austerity measures in Britain[186], France, and Germany, while the OECD and European Central Bank (ECB) have in recent years urged a package of policies including a substantial increase in the retirement age, and measures to force more older people to pay towards the health care they receive (ECB 2003, Hennessy 1995).

In Britain, the long-term care of frail older people has since 1993 been excluded from the NHS, where services are delivered free of charge at point of use, and transferred to the control of local government social services, where means-tested charges apply. In Spain the government decided that pensioners, some with very low incomes, should have to pay for their (previously free) prescriptions to raise an additional £150 million a year (Bosch 2000).

The removal of elderly care from the mainstream publicly-provided health care system in Britain and other countries has represented a significant step towards 'recommodifying' services which had previously been excluded from the market. Hiving off older people into long term care in privately-owned, for-profit nursing and residential homes, or consigning them to the attentions of private, for-profit domiciliary services results – even where the state continues to foot the full cost of treatment – in care being measured in cash terms in which each patient is a potential source of surplus value to a provider (Leys 2001).

The offensive against welfare provision for the elderly is relatively recent in origin. In 1995, when the OECD launched a debate on the wider economic and policy implications of an 'ageing society', its own research staff pointed out that the concern over future provision of care for the older population was 'a marked departure from debates about welfare policies as recently as the early 1980s':

> OECD countries did not ...highlight this as a significant problem during a conference in 1980 on The Welfare State in Crisis (Hennessy 1995:7).

Hennessy's report goes on to show that even where the care of older people has appeared to take a higher position on the political agenda, the driving force has often been the economic and financial implications of the cost of their care, rather than concern for the older people and their health needs. Hennessy goes on to argue that the package of policies which many OECD countries have imposed on services for older patients, which allow the potential for 'catastrophic' costs to arise for a family which has to pay for long-term care, have been deemed

---

186 Margaret Thatcher's government struck an early blow for neoliberalism by cutting the cherished link between the state pension and average earnings. Since 1997 the New Labour government has angered trade unions and pensioners' organisations by breaking with decades of tradition and refusing to restore the link.

acceptable for older people – even though they fail to uphold the principles of adequacy, equity and income protection that apply to other welfare provision (Hennessy 1995:9).

Semi-detached care

In many wealthier countries, even where large and well-resourced health care systems have developed in the post-war period, long-term care of the frail elderly has remained semi-detached from mainstream health care, in the domain of private or charitable nursing and residential homes. Some of these homes exploit their arms' length separation from the public sector and the patchy level of regulation and inspection of standards to offer a questionable quality of care.

In the USA in 1997 a quarter of all the country's nursing homes (two-thirds of them profit-making) were cited for deficiencies on food hygiene, while one in five failed to make a comprehensive assessment of their residents' needs. There has been an unresolved battle over the possible deregulation of nursing homes dating back to the 1980s, while numbers of older Americans in nursing home beds are expected to rise to 5.7 million by 2040, a 350% increase on 1990 (Abt 1999b). By 2001 as many as 33% of US nursing homes were reported to be raising serious or potentially life-threatening problems or harming residents – yet 62% of the $87 billion revenue earned by US nursing homes comes from the government through Federal Medicare payments. Despite its strong bargaining position, the government has chosen not to use powers given by 2000 legislation to set minimum nurse staffing requirements (Harrington 2001).

One of the largest US operators also runs long term care beds in the UK, Spain Germany and Australia, and concerns over the quality of nursing home provision in Britain and over the adequacy of training of nursing staff for such tasks have also been raised (Kerrison and Pollock 2001, UKCC 1997). There are also similar examples of poor standards in other countries where provision is in the hands of private, often for-profit companies. In Spain in 1998 around one in ten of the homes offering residential care were not officially accredited (European Observatory 2000).

'Community care'

Despite these question marks over the quality of alternative sources of care, and the fact that nursing homes are themselves often simply smaller and less well-staffed institutions, since the 1950s the developing concept of 'community care' (described by Jones (1994:140) as a convenient 'shorthand' for 'outside the hospital') has become increasingly popular with reformers and managers alike. Its emphasis on keeping people in their own homes while scaling down and closing the larger institutions which previously offered care services – albeit often of poor quality, in crumbling and neglected buildings, with a minimum of staffing and resources and little if any systematic therapeutic input – has been selectively developed as a means to devolve increasing levels of caring responsibility to families, with or without external support, and the private sector.

In Britain, despite the establishment of the National Health Service as a universal, tax-funded service free at point of use, the British state has never supported the majority of disabled and older people (Parker and Clarke 1995). And it was under the banner of 'community care' that from the 1980s onwards continuing care of frail older people became the first substantive area of care in the NHS to be effectively privatised. The final stages of that privatisation were a result of the changes proposed in the Griffiths Report (1988), which having noted that a growing number of older people had savings and property assets that could be used to pay for care, urged the Thatcher government to transfer responsibility for continuing care from the NHS to local government, where it became as a result subject to means-tested charges (Lister and Martin 1988).

The local authorities have never provided nursing home provision, and were therefore obliged to buy in the necessary services from an expanding private sector: any possibility that the policy might possibly lead to an expansion of public sector provision was excluded by the requirement that over 70% of funding allocated to councils for this 'community care' had to be spent in the private and 'independent' sector (Ham 1999, Lister 1989a, 1989b).

A simultaneous process of change began in the NHS hospital sector, where a rapid closure of over 40% of elderly care beds ensued, coupled in the mid 1990s with the elaboration of new 'eligibility criteria' designed to draw a firm line between those eligible for admission as hospital patients for health care treatment, and those to be excluded (DoH 1995, Lister 1996b, 1997b, Ivatts and Millard 2002). The 1990s also saw a rapid privatisation of over 70% of council-funded domiciliary services for frail older people. One subsequent study suggests that Britain might be the only advanced industrialised country in which health spending on people aged over 65 has fallen since 1985 (Dobson 2002).

Despite the Labour Party's commitment in opposition to set up a Royal Commission study on long-term care for the elderly, Labour in government ignored the Commission's recommendation that such care in nursing homes should be funded from taxation. The essential framework of the Griffiths structure has remained largely intact, leaving a system in which the public sector lacks any strategic planning capacity over provision or a largely privatised service. But Britain is not unique: the general complexity of financial and professional structures involved with health and social care of older people in the EU countries have been criticised by Age Care Research Europe as making a coherent and integrated policy 'difficult if not impossible' (Kroger 2001:16).

Policy convergence in the EU?

Processes of change have run differently in different EU countries, but appear to be converging towards a model of a relatively low-level of state-funded – largely private – provision of continuing care services, supplemented by low-cost care delivered 'informally' by unpaid family members. Yet Kroger argues that despite this general trend towards a common pattern, the actual levels of provision for older people do not appear to be harmonising between different member states (Kroger 2001:21). In the early 1990s the EU countries offered a varying level of 'institutional' (hospital, residential and nursing home) care, ranging from over 10% of over-65s (UK, Netherlands and Denmark) to fewer than 3% (Greece, Italy, Portugal and Spain). The most recent OECD data show that the highest level of institutional care is now Sweden (8.9%), while provision has increased relatively slowly in Italy and Spain[187]. One common factor is the extent of privatisation: only in Denmark is the public sector still the biggest provider of long-term care and home-care services for older people (Kroger 2001).

Concern over the forecast further growth in the ratio of older people to those of working

---

[187] Across the much more varied OECD countries the average level of institutional care for older people was around 5% (Hennessy 1995).

age has triggered a debate in the OECD on a market-driven 'reform' – seeking to minimise pension eligibility by raising the retirement age to 70 or beyond:

> The public pension accounts in most Member countries will start to go into sustained deficit in about ten years time. Public provision of health and long term care for retirees will add to the burden. Countries could finance future social spending obligations by raising payroll taxes to whatever level was necessary, but these would be so high as to discourage work effort and would cut deeply into working people's living standards. These considerations point to the overriding importance of curbing the growth of spending on public pensions, health and long term care (OECD 1998:13).

A context of panic

There seems little hint here of the 'demographic triumph' that was hailed by the UN in Madrid in 2002. It is worth noting the deliberate counterposition in this OECD analysis between those receiving pensions, health care and long-term care on the one hand (the previous generation of workers, whose needs are now described as a 'burden'), and 'working people's living standards' on the other. This approach has no room for inter-generational solidarity.

Nor does the OECD question whether other possible sources of taxation revenue – such as taxing top earnings, or company profits (possibly through a turnover tax), or taxing the $1 trillion daily turnover in international currency transactions (the 'Tobin Tax' proposal, Hayward 2002) – might be fairer and more politically acceptable to the majority than landing the bill on to working people[188].

It is from this context of growing panic over the inability of the capitalist system – even in the most advanced capitalist states – to care properly for its older population that the OECD argues for a new attitude to the elderly. In place of the notion that the reward for increased productivity, an expanding economy and a lifetime of hard work would be a future of increased leisure and earlier retirement has come the proposal that – to keep the system solvent – working lives should be prolonged, at least to 70 years of age.

> There is no economic or biological basis for retirement when people are in their 50s or 60s, yet the length of leisure in retirement is increasing rapidly (OECD 1998:11).

The OECD began an earnest debate to formulate a plan to persuade older people to stay at work, seeking:

> ...a coherent set of policy measures providing appropriate financial incentives for people to work beyond current retirement ages in most OECD countries. Existing financial incentives for early retirement should be withdrawn or scaled back significantly (OECD 1998 b).

Though life expectancy has risen in the last century, such a proposal echoes the first state pension plans in Europe, introduced in Germany by Bismarck, which also fixed the retirement age at 70, on the relatively safe assumption that few workers who paid in to the scheme would survive long enough to claim much – if any – of their entitlement after they finished work. The

---

188 Oxfam has calculated that simply ending the massive tax evasion by multinational companies operating in developing countries could generate as much as $50 billion per year for investment in health care and other services, without taxing local people at all (Labonte et al 2004, citing Oxfam (2000)).

OECD debate on health and social care policies for older people began with 'a high level of agreement' across the OECD countries that ideally they should be 'enabled' to continue living in their own homes, or, if that can't continue they should be supported in:

> ...a sheltered and supportive environment that is as close to their community as possible (Hennessy 1995:8).

Eschewing the customary – if vague and widely misused – phrase 'community care' to describe such a policy objective, Hennessy offers instead the intriguing and equally ambiguous term 'ageing in place', which appears to have been embraced by the OECD and by the UN (OECD 1998:99, UN 2002).

It is clear that the majority of the policy that exists so far on the care and health of older people begins more or less explicitly from the standpoint that they are an expensive 'burden' on taxpayers and the working population, who need to be maintained as cheaply as possible.

Older people in developing countries

United Nations figures show that life expectancy on a world scale has increased from an average of just 45 years for men and 48 for women in 1945, to 62 and 66 respectively in 1990-95 and an estimated 63 and 68 by 2000. By 2020 the average life expectancy at birth in the developing countries is projected to reach 70 years. Over 20 developing countries have already exceeded this level.

Only Africa, where falling life expectancy has been projected for the first ten years of the 21st century, had been expected to buck the trend towards an increasing proportion of elderly within the population. But numbers of Africans aged over 60 are expected to more than double from 40 million in 2002 to 102 million by 2050, almost a fifth of whom will then be aged over 80 (Help Age International (HAI) 2002a).[189]

Of course these global figures also conceal sharp divergences between the poor and the rich. A World Bank commissioned study found that in 1990, 75% of the poorest 20% were dead by the age of 60, compared with fewer than 22% of the richest 75% (Murray and Lopez, 1996). Nevertheless, according to WHO projections, the world will have over 1 billion citizens aged 60 and over by 2020: 70% of them (700 million) will be living the poorer, developing countries, many of which have little, if any, developed infrastructure of health care services to support frail elderly people (WHO 1998).

Numbers of the more dependent over-75 age group are also on the increase throughout the world, but at a slower pace, with the biggest growth concentrated in the wealthiest countries. However, the pace of change is especially challenging for the less developed economies. The rising numbers of older people are significant because, as might be expected, international comparisons show sharp increases in the average cost of health care for older age groups, with average expenditure levels from three to five times higher than for people aged under 65 (Anderson & Hussey 2001).

---

189 Life expectancy has actually *declined* since 1980 in 15 African countries, in a trend now exacerbated by the ravages of the AIDS virus (UN 1997). Many sub-Saharan African countries have current life expectancy well below 50 for both men and women, with Sierra Leone the lowest at 35 for men and 39 for women. Other areas hit by poverty and lack of developed health care systems include Afghanistan (life expectancy 45-46), Cambodia (51-55), Haiti (51-56) and Bangladesh (58).

The expansion of the most potentially vulnerable age group, with the highest levels of morbidity use of health services, will place huge new demands on available health care resources (UN 2002). But until recently the issue of health policy for older people rated relatively low on the scale of political priorities for health system reformers: even now the leading NGO raising the demands of older people on an international level argues that despite 'an era of unprecedented, rapid and inexorable global ageing', the older population is a largely 'invisible' factor on the policy agenda (HAI 2002a).

Lloyd Sherlock shows that the World Bank's limited interest in care of the elderly only developed during the mid 1990s. Indeed its new-found interest in the issues of ageing came too late to influence the Bank's input to the 1994 Cairo International Conference on Population and Development, where its submission, in line with much of the discussion, was largely focused on issues of reproductive health (World Bank 2001a).

The Bank now admits that it was slow to recognise the scale of poverty amongst the older population. But even when it did begin to take up issues of ageing, the Bank's initial focus centred on the establishment of pension schemes for workers employed in the formal economy. This would cover only 10-20% of people in the Bank's poorest client countries, while the large majority of the current and previous generations of working people in those countries have been employed outside the formal sector. In 1999, five years after the Cairo conference, when the Bank prepared a follow-up paper on the changing demographics of the world, issues of ageing and the implications 'were mentioned' – though once again ageing 'was not the central focus' (ibid).

Misconceptions on needs and costs

Part of the Bank's reluctance to discuss expanded and improved services for older people in developing counties is due to the false impression that very large numbers of older people are likely to require expensive and complex treatment. Yet many of the treatments most needed are relatively cheap and effective. An expansion of treatment for cataracts could prevent blindness in up to 150 million people, two-thirds of them aged over 60. In fact quality data on the health problems and needs of older people in developing countries is remarkable by its absence, again underlining the lack of priority that has been accorded this area of health policy (Lloyd Sherlock 2002:200, HAI 2002a).

Instead, governments and international agencies are increasingly looking to reforms based on market models, or promoting insurance-based systems and user charges, or seeking ways of maximising 'efficiency', containing costs, and restricting public spending.

With media headlines focused on high levels of child mortality and the grim toll of HIV/AIDS, the agenda of issues relevant to the care of older people has been seen as tangential even to the campaign for Health for All 2000 (HFA) promoted by the WHO in the world's poorest countries. The focus of HFA and other WHO programmes, and much of the rationale of World Bank 'targeted' measures, has generally centred on mothers, reducing child mortality, promoting health through vaccination of the young, and buttressing the health of the working population.

While these are perfectly legitimate goals, they appear to leave little in the way of resources for care of older people. As Lloyd Sherlock (2002:197) argues, the primary health care (PHC) focus of the WHO reform campaign effectively sidelined the needs of the elderly:

> Whilst age discrimination was never an explicit goal of PHC, it inevitably entailed a reduced prioritisation of services which principally benefited older age groups.

This generalised, tacit downgrading of the priority of care for the elderly can be compounded at local level by ageist, discriminatory policies including age limits, and sometimes by the prejudices and negative stereotypes which may shape the attitudes of health service workers to older people seeking treatment (UN 2002:§70, HAI 2002a:13).

Overview: the economics of elderly care

Much of the focus of World Bank and WHO policies which seek to establish an infrastructure of basic health care in developing countries, starts from a calculation of the economic costs of ill-health in terms of lost production. The WHO argues that Africa's GDP would have been £100 billion higher in 2001 if not for malaria (dwarfing the direct economic costs of treating the disease itself, which has risen more than four-fold from an estimated $800 million in 1995 to $3.5 billion in 2000 (WHO 2001b).

For those who seek an economic justification for investment in health care, there is therefore the argument that securing a healthier workforce will reduce poverty through enabling economic growth, or as Cohen argues:

> A healthy population is an engine for economic growth. [...] Healthier workers are physically and mentally more energetic and robust, more productive and earn higher wages. A healthy workforce is important when attracting foreign direct investment. [...] Ill health may leave persons able to work, but reduce their productivity, shorten their working lives, and increase the numbers of days lost to illness (Cohen 2002).

From this standpoint, health promotion among younger adults is a sound business investment. By contrast providing health care and decent living standards to the older population is not only an irrelevance, but potentially a drag on the potential expansion of the economy. Indeed the World Bank's favoured statistical device for measuring the cost-effectiveness of health interventions, the Disability Adjusted Life Year (DALY) attributes substantially less value to the health gains experienced by those aged over 55 compared with the 'working age' population (aged 9-55) (Lloyd Sherlock 2002:198, Labonte et al 2004:75fn).

Following this same logic, four of the five main 'agency goals' set out in the USAID Strategic Plan 1998-2003 relate to issues of unwanted pregnancy, childbirth, child nutrition and HIV transmission – none of which relates to older people (USAID 1999).

Older people are in many cases seen as having finished their productive working lives – even though research shows that many remain economically active in developing countries well into their seventies (HAI 2002a:31, Lloyd Sherlock 2002:199). But as Lloyd Sherlock argues, the fundamental factor is that older people are simply seen as consumers of health care and social support, ignoring the significant – if invisible – role they play in sustaining the current workforce and caring for younger generations:

> When ageing is mentioned by proponents of sectoral reform, it is primarily in terms of a pressure on health spending and is used as a justification for change (Lloyd Sherlock 2002:199).

The evident lack of concern for reforming the care of older people demonstrates that the pattern of health care reform is not driven by the progress in medical and pharmaceutical technology; nor does it flow organically from attempts to tackle problems and pressures within health care. Instead, the menu of health care reforms is derived from a separate political and ideological agenda. This approach, as chapters above seek to show, starts from the wrong questions, and almost inevitably winds up advocating the wrong answers.

References

AAWH (American Association for World Health) (1997) *Denial of food and medicine: the impact of the US embargo on health and nutrition in Cuba*, New York, http://ifconews.org/aawh.html, accessed 23.10.03

Abbasi, K (1999a) 'The World Bank and world health: Healthcare strategy', *British Medical Journal* 318:865-869

Abbasi, K (1999b) 'The World Bank and world health: Changing sides', *British Medical Journal* 318:933-936

Abbasi, K (1999c) 'The World Bank and world health: Under fire', *British Medical Journal* 318:1003-1006

Abbasi, K (1999d) 'The World Bank and world health: Focus on South Asia – I: Bangladesh', *British Medical Journal* 1066-1069

Abbasi, K (1999e) 'The World Bank and world health: Focus on South Asia – II: India and Pakistan', *British Medical Journal* 318:1132-1135

Abbasi, K (1999f) 'The World Bank and world health: Interview with Richard Feachem', *British Medical Journal* 318:1206-1208

Abbasi, K (2004) 'The Mexico Summit on Health Research 2004', *British Medical Journal* 329:1249-50

Abel-Smith B (1994) *An introduction to health policy planning and financing*, Longman, London

Abrantes A (1999) *Contracting public health care services in Latin America*, June, World Bank, Washington

Abrantes A (2003) 'Contracting public health care services in Latin America', in Preker and Harding (2003)

Abt Associates (1999a) 'Health insurance and access to care', *Healthwatch* Fall 1999, Volume IV No.1, pages 1,2,6

Abt Associates (1999b) 'Regulating Quality in US nursing homes', *Healthwatch* Winter 1999, Volume IV No.2, pages 3-4, accessed 12.7.03

Achieng J (2001) Kenya: 'NGOs seek to import generic drugs from India', *Third World Network*, www.twnside.org.sg/title/generic.htm, Feb 22 2001, accessed 06.10.02

Adams R (2004) 'Policy by numbers', *The Guardian* Analysis, June 1

Adler A (ed) (1980) *Theses, Resolutions and Manifestos of the first four Congresses of the Communist International*, Ink Links, London

Agasi S (2002) 'Cross border healthcare in Europe: a perspective from German patients', *eurohealth* 8:1 37-40 (Winter 2001-2002)

AHA (American Hospital Association) (2004a) 'The economic contribution of hospitals', *Trendwatch* 6 (1), May

AHA (American Hospital Association) (2004b) 'Impact of limited-service providers on communities and full-service hospitals', *Trendwatch* Vol 6, No2, September

AHA (American Hospital Association) (2005) 'Senate budget plan targets Medicaid spending cuts', *NewsNow* March 10, www.aha.org

Ahmed K (2001) 'Asians still trail in hunt for health jobs', *The Observer* June 17

AIHW (Australian Institute of Health and Welfare) (2001) *Australian Hospital Statistics 2000-01*, Australian Institute of Health and Welfare, Canberra

AIHW (Australian Institute of Health and Welfare) (2002) *Australia's health 2002*, Australian Institute of Health and Welfare, Canberra

Akumu W (2004) 'Lobby puts forward proposals to streamline costly health scheme', *The Nation* September 7

Alarcon RD and Aguilar-Gaxiola SA (2000) 'Mental health policy developments in Latin America', *Bull WHO* 78(4) 483-490

Alcock P and Craig G (eds) (2001) *International Social Policy*, Palgrave, Basingstoke

Ali T (2003) 'The same old racket in Iraq', *The Guardian* 13 December

Almeida C (1998) 'New health care models: conceptual basis and experiences in health sector reform', *Informing and Reforming*, No 6: 2-7 ICHSRI Apr-Jun

Almeida C (2001) 'Research on health sector reform policies in Latin America: regional initiatives and state of the art', *Paper for International Forum on Health Sector Reform in the Americas* International Development Research Centre, Montreal, www.idrc.ca/lacro/docs/conferencias/almeida_e.html, accessed 17.09.03

Almeida C and 17 other international academics (2001) 'Methodological concerns and recommendations on policy consequences of the World Health Report 2000', *The Lancet* 357: 1692-1697 May 26

Almeida C, Travassos C, Labra ME and Porto S (1997) 'Health sector reform in Brazil', *Informing and Reforming* No 4: 10-13 ICHSRI Oct-Dec

Amrith S (2001) *Democracy globalisation and health: the African dilemma*, December, Centre for History and Economics, Cambridge www.kings.cam.ac.uk/histecon/papers.htm, accessed 07.07.03

Anderson GF and Hussey PS (2001) 'Trends in expenditures, access and outcomes among industrialised countries', in Wieners (2001)

anon (2004) 'Weiss Ratings: HMO profits reach $6.7B', *The South Florida Business Journal*, http://southflorida.bizjournals.com/southflorida/stories/2004/05/03/daily5.html?t=printable, accessed 29.05.04

anon (2005) 'Policy shift sees costs rise and beds reduced', *Health Service Journal* March 24:9

Appleby J (1998) 'Economic perspectives on markets and health care', in Ranade (1998)

Appleby J (2002) 'Japan's social insurance', *Health Service Journal* 30 May, p30

Arhin-Tenkorang D (2000) 'Mobilising resources for health: the case for user fees revisited', CMH *Working Paper series*, WHO Commission on Macroeconomics and Health, WG3: 6, November

Arias J and Yepes F (1997) 'Research in Public Health and health systems in Latin America in the light of the reforms', *IDRC/CRDI: CIID Montivideo* www.idrc.ca/lacro/publicaciones/948756_e9.html, accessed 17.09.03

Arie S (2002) 'Malnutrition spreads in Argentina, once the "breadbasket" of the world', *British Medical Journal* 325: 1261

Armey D (2001) *Just gotta learn from the wrong things you done*, Heartland Institute, 9 Jan 2001, www.heartland org

Armstrong P, Armstrong H and Coburn, D (2001) *Unhealthy Times, Political Economy Perspectives on Health and Care in Canada*, Oxford University Press

Armstrong P, Glyn A and Harrison J (1984) *Capitalism since World War II, The making and breakup of the long boom*, Fontana Original, London

Asian Development Bank (1995) 'Korean health experience has lessons for Philippines and other countries', *ADB website* May 22: news release No.047/95

Asian Development Bank (1997) 'Health Sector Development Program: Mongolia', *ADB website* www.adb.org/documents/news

Asian Development Bank (1999) 'Policy for the Health Sector', February, *ADB website*, Manila, Philippines

Aubrey ME (2001) 'Canada's fatal error -- health care as a right (part 1)', *Medical Sentinel* 6(1): 26-28, Ass of American Physicians and Surgeons, Macon Georgia

Audit Commission (1992) *Lying in wait: the use of medical beds in acute hospitals*, January, HMSO, London

Auerbach L (2002) P3: *Issues raised by Public Private Partnerships in Ontario's hospital sector*, CUPE, Toronto, December

Aviles LA (2001) 'Epidemiology as discourse: the politics of development institutions in the Epidemiological Prifile of El Salvador', *Journal of Epidemiological and Commmunity Health* 55: 164-171

Ayonrinde OA, Sauer J and Macdiarmid F (2000) 'Letter: PACT to the future', *British Journal of Psychiatry* April, 176: 397-8

Bach S (2000) 'Decentralisation and privatisation of municipal services: the case of health services', *Sectoral activities programme Working Paper* ILO, Geneva, November 2000

Baggott R (2000) 'Understanding the New Public Health: towards a policy analysis', in Hann (2000)

Bale M and Dale T (1998) 'Public sector reform in New Zealand and its relevance to developing countries', *World Bank Research Observer* Vol 13; 1: 102-21 (February)

Balls A and Sevastopulo D (2005) 'Bush's man at the World Bank: can Wolfowitz put poverty before politics?' *Financial Times* March 30:15

Bambas A, Casas JA, Drayton HA and Valdés A (eds) (2000) *Health and human development in the new global economy: the contributions and perspectives of civil society in the Americas*, PAHO, Washington DC

Banerji D (1999) 'A fundamental shift in the approach to international health by WHO UNICEF and the World Bank: instances of the practice of "intellectual fascism" and totalitarianism in some Asian countries', *International Journal of Health Services* 29(2): 227-59

Barlow M (2000) *The Free Trade Area of the Americas and the threat to social programs, environmental stability and social justice in Canada and the Americas*, The Council of Canadians, www.canadians.org

Barlow M (2002) *The right choice to make*, Council of Canadians, release Dec 9 2002 council-of-canadians@topica.email-publisher.com, accessed 09.12.02

Barnum H, J Kutzin and H Saxenian (1995) 'Incentives and Provider Payment Methods', *International Journal of Health Planning and Management* 10: 23-45

Barraza-Llorens M, Berozzi S, Gonzalez-Pier E and Gutierrez JP (2002) 'Addressing inequity in health and health care in Mexico', *Health Affairs* Vol 21, No 3, p47-56 May-June

Barrientos A and Lloyd-Sherlock P (2000) 'Reforming health insurance in Argentina and Chile', *Health Policy and Planning* 15(4): 417-423

Bayliss K and Hall D (2002) *Glimpses of an alternative – the possibility of public ownership in the World Bank's latest PSD strategy paper*, January, Public Services International Research Unit, Greenwich, UK

Beecham L (1994) 'OECD backs NHS Reforms', *British Medical Journal* 309 (6949) 221-222

Beeharry GK (1999) *Decentralization of Health Services in Latin American Countries: Issues and Some Lessons*, September, World bank, Washington

Bell G (2003) 'Manuel upbeat on peer review but others wary', *Independent Day* June 12, www.avmedia.at/nepad/indexgb.html, accessed 09.07.03

Belmartino S (2000) 'The context and process of health care reform on Argentina', in Fleury et al (2000)

Bennett S, Quick JD and Velasquez G (1997) *Public-private roles in the pharmaceutical sector: Implications for equitable access and rational drug use*, WHO, Geneva

Bennett S (1989) 'The Impact of the Increase in User Fees', *Lesotho Epidemiological Bulletin* 4

Bentes M, Dias CM, Sakellarides C and Bankauskaite V (2004) *Health Care Systems in Transition: Portugal*, European Observatory on Health Systems, Copenhagen

Berliner H (1999a) 'State of the union', *Health Service Journal* August 12: 27

Berliner H (1999b) 'Profits of doom', *Health Service Journal* November 4: 30

Berliner H (2002) 'United Straits', *Health Service Journal* 27 June, p 32

Berliner HS (1983) 'Starr Wars', *International Journal of Health Services* 13(4): 671-5

Berman P (1995) 'Health sector reform: making development sustainable', *Health Policy* 37: 13-28

Berman P, Nwuke K, Hanson K, Kariuki M, Mbugua K, Ngugi J, Omurwa T and Ong',ayo S (1995) 'Kenya: non-governmental health care provision', April, *Data for Decision Making Project*, Harvard School of Public Health

Bernal S (2001) *Women's Health Care in Cuba: Observations of Medical Facilities in Cerro, Havana*, http://ii.csusb.edu/journal/cuba/women.html

Berndt ER (2001) 'The US pharmaceutical industry: why major growth in times of cost containment?' *Health Affairs* 20 (2): 100-114, March-April

Bertranou FM (1999) 'Are market oriented health reforms possible in Latin America? The cases of Argentina, Chile and Colombia', *Health Policy* Apr 47 (1) 19-36

Berwick DM (2004) 'Lessons from developing nations on improving health care', *British Medical Journal* 328: 1124-9

Bevan G, France G and Taroni F (1992) Dolce Vita: Healthcare in Italy, *Health Service Journal* 20-23, February 27

Bhushan I (2001) 'Health sector challenges in Asia and the Pacific: the Strategy of the Asian Development Bank', in Molina and del Arco (2001)

Bilous A (1997) 'Strikes in the hospital sector', *EIRO online* April, European Industrial Relations Observatory, Dublin, www.eiro.eurofound.eu.int/1997/04/feature/FR9704139F.htm, accessed 08.06.03

Birdsall N and James E (1992) 'Health, government, and the poor: the case for the private sector', *Policy Research Working Paper* July, World Bank, Washington DC

Birn AE, Zimmerman S and Garfield R (2000) 'To Decentralize or not to Decentralize; is that the Question? Nicaraguan Health Policy under Structural Adjustment in the 1990s', *International Journal of Health Services* Dec 30(1) 111-128

Birrell B, Hawthorne L and Rapson V (2003) *The outlook for surgical services in Australasia*, June, Centre for Population and Urban Research, Monash University

Birungi H, Mugisha F, Nsabagasani X (1999) 'Uganda: a new public-private mix', *Informing and Reforming*. 10-11, Jan-Jun 1999, 6-7

Bitran R and Yip WC (1998) 'A review of health care provider payment reform in selected countries in Asia and Latin America', *Major Applied Research 2, Working Paper 1* August PHR, Abt Associates Inc, Bethesda

Bitran R and Yip WC (1999) 'Reform of provider payment systems in Latin America', *Informing and Reforming*, 10-11 Jan-Jun 1999, 3-4

Bitran R, Munoz J, Aguad P and Navarete M (2000) 'Equity in the financing of social security for health in Chile', *Health Policy* Jan 1 50(3): 171-196

Bitran y Asociados (Ubilla G, Espinosa C and Bitran R) (2000) 'The use of capitation payment by the Social Security Institute and previsional medical enterprises in Nicaragua', *Major Applied Research 2, Working Paper 3* PHR, Abt Associates, Bethesda Ma

Black D (1980) *Inequalities in Health (the Black Report)*, DHSS London

Black R (1970) *Stalinism in Britain*, New Park Publications, London

Blair T (2001) *The power of community can change the world*, Labour Party, October 3

Blair T (2002) 'The power of community can change the world', *Speech to Labour Party Conference* 2001 http://www.ppionline.org/ppi_ci.cfm?knlgAreaID=128&subsecID=187&contentID=3881, accessed 08.09.02

Blair T (2003) 'Where the third way goes from here', *Progressive Governance* www.progressive-governance.net/php/print_preview.php?aid=35, accessed 12.05.03

Bloom BSI, de Pouvourville N, Libert S and Fendrick AM (2000) 'Surgeon predictions on growth of minimal invasive therapy; the difficulty of estimating technologic diffusion', *Health Policy* Dec 54(3) 201-207

Bloom DB, Craig P and Mitchell M (2000) 'Public and Private Roles in Providing and Financing Social Services: Health and Education', in Wang (2000)

Bloom FE (2003) 'AAAS president calls to restore American health system', *Press Release* Feb 13, American Association for the Advancement of Science, Denver Colorado

Bloom G (1998) 'Primary health care meets the market in China and Vietnam', *Health Policy* 44(3): 233-252

Bloom G (2001) *China's rural health system in transition: towards coherent institutional arrangements?* September 13, Centre for Business and Government, Harvard, www.ksg.harvard.edu/cbg/Conferences/financal_sector/home.htm, accessed 10.7.03

Bloom G, Lu Y and Chen J (2002) 'Financing health care in China's cities: balancing needs and entitlements during rapid change', *IDS Working Paper* 176 December, Institute of Development Studies, Brighton

Bloor K and Maynard A (1994) 'An outsider's view of the NHS reforms', *British Medical Journal* 309: 352-3

Bloor K, Maynard A and Street A (2000) 'The cornerstone of Labour's "new NHS": Reforming primary care', in Smith (2002)

BMA (British Medical Association) (1997) *Leaner & Fitter*, October BMA Health Policy & Economic Research Unit, London

BMA (British Medical Association) (2003) *Memorandum to Health Select Committee inquiry into foundation hospitals*, January, www.bma.org.uk/ap.n...current&Highlight=2.foundation.hospitals, accessed 13.01.0

Boehmer U (2002) 'Twenty years of public health research: inclusion of Lesbian, Gay, Bisexual and Transgender populations', *American Journal of Public Health* 92(7) 1125-1130, July

Bond P (2003) 'The new apartheid: South Africa's trade unions loudly oppose the Government's sell-off of basic services', *New Internationalist* April

Bosch X (2000) 'Spain to charge elderly for drugs', *British Medical Journal* 321: 10

Bosch X (2001) 'Milburn visits Spain for doctors and ideas', *British Medical Journal* 323: 11

Bosch X (2002) 'Spain decentralises its healthcare system', *British Medical Journal* 324: 68.

Boseley S (2003a) 'Aids drugs scandal: toll soars', *The Guardian* July 3

Boseley S (2003b) 'Diabetes creating world health catastrophe, warns leading doctor', *The Guardian* 25 August

Boseley S (2003c) 'Huge NHS bill for infertility rights', *The Guardian* August 26

Boseley S (2003d) 'UK backs poor nations over medicine patents', *The Guardian* May 8

Bossert TJ (2000) 'Decentralisation of Health Systems in Latin America: A comparative study of Chile, Colombia and Bolivia', *Data for Decision Making Project*, Harvard School of Public Health, June

Bossert TJ, Beauvais J and Bowser D (2000) 'Decentralization of Health Systems: Preliminary Review of Four Country Case Studies', *Major Applied Research 6, Technical Report* No1, January 2000, Partnerships for Health Reform Project, Abt Associates Inc. Bethesda, MD

Boulle A, Blecher M and Burn A (2000) 'Hospital Restructuring', *South African Health Review* Health Systems Trust, Durban, www.hst.org.za/sahr, accessed 08.07.03

Bourdieu P (1998) 'Utopia of Endless Exploitation - the essence of neoliberalism', *Le Monde Diplomatique* December, Translated by JJ Shapiro, http:/www.forum-global.de/soc/bibliot/b/bessenceneolib.htm, accessed 24.08.03

Boyer R and Drache D (eds) (1996) *States Against Markets: the Limits of Globalisation*, London, Routledge

Boyle D, Conisbee M and Burns S (2004) *Towards an asset-based NHS. The missing elements of NHS reform* February, New Economics Foundation, London

Brandon RM, Podhorzer M and Pollak TH (1991) 'Premiums without benefits: waste and inefficiency in the commercial health insurance industry', *International Journal of Health Services* Vol 21 No. 2 265-283

Braveman P (1998) *Monitoring Equity in Health: a policy-oriented approach in low- and middle-income countries*, WHO, http://whqlibdoc.who.int/hq/1998/WHO_CHS_HSS_98.1.pdf, accessed 06.12.03

Braveman P, Starfield B and Geiger HJ (2001) 'World Health Report 2000: how it removes equity from the agenda for public health monitoring and policy', *British Medical Journal* 323: 678-681

Breitman G and Stanton F (eds) (1977) *The Transitional Program for Socialist Revolution*, Pathfinder Press, New York

Breman A and Shelton C (2001) *Structural Adjustment and Health: a literature review of the debate, its role players and presented empirical evidence*, CMH Working Paper series WG6:6, June, WHO, Geneva

Brown, A (2000a) *Current issues in sector-wide approaches to health development: Mozambique case study*, WHO Geneva

Brown, A (2000b) *Current issues in sector-wide approaches to health development: Uganda case study*, WHO Geneva

Brown, P (2002) 'WHO to revise its method for ranking health systems', *British Medical Journal* 324: 190

Brugha R and Walt G (2001) 'A global health fund: a leap of faith?' *British Medical Journal* 323: 152-154

Brugha R and Zwi A (2002) 'Global approaches to private sector provision: where is the evidence?' in Lee et al (2002)

Brundtland GH (1998a) *Address to the Regional Committee for Africa (48th session, Harare)*, August 31, WHO

Brundtland GH (1998b) *Dr Gro Harlem Brundtland: entry on duty in Geneva*, WHO: office of Director General, July 21

Brundtland GH (1999c) 'Raising awareness, fighting stigma, improving care: Brundtland unveils new WHO global strategies for mental health', *Press Release*, WHO Geneva, Nov 12 1998

Brundtland GH (2001a) 'Globalisation as a force for better health', *Lecture at LSE* 16 March, WHO

Brundtland GH (2001b) 'WHO/WTO workshop on differential pricing and financing of essential drugs', Speech 8 April, Norway

Brundtland GH (2001c) 'Scaling up action to tackle illness associated with poverty: the global fund for AIDS and health', *World Health Assembly Technical Briefing* February 18, Geneva

Buchan J (2005) 'International recruitment of health professionals', *British Medical Journal* 330:210

Bukharin NI and Preobrazhensky EA (1919) *The ABC of Communism*, (ed EH Carr) Pelican Classics, London 1970

Burgermeister J (2004a) 'Sweden bans privatisation of hospitals', *British Medical Journal* 328: 484

Burgermeister J (2004b) 'Exodus of Polish doctors could threaten health system', *British Medical Journal* 328: 1280

Burgermeister J (2004c) 'Japan's doctors say low fees are driving many to ruin', *British Medical Journal* 329:531

Burki SJ, Perry GE and Dillinger WR (1999) 'Beyond the Center: Decentralizing the State', *Latin American and Caribbean Studies*, World Bank, Washington

Burrows R & Loader B (eds) (1994), *Towards a Post Fordist Welfare State*, Routledge

Buse K and Walt G (2000a) 'Global public-private partnerships part I – a new development in health?' *Bull WHO* 78(4), 549-561

Buse K and Walt G (2000b) 'Global public-private partnerships part II – what are the health issues for global governance?' *Bull WHO* 78(5) 699-709

Buse K and Waxman A (2001) 'Public-private health partnerships: a strategy for WHO', *Bull WHO* 79(8) 748-754

Busse R (1999) 'Priority setting and rationing in German health care', *Health Policy* Dec50(1-2): 71-90

Busse R (2000) 'Health in Transition: Czech Republic', *Health Care Systems in Transition*, WHO, Copenhagen

Busse R and Riesberg A (2000) 'Health in Transition: Germany', *Health Care Systems in Transition*, WHO Euro Observatory

Busse R and Riesberg A (2004) 'Health in Transition: Germany', *Health Care Systems in Transition*, WHO Euro Observatory

Busse R, van der Grinten T and Svensson PG (2002) 'Regulating entrepreneurial behaviour in hospitals: theory and practice', in Saltman et al (2002)

Caballero JTG and Lopez HG (1997) 'Decentralisation of health services in Bolivia', *Informing and Reforming* 4: 8-10, Oct-Dec

Calamitsis E (1999) 'Adjustment and growth in sub-Saharan Africa: The Unfinished Agenda', *Finance and Development* 36(1), March, IMF, Washington

Caldwell K, Francome C and Lister J (1998) *The Envy of the World*, NHS Support Federation, London

Campbell D (2004) 'Havens that have become a tax on the world's poor', *The Guardian* 21 September

Campbell P, Quigley K, Collins A, Yeracaris P and Chaora M (2000) 'Applying managed care concepts and tools to middle and lower income countries: the case of Medical Aid Societies in Zimbabwe', June, *Data for Decision Making*, Harvard

Cancer Care Advocacy Coalition (2003) 'Deadly silence meets growing cancer crisis', January 16, *News Release*, Cancer Care Advocacy Coalition

Canter C (2001) 'Commitment to care: nurses in Cuba offer a glimpse into the island republic's health system', *Nurseweek.com* June 11

Cardelle AJF (2000) *Democratization, Health Care Reform, and NGO-Government Collaboration*, Status of Women Canada, Ottawa

Carlisle D (2003) 'Deals and costs yet to be finalised', *Health Service Journal* 18 September: 6-7

Cartwright WS (1999) Book Review: Methods for the Economic Evaluation of health care programmes, Drummond MF et al *Journal of Mental Health Policy and Economics* 2: 43

Carvel J (2004) 'NHS Trusts bullied into private contracts: Chairman lost job for resisting cataracts deal with foreign firm', *The Guardian* 1 June

Casas JA and Casco RD, Torres-Parodi C (2000) 'Governability and governance: toward health and human development', in Bambas et al (2000)

Castano R, Bitran R and Giedion U (2004) *Monitoring and evaluating hospital autonomization and its effects on priority health services*, The Partners for Health Reformplus Project, Abt Associates Inc, Bethesda

Castles, F and Mitchell D (1991) 'Three Worlds of Welfare Capitalism or Four?' *Discussion Paper* 21, Australian National University

Catan T (2004) 'Big spender: what happened to $20 billion of Iraqi funds?' *Financial Times* December 9

Caufield C (1997) *Masters of Illusion, The World Bank and the Poverty of Nations*, Pan Books

Central Bureau of Statistics (2003) *Health statistics*, http://www.cbs.go.ke/health_summary.htmil, accessed 27.03.05

Chaco Sosa FJ (1997) 'Pan American Health Organisation: Progress of activities in Health Sector Reform', *Informing and Reforming* 4: 17, Oct-Dec

Chambaud L (1993) 'A la carte', *Health Service Journal* March 18, 24- 27

Chanda R (2002) 'Trade in health services', *Bull WHO* 80(2): 158-163

Chandrasekhar CP and Ghosh J (2003) 'WTO drugs deal: Does it really benefit developing countries?' *Business Line - India* September 9, http://www.thehindubusinessline.com/bline/2003/09/09/stories/2003090900140900.htm, accessed 24.01.04

Charatan F (2002) 'US report blames poor quality control for soaring healthcare costs', *British Medical Journal* 324:1478

Charatan F (2003) 'Governors resist Bush plan to rein in Medicaid costs', *British Medical Journal* 326: 1230

Chinitz D, Preker A and Wasem J (1998) 'Balancing solidarity and competition in health care financing', in Saltman et al (1998)

Chisholm A and Ford R (2004) *Transforming mental health care*, Sainsbury Centre for Mental Health, London

Christian Aid (2003) *Struggling to be heard. Democratising the World Bank and IMF*, Christian Aid, London

Clarke J, Langan M and Williams F (2001) 'Remaking welfare: the British welfare regime in the 1980s and 1990s', in Cochrane et al (2001)

Clarke R (2001) 'How healthy is our healthcare?' *OECD Observer* Dec 18, OECD, Paris

CMA (Canadian Medical Association) (1998) 'Looking toward tomorrow: health, health care and medicine', *Background paper for 131st Annual Meeting*, www.cma.ca/inside/annmeet/131/bg/bg%2D01.htm, accessed 26.09.00

CMMC (Central Manchester and Manchester Children's University Hospitals NHS Trust) (2004) *New Hospitals Development Executive Summary (technical)*, CMMC, Manchester, February

CMMH (Central Manchester and Manchester Children's University Hospitals NHS Trust) (2003) *Outline agreement of the Trust, Manchester Primary Care Trusts, the Strategic Health Authority, Private Finance Unit and the Review team*, Nov 14, http://www.cmmc.nhs.uk/your_trust/trustboard/dec2003/agenda_item8.pdf, accessed 29.5.04

Coast J, Inglis A and Frankel S (1996) 'Alternatives to hospital care: what are they and who should decide?' *British Medical Journal* 312: 162-166

Coburn D (2000) 'Income inequality, lowered social cohesion and the poorer health status of populations: the role of neo-liberalism', *Social Science and Medicine* 51: 135-146.

Coburn D (2001) 'Health, Health care and neoliberalism', in Armstrong (2001)

Cochrane A, Clarke J and Gewirtz S (eds) (2001) *Comparing Welfare States* (Second Edition), Open University and Sage, London

Cohen A (2001) 'The effectiveness of mental health services in primary care: the view from the developing world' Nations for Mental Health, WHO, Geneva

Cohen, D (2002) 'Health and Economic Growth' Future, *The Aventis Magazine* February http://www.aventis.com/future/downloads/PDF/fut0202/En_2_2002_health_and_wealth.pdf accessed 21.02.03

Coker N (ed) (2001) *Racism in Medicine: An Agenda for Change*, Kings Fund London

Colgan AL (2002) 'Hazardous to Health: the World Bank and IMF in Africa', Africa Action Position Paper, April www.africaaction.org/action/sap0204.htm, accessed 29.06.02

Collins CD and Green AT (1994) 'Decentralisation and primary health care: some negative implications in developing countries', *International Journal of Health Services* Vol 24 No.3 459-475

Collins CD and Green AT, (1999) 'Public sector hospitals and organisational change: an agenda for policy analysis', *International Journal of Health Planning and Management* 14: 107-128

Collins CD and Green AT, Hunter DJ (1994) 'International transfers of National Health Service reforms; problems and issues', *The Lancet* Jul 23 344(8917): 248-50

Collins CD, Green AT and Hunter DJ (1999) 'Health Sector reform and the interpretation of policy context', *Health Policy* 47: 69-85

Collins D, Njeru G and Meme J (1996) 'Hospital Autonomy in Kenya: the experience of Kenyatta National Hospital', June, *Data for Decision Making Project*, Harvard School of Public Health

Collins DH, Quick JD, Musau SN and Kraushaar DL (1996) *Health financing reform in Kenya: the fall and rise of cost sharing 1989-94*, Management Sciences for Health, Boston

Colombo F and Hurst J (2003) OECD *Reviews of Health Care Systems*: Korea, OECD, Paris

Commons Health Committee (2002) *Public expenditure on health and social services*, October, HC 1210, session 2001-2, House of Commons, London

Commons Social Services Committee (1985) *Session 1984-85 Community Care Vol 1*, London HMSO

Connolly C (2002) 'Health care's soaring cost takes a toll', *Washington Post* July 9 2002 page A01

Connolly G (2002) 'South African Health Care a system in transition', *Background paper for Asian Social Forum Hyderabad*, January 2003, www.cehat.org/rthc/paper6.htm

Conrad M (2005) 'Expert warns of more delays on PBR rollout', Public Finance March 18-24:8

Coombes R (2005) 'Private providers must be stopped from skimming off easy cases', *British Medical Journal* 330:691

Coopers and Lybrand (1995) *European healthcare trends: towards managed care in Europe*, May, Cooper and Lybrand, London

Coovadia H (2004) 'Building partnerships to respond to the AIDS epidemic', Paper delivered at *Public Health* 2004 Conference, June 8, Durban www.mrc.ac.za/conference

Cope S and Goodship J (1999) 'Comparing regulatory regimes in the new governance', *Nottingham Conference papers*, Political Studies Association http://www.psa.ac.uk/cps/1999/cope.pdf

COSATU (Congress of South African Trade Unions) (2000) 'NEHAWU: improving health and management', April *Campaigns* Report, www.cosatu.org.za/docs/2000/sdcamp.htm, accessed 07.07.03

COSATU (Congress of South African Trade Unions) (2002) *Initial submission on the Draft National Health Bill*, Cosatu, March 8, www.cosatu.org.za/docs/2002/initial.htm, accessed 11.06.04

Costello A, Osrin D and Manandhar D (2004) 'Reducing maternal and neonatal mortality in the poorest communities', *British Medical Journal* 329:1166-1168

Cotlear, D (2000) 'Peru: Reforming health care for the poor', *Human Development Department LCSHD Paper*, Mar, Paper No. 57 World Bank, Washington

Coulter A (1998) 'Managing demand at the interface between primary and secondary care', *British Medical Journal* 316: 1974-6

Coulter A and Ham C (eds) (2000) *The Global Challenge of Health Care Rationing*, Open University Press, Buckingham

Council of Canadians (2002) *Why profit is not the cure*, Council of Canadians www.Canadians.org, accessed 14.11.03

Court J and Smith F (1999) *Making a killing: HMOs and the threat to your health*, Common Courage Press, Monroe ME USA

Crawford L (2003) 'Spanish law gives hospitals broader powers', *Financial Times* May 7

Creed F, Mbaya P, Lancashire S, Tomenson B, Williams B and Holme S (1997) 'Cost effectiveness of day and inpatient psychiatric treatment: results of a randomised controlled trial', *British Medical Journal* 314: 1381

Creese A (1997) 'User fees: they don't reduce costs, and they increase inequity', *British Medical Journal* 315: 202-203

Creese A and J Kutzin (1995) 'Lessons From Cost-Recovery in Health, Forum on Health Sector Reform', *Discussion Paper No. 2* Division of Strengthening Health Services, WHO, Geneva

Cullinan K (2003) 'Legal vacuum hampers health for all', March 31, *HIVAN* (Centre for HIV/AIDS Networking www.hivan.org.za, accessed 11.6.04

Cullinan T (2001) 'Drug resistant TB treatment in Siberia: a window out of Russia's misery?' *eurohealth* Vol 7; No 4: 24-25, Autumn

D'Amato E (2000) 'New Frontiers: A healthy choice', *Impact*, International Finance Corporation www.ifc.org/publications/pubs/impact/winter00/frontiers/frontiers.htm, accessed 26.5.03

Dahlgren, G (2000) 'Efficient equity-oriented strategies for health', *Bull WHO* 78(1) 79-81

Danzon M (2002) 'Foreword' in Mossialos et al (2002)

David DS (2002) Letter: 'Working knowledge would have been needed for comparison', *British Medical Journal* 324: 1332

Day K (2005) 'Major report on health service finances could be delayed until after election', *Public Finance* March 11-17:6

De Ferranti D (1985) 'Paying for health services in developing countries: an overview', *World Bank Staff Working Papers* No 721, Washington DC

De Ferranti D and Feachem RGA (1997) *Sector Strategy, Health Nutrition and Population*, World Bank, Washington

De Ferranti D, Perry GE, Ferreira FHG, Walton M, Coady D, Cunningham W, Gasparini L, Jacobsen J, Matsuda Y, Robinson J, Sokoloff K and Wodon Q (2003) 'Inequality in Latin America and the Caribbean: Breaking with history?' *World Bank Latin American and Caribbean Studies*, World Bank, Washington

De la Jara JJ and Bossert T (1995) 'Chile's health sector reform: lessons from four reform periods', *Health Policy* Apr-Jun 32(1-3): 155-66

Deacon B (2001) 'International Organisations, the EU and global social policy', in Sykes et al (2001)

Deacon B, Hulse M and Stubbs P (1997) *Global Social Policy: International organisations and the future of welfare*, London: Sage

Deber R (2000a) 'Thinking before rethinking: some thoughts about babies and bathwater', *Healthcare Papers* Vol 1 (3) 25-32 (Summer 2000), www.longwoods.com/hp/summer00/2.html, accessed 07.05.03

Deber R (2000b) 'Getting what we pay for: myths and realities about financing Canada's health care system', *Background papers for the Dialogue on Health Care reform* http://www.utoronto.ca/hpme/dhr/4.html, accessed 11.05.03

Deber R and Baranek P (1998) 'Canada; markets at the margin', in Ranade (1998)

Deber R, Forget E, Roos L and Shortt SED (Deber et al 2002a) 'Medical Savings Accounts: an idea that just won't die', *Globe and Mail* July 26 Toronto

Deber R, Forget E and Roos L (Deber et al 2002b) 'Return of the "zombie": Are medical savings accounts a better way to meet health-care needs, or will they simply increase costs?' *National Post* August 7, Toronto

Deber R, Forget E and Roos L (Deber et al 2002c) 'MSAs: even less than meets the eye', *Technical Report* University of Mainitoba, http://www.umanitoba.ca/centres/mchp/hot_topic/msa.html, accessed 14.11.03

Deeming C (2001) 'The decentralisation dream', *Public Finance* Nov 23-29: 28-29

Defever M (1995) 'Health care reforms: the unfinished agenda', *Health Policy* Oct 34(1): 1-7

Deininger K, Den Exter A, Hermands H, Dosljak M and Busse R (2004) Netherlands *Health Care Systems in Transition*, European Observatory on Health Systems, WHO Copenhagen

Despeignes P (2003) 'Cash-strapped US states boost borrowing', *Financial Times* May 13

Development GAP (1999) *Statement of the Development GAP on the proposed multilateral and G7 debt-reduction plan*, http://www.developmentgap.org/debtstatement.html, accessed 22.09.03

Devers KJ (2003) 'Specialty Hospitals: focused factories or cream skimmers?' *Speech and conference paper* April 15, Center for Studying Health System Change (HSC), Washington DC www.hschange.org

Devlin N, Maynard A and Mays N (2001) 'New Zealand's new health sector reforms: back to the future?' *British Medical Journal* 322: 1171-4

Diderichson F (1993) 'Market reforms in Swedish health care: a threat to or salvation for the universalistic welfare state?' *International Journal of Health Services* Vol 23, No. 1 185-188

Diderichson F (1995) 'Market reforms in health care and sustainability of the welfare state: lessons from Sweden', *Health Policy* 32: 141-153

Diop FP (1996) 'Assessment of Niger's cost recovery policy in the primary health care sector', Dec, *Technical Report* 6, PHR, Harvard

Diop FP, Seshamani V and Mulenga C (1998) 'Household health seeking behaviour in Zambia', June, *Technical Report* 20, PHR, Harvard

Dixion J (1997) 'France seeks to curb health costs by fining doctors', *British Medical Journal* 315: 895-896

Dixon A (2002) 'Dilemmas in financing mental health', *eurohealth* 8:1 25-28 (Winter 2001-2002)

Dixon A and Mossialos E (eds) (2002) *Health care systems in eight countries: trends and challenges*, European Observatory on Health Care Systems and London School of Economics, London

Dixon A, Langenbrunner J and Mossialos E (2002) *Facing the challenges of health care financing*, July, USAID, Washington

Dixon J and Welch H (1991) 'Priority setting: lessons from Oregon', The Lancet 337: 891-4, April 13

Dmitriev M, Potapchik Y, Solonieva O and Shishkin S (2000) *Economic problems of health services system reform in Russia.* www.imf.org/external/pubs/ft/seminar/ 2000/invest/pdf/dmitriev2.pdf

Dobson R (2002) 'Proportion of spending on care for older people falls', *British Medical Journal* 325: 355

Docteur E and Oxley H (2003) Health Care Systems: *Lessons from reform experience.* December 5, OECD, Paris

Docteur E, Suppanz H and Woo J (2003) 'The US Health System: an assessment and prospective directions for reform', *Economics dept Working Papers* No. 335 February 27, OECD, Paris

Doctors without Borders (2004) 'CAFTA Provisions Restrict Access to Miedicines', *Press Release* February 3, New York, www.doctorswithoutborders.org, accessed 01.03.05

DoH (Department of Health) (1989a) *Working for Patients*, January, HMSO, London

DoH (Department of Health) (1989b) *Caring for People: Community Care in the next decade and beyond*, November, HMSO, London

DoH (Department of Health) (1992) *The Health of the Nation*, HMSO, London

DoH (Department of Health) (1993) *Making London Better*, DoH Lancashire Publications Unit

DoH (Department of Health) (1995) *NHS responsibilities for meeting continuing health care needs*, HSG (95) 8, LAC (95) 5 February, HMSO, London

DoH (Department of Health) (1997a) *Our Healthier Nation*, HMSO, London

DoH (Department of Health) (1997b) *The new NHS, Modern, Dependable*, HMSO, London

DoH (Department of Health) (1998a) *KIGS (Key Indicators Graphical System.)* HMSO, London

DoH (Department of Health) (1998b) *The Government's Expenditure Plans 1998/99*, HMSO, London

DoH (Department of Health) (1998c) *The Health of the Nation – a policy assessed*, HMSO, London

DoH (Department of Health) (1999a) 'New figures give picture of clinical care in the NHS', *Press Release* June, HMSO, London

DoH (Department of Health) (1999b) 'NICE proposals launched today', *Press Release* February, HMSO, London

DoH (Department of Health) (2000a) *National Beds Inquiry*, February 10, HMSO, London

DoH (Department of Health) (2000b) *Shaping the future NHS: long-term planning for hospitals and related services. Consultation document on the findings of the National Beds Inquiry*, HMSO, London

DoH (Department of Health) (2002a) *Growing capacity: Independent Sector Diagnosis and Treatment Centres*, HMSO, London

DoH (Department of Health) (2002b) 'New generation surgery-centres to carry out thousands more NHS operations every year', *Press release* 2002/00529 December 23, HMSO, London

DoH (Department of Health) (2002c) *Reforming NHS financial flows*, October, HMSO, London

DoH (Department of Health) (2002d) 'Seminar on Foundation Trusts: learning from European organisations', *Summary of messages*, European chief executives May 22, www.doh.gov.uk/conference/foundtrustsmau021execs.htm, accessed 04.12.02

DoH (Department of Health) (2002e) *A Guide to Foundation Trusts*, December, HMSO, London

DoH (Department of Health) (2003a) *Chief Executive's Report to the NHS*, December, HMSO, London

DoH (Department of Health) (2003b) *Chief Executive's Report to the NHS*: Statistical supplement, December, HMSO, London

DoH (Department of Health) (2003c) *Departmental report 2003*, July, HMSO, London

DoH (Department of Health) (2003d) *Agenda for Change proposed agreement*, January, Department of Health www.dh.gov.uk

DoH (Department of Health) (2004a) *Hospital Episode Statistics* 2002-3, http://www.dh.gov.uk/PublicationsAndStatistics/Statistics/HospitalEpisodeStatistics/HESFreeData/HESFreeDataList/fs/en?CONTENT_ID=4028328&chk=6HBoYS, accessed 23.05.04

DoH (Department of Health) (2004b) *NHS Hospital, Public Health Medicine and Community Health Service Medical and Dental Workforce census, England, 30 September 2003 - Detailed statistics*, http://www.publications.doh.gov.uk/public/work_workforce.htm, March 19 2004, accessed 16.05.04

Doherty J, Thomas S, Muirhead D and McIntyre D (2002) 'Health Care Financing and Expenditure', *South African Health Review* 13-39, March, Cape Town

Donatini A, Rico A, D',Ambrosio MG, Lo Scalzo A, Orzella L, Americo Cicchetti A and Profili S (2001) *Italy. Health Care Systems in Transition*, WHO European Observatory, Denmark

Donnan S (2005) 'Indonesian initiation wins mixed reviews', *Financial Times* March 30:15

Dorozynski A (1994) 'Report criticises French hospitals', *British Medical Journal* 308: 1257-1258

Dorozynski A (1995a) 'France gears up to fight health insurance debts', *British Medical Journal* 311: 967-968

Dorozynski A (1995b) 'France faces radical health insurance reforms', *British Medical Journal* 311: 1386

Dorozynski A (1996) 'New battle looms for France over health reforms', *British Medical Journal* 312:9

Dorozynski A (1997a) 'French doctors' strike enters third week', *British Medical Journal* 314: 993

Dorozynski A (1997b) 'New French government will try to reduce health costs', *British Medical Journal* 314: 1709

Dorozynski A (1998a) 'France launches plan to control health costs', *British Medical Journal* 317: 164

Dorozynski A (1998b) 'France moves towards a GP system', *British Medical Journal* 317: 1545

Dorozynski A (1998c) 'French doctors grumble at healthcare reforms', *British Medical Journal* 316: 1407

Dorozynski A (1999) 'France abandons fines to control health costs', *British Medical Journal* 318: 76

Dorozynski A (2000a) 'French health staff strike over budget cuts', *British Medical Journal* 320: 333

Dorozynski A (2000b) 'French health costs rising rapidly', *British Medical Journal* 321: 528

Dorozynski A (2001) 'French government agrees to subsidise private clinics by £300 million', *British Medical Journal* 323: 1148

Dorozynski A (2002a) 'French healthcare system beset by strikes', *British Medical Journal* 324: 258

Dorozynski A (2002b) 'French emergency services reach crisis point', *British Medical Journal* 325: 514

Dorozynski A (2003a) 'French government cuts payments for "moderately useful" drugs', *British Medical Journal* 326: 951

Dorozynski A (2003b) 'France offers E800 reward for each new baby', *British Medical Journal* 326: 1002

Doyal L (1979) *The Political Economy of Health*, Pluto Press, London

Doyal L (1998) 'Gender and health', *WHO Technical paper* WHO/FRH/WHD/98.16, WHO Geneva

Doyal L (2004) 'Why health research needs to be more sesnistive to sex and gender differences', *Global Forum Update on Research for Health 2005* http://www.globalforumhealth.org/Site/002__What%20we%20do/005__Publications/002__Global%20Forum%20Update%20on%20Research%20for%20Health.php, accessed 21.03.05

Drache D, and Sullivan T (eds) (1999) *Health Reform: public success, private failure*, Routledge, London

Du Gay P (2000) 'Entrepreneurial governance and public management: the anti-bureaucrats', in Clarke et al (2001)

Dufour C (2001) 'Midwives take lengthy strike action', *EIRO online* May, European Industrial Relations Observatory, Dublin, www.eiro.eurofound.eu.int/2001/05/inbrief/FR0105151F.htm, accessed 08.06.03

Dunlop DW and Martins JM (eds) (1996) *An International Assessment of Health Care Financing: Lessons for Developing Countries*, World Bank, Washington

Dunne N (2000) *Fees issue entangles US debt relief plan*, www.ft.com October 17, accessed 09.02.03

Dunnigan MG and Pollock AM (2003) 'Downsizing of acute inpatient beds associated with private finance initiative: Scotland's case study', *British Medical Journal* 326: 905

Durand-Zaleski I, Colin C and Blum-Boisgard C (1997) 'An attempt to save money by using mandatory practice guidelines in France', *British Medical Journal* 315: 943-946

Dyer G (2003a) 'As the pandemic spreads, developed nations must respond to a new challenge from the White House', *Financial Times* June 2

Dyer G (2003b) 'Analysts count the cost of AIDS as it hits the money-earning generation', *Financial Times* July 18

Dyer O (2003a) 'Eye surgeon claims that new treatment centre is a threat to NHS' *British Medical Journal* 327:580

Dyer O (2003b) 'New health secretary vows to continue NHS reform agenda' *British Medical Journal* 326:1347

Dyer O (2004) 'NHS overcharged for private surgery' *British Medical Journal* 328: 1158

Dyer O (2004) 'Infectious diseases increase in Iraq as public health service deteriorates', *British Medical Journal* 329:940

ECB Economic Policy Committee (2003) 'The need for comprehensive reforms to cope with population ageing', *Monthly Bulletin* European Central Bank, Frankfurt

Editorial (2003) 'In need of health infrastructure', *The Times of Zambia (Ndola)* June 18 http://allafrica.com/stories/200306180236.html, accessed 22.06.03

Edwards N and Hensher M (1998) 'Managing demand for secondary care services: the changing context', *British Medical Journal* 317: 135-138

Edwards N, Hensher M and Wernecke U (1998) 'Changing Hospital Systems', in Saltman et al (1998)

EIROonline (1997a) 'Hospitals faced with strikes', *EIRO online* March, European Industrial Relations Observatory, Dublin, www.eiro.eurofound.eu.int/1997/03/inbrief/FR9703132F.htm, accessed 08.06.03

EIROonline (1997b) 'Sweeping changes in social insurance contributions', *EIRO online* September, European Industrial Relations Observatory, Dublin, www.eiro.eurofound.eu.int/1997/09/inbrief/FR9709164F.htm, accessed 08.06.03

Elliott L (2003a) 'NHS is being railroaded', *The Guardian* 5 May

Elliott L (2003b) 'Third-way addicts need a fix', *The Guardian* 14 July

England S, Kaddar M, Nigam A, and Pinto M (2001) *Practice and policies on user fees for immunization in developing countries*, Department of vaccines and biologicals, World Health Organization Geneva

Engler M (2003) 'CAFTA: Free trade vs democracy', *Oneworld.net* April 1, http://amlat.oneworld.net/article/view/53430/1/1730, accessed 02.06.03

Enthoven AC (1985) 'National Health Service: some reforms that might be politically feasible', *The Economist* June 22, p19

Enthoven AC (1997) 'Market-based reform of US health care financing and delivery: managed care and managed competition', in Schieber (1997)

Enthoven AC (2003) 'Employment-based health insurance is failing: now what?' *Health Affairs web exclusive* www.healthaffairs.org/WebExclusives/Enthoven_Web_Excl_052803.htm May 28, accessed 19.06.03

Equinet (2000) 'Equity in health in Southern Africa: Turning values into practice' *Paper for the Regional Conference Building Alliances for Equity in Health*, Equinet, Harare

Equinet (2003) 'Resource Allocation and Deprivation Issues For Health Equity', *Report of the EQUINET Regional Meeting*. Equinet, Harare, http://www.equinetafrica.org/confs.html

Ernst & Young (2003) 'Health care systems and health market reform in the G20 countries', *Paper for World Economic Forum*, http://www.ey.com/global/download.nsf/International/G20_Health_System_SummariesWEF2003/$file/G20%20Health%20System%20SummariesWEF2003.pdf, accessed 28.03.05

Esmail A and Everington S (1997) Letter: 'Asian doctors are still being discriminated against', *British Medical Journal* 314:1619

Esmail N and Walker M (2002) 'Waiting your turn', *Critical Issues Bulletin*, September Fraser Institute, Vancouver

Esping-Andersen G (1990) *The Three Worlds of Welfare Capitalism*, Polity Press

Esping-Andersen G (ed) (1996) *Welfare states in transition: national adaptations in global economics*, Sage

Essif M (2001) *Health Care in Cuba*, Kaiser Family Foundation Online http://www.kff.org/docs/fellowships/essifcubareport.html, accessed 23.10.03

European Observatory (2000) *Health Care Systems IN Transition: Spain*, European Observatory, WHO Regional Office, Denmark

Evans RG (1997) 'Going for the gold: The redistributive agenda behind market-based health care reform', *Journal of health policy, politics and law* 22: 2 (April 1997)

Ewing D (2001) *Reality check: could China have picked a worse time to join the WTO?* December 21, The Nixon Centre, www.nixncenter.org/publications, accessed 10.07.03

Fabricus P (2003) 'Many governments are not promoting NEPAD', *The Star* June 13, www.avmedia.at/nepad/indexgb.html, accessed 09.07.03

Fairfield G, Hunter DJ, Mechanic D and Rosleff F (1997) 'Managed care: origins, principles, and evolution', *British Medical Journal* 314: 1823

Families USA (2003a) 'Individual tax credits do not work', *Factsheet* May, Washington DC

Families USA (2003b) 'Private plans: a bad choice for Medicare', *Factsheet* June, Washington DC

Families USA (2003c) 'Tax free savings accounts for medical expenses: a tax cut masquerading as help for the uninsured', *Issue Brief* July 22, Washington, www.familiesusa.org

Farrant W (1991) 'Addressing the contradictions: Health promotion and community health action in the United Kingdom', *International Journal of Health Services* Vol 21 No.3, 423-439

Feachem R. (1999) 'A new role for the Bulletin', *Bull WHO* 77(1) p2

Feachem RGA, Sekhri NK and White KL (2002) 'Getting more for their dollar: a comparison of the NHS with California's Kaiser Permanente', *British Medical Journal* 324: 135-43

Ferge Z (2001) 'Welfare and "Ill-Fare" systems in Central-Eastern Europe', in Sykes (2001)

Fiedler JL (1996) 'The privatisation of health care in three Latin American social security systems', *Health Policy Planning* Dec 11(4): 406-17

Fiedler JL and Suazo J (2002) 'Ministry of Health user fees, equity and decentralisation: lessons from Honduras', *Health Policy and Planning* 17(4): 362-377

Figueras J, Saltman RB and Sakellarides C (1998) 'Introduction', to Saltman, et al (1998)

Filmer D, Hammer J and Pritchett L (1997) *Health Policy in Poor Countries: Weak Links in the Chain*, October 22, World Bank, Washington DC

Flanagan J (2003) 'Patients pay for HMO profits with their health', *Press Release*: Foundation for Taxpayer and Consumer Rights, December 12

Fleury S (2000) 'Reshaping health care systems in Latin America: towards fairness?' in Fleury et al (2000)

Fleury S (2001) 'Dual, Universal or Plural? Health care models and issues in Latin America: Chile, Brazil and Colombia', in Molina and del Arco (2001)

Fleury S, Belmartino S and Baris E (eds) (2000) *Reshaping Health Care in Latin America: a comparative analysis of health care reform in Argentina, Brazil and Mexico*, International Development Research Centre, Ottawa

Flood CM (2000) *International Health care Reform*, Routledge, London

Forget EL, Deber R and Roos LL (2002) 'Medical Savings accounts: will they reduce costs?' *Canadian Medical Association* Journal 167(2) 143-7, July 23

France G (2001) 'Devolution in the Italian health service: balancing diversity and equality', *eurohealth* 7:4, 26-28, Autumn

Francome C and Marks S (1996) *Improving the Health of the Nation*, Middlesex University Press

Frank M (2004) 'Cuba arms against shrill US voices', *Financial Times* February 11

Frankel, Ebrahim and Davey Smith (2000) 'The limits to demand for health care', *British Medical Journal* 321: 42-45.

Freeman R (1998) 'Competition in context: the politics of health care reform in Europe', *International Journal of Quality Health Care* Oct 10(5): 395-401

Freeman R (2000) *The politics of health in Europe*, Manchester University Press, Manchester

Frenk J, Bobadilla JL, Sepulveda J and Lopez-Cervantes M (1989) 'Health transition in middle-income countries: new challenges for health care', *Health Policy and Planning* 4: 29-39

Frenk J, Bobadilla JL, Stern C, Frejka T and Lozano R (1991) 'Elements for a theory of the health transition', *Health Transition Review* 1: 21-38

Furuholmen C and Magnussen J (2000) 'Norway', *Health Care Systems in Transition*, WHO European Observatory, Denmark

Gaál P, Rékassy B and Healy J (1999) 'Hungary', *Health Care Systems in Transition*, WHO, Copenhagen

Gaffney D and Pollock AM (1997) *Can the NHS afford the Private Finance Initiative?* December, BMA Health Policy and Economic Research Unit, London

Gamkrelidze A, Atun R and Garcia A (2001) *Healthcare reform in Germany: the search for efficiency and cost control*, 30 November, www.frost.com/prod/news.nsf

Garrett L (2001) *Betrayal of Trust*, Oxford University Press

Gatheru W and Shaw R (eds) (1998) *Our problems our solutions*, Institute of Economic Affairs, Nairobi

Gauri V (2001) *Are incentives everything? Payment mechanisms for health care providers in developing countries*, World Bank, Washington

Geddes J, Reynolds S, Streiner D and Szatmari P (1997) 'Evidence based practice in mental health', *British Medical Journal*, 315: 1483-1484

George S (1999) 'A short history of neo-liberalism', *Conference on Economic Sovereignty in a Globalising World* http://www.globalexchange.org/economy/econ101/neoliberalism.html, accessed 20.01.01

George V and Wilding P (1994) *Welfare and Ideology*, Harvester Wheatsheaf, Hemel Hempstead

Gertler PJ and Hammer JS (1997) 'Strategies for pricing publicly provided health services', in Schieber (1997)

Gertler PJ and Molyneaux J (1997) *Experimental evidence on the effect of raising user fees for publicly delivered health care services: utilization, health outcomes, and private provider response*, RAND, Santa Monica, CA

Geyman JP (2002) 'Family practice in a failing health care system: new opportunities to advocate for system reform', *Journal of American Board of Family Practice* 15; 5, 407-416 (Sept-Oct)

GFHR (Global Forum for Health Research) (2002) *The 10/90 Report on Health Research 2001-2002*, GFHR, Switzerland

GFHR (Global Forum for Health Research) (2004) *Health Research for equity in global health*, November http://www.globalforumhealth.org/forum8/Statement.html

Gilson L (1999) 'Implementing and evaluating health reform processes: lessons from the literature', *Informing and Reforming* 10-11, Jan-Jun 1999, 2-3

Gilson L and Mills A (1995) 'Health sector reforms in sub-Saharan Africa: lessons of the last 10 years', *Health Policy* Apr-Jun 32(1-3): 215-43

Gilson L, Doherty J, McIntyre D, Thomas S, Briljal V and Bowa C (1999) 'The Dynamics of Policy Change: health care financing in South Africa 1994-1999', Major Applied Research 1, *Technical Paper* 1 November, Partnerships for Health Reform, Bethesda

Ginsburg PB (2004) 'Controlling health care costs', *New England Journal of Medicine* 351:1591-1593

Glennerster H and Midgley J (eds) (1991) *The Radical Right and the welfare state: an international assessment*, Harvester Wheatsheaf, Hemel Hempstead

Global Fund to Fight AIDS, Tuberculosis & Malaria (2003) *A Partnership to Prevent and Treat AIDS, Tuberculosis and Malaria*, http://www.globalfundatm.org/qa.html, accessed 03.05.03

Godlee F (1994a) 'The World Health Organisation', (series) *British Medical Journal* 309: 1424-142

Godlee F (1994b) 'WHO in retreat: is it losing its influence?' *British Medical Journal* 309: 1491-1495

Godlee F (1994c) 'WHO at country level -- a little impact, no strategy', *British Medical Journal* 309: 1636-1639

Godlee F (1998) 'Change at last at WHO', *British Medical Journal* 317: 296

Goldberg R (1993) 'Pharmaceutical Price Controls: saving money today or lives tomorrow?' *IPI Policy Report* No. 123 Institute for Policy Innovation

Goldberg R (2003) 'Political parties take opposing sides in health care debate', Feb 1 2003, Heartland Institute, 9 Jan 2001, www.heartland org

Gonzalez Block MA (1997) 'Health reforms in a comparative perspective', *Informing & Reforming* April, No 2, 2-4

Gonzalez Block MA (2004) 'Health policy and systems research agendas in developing countries', *Health Policy and Systems* August 2:6

Gonzalez Block MA and Frenk J (1997) 'Mexico: the fight against poverty in health', *Informing and Reforming* 4: 13-15, Oct-Dec

Gordon D (2002) 'The international measurement of poverty and anti-poverty policies', in Townsend & Gordon (2002)

Gotsadze G, MacLehose L (2002) Georgia. *Health Care Systems in Transition*, WHO, Copenhagen

Gould BS (2001) 'When Managed Care doesn't travel well', in Wieners (2001)

Gould M (2005) 'Managers move to quell protest over bed cuts', *Health Service Journal* March 24:8

Govindaraj R and Chawla M (1996) 'Recent experiences with hospital autonomy in developing countries: what can we learn?' September, *Data for Decision Making Project*, Harvard School of Public Health

Govindaraj R, Obuobi AAD, Enyimayew NKA, Antwi P and Ofusu-Amaah S (1996) 'Hospital autonomy in Ghana: the experience of Korle Bu and Komfo Anyoke teaching hospitals', August, *Data for Decision Making Project*, Harvard

Graham R (2003) 'OECD berates France over budget deficit', *Financial Times* July 9

Grant J (2003) 'GM pumps $3 billion into employee health fund', *Financial Times* August 11

Gratzer D (2002) 'It's time to consider Medical Savings Accounts', *Canadian Medical Association Journal* 167(2) 151-2

Gribble JN and Preston SH (eds) (1993) *The Epidemiological Transition, policy and planning implications for developing countries*, National Academy Press, Washington DC

Griffin CC and Shaw RP (1995) 'Health Insurance in Sub Saharan Africa: Aims, Findings and Policy Implications', in Shaw & Ainsworth (1995)

Griffiths R (1988) *Community Care, Agenda for Action* HMSO, London

Guichard S (2004) 'The reform of the health care system in Portugal', *Economics Department Working Papers* No. 405, October, OECD, Paris

Gulland A (2001) 'Doctor wins seat in fight to save hospital', *British Medical Journal* 322:1443

Gulland A (2002) 'Health professionals question "star ratings" for NHS', *British Medical Journal* 325: 236

Gureje O and Alem A (2000) 'Mental health policy development in Africa', *Bull WHO* 78; 4: 475-482

Gwatkin DR and Guillot, M (2000) 'The Burden of Disease among the Global Poor', *Global Forum for Health Research*, World Bank, Washington

Hadley J and Holahan J (2003) 'How much medical care do the uninsured use, and who pays for it?' *Health Affairs web exclusive* February 12, W3-66-W3-81

Hadley TR and Goldman H (1995) 'Effect of recent health and social service policy reforms on Britain's mental health system', *British Medical Journal* 311: 1556-1558, December 9

HAI (Help Age International) (2002a) *State of the World's Older People 2002.* www.helpage.org, accessed 22.02.03

HAI Help Age International (2002b) *HIV/AIDS and older people: the African situation*, www.helpage.org, accessed 22.02.03

Hall D (2003) 'Multinational corporations and the pattern of privatisation in healthcare', in Sen, 2003

Hall D and de la Motte R (2004) 'Dogmatic development. Privatisation and conditionalities in six countries', *A PSIRU report for War on Want* February, www.waronwant.org, accessed 03.03.04

Hall J and Maynard A (2005) 'Healthcare lessons from Australia: what can Michael Howard learn from John Howard?' *British Medical Journal* 330:357-9

Hall PA (1993) 'Policy paradigms, social learning and the state: the case of economic policymaking in Britain', *Comparative Politics* 25: 275-29.

Ham C (1997) 'Why rationing is inevitable in the NHS', in New (1997)

Ham C (1998) 'Retracing the Oregon trail: the experience of rationing and the Oregon health plan', *British Medical Journal* 316: 1965-9

Ham C (1999) *Health Policy in Britain* (4th edition) Macmillan, London

Ham C and Coulter A (2000) 'Conclusion: where are we now?' in Coulter and Ham (2000)

Ham C and Honigsbaum F (1998) 'Priority setting and rationing health services', in Saltman (1991)

Hammond R (1998) *Addicted to Profit: Big Tobacco's Expanding Global Reach*, Essential Action, Washington

Hann A (ed) (2000) *Analysing Health Policy*, Ashgate, Aldershot

Hanson K and Berman P (1998) 'Private health care provision in developing countries: a preliminary analysis of levels and composition', *Health Policy and Planning* 13(3): 195-211

Harrington C (2001) 'Residential nursing facilities in the United States', *British Medical Journal* 323: 507-510

Harrington C, Woolhandler S, Mullan J, Carrillo H and Himmelstein DU (2001) 'Does investor ownership of nursing homes compromise the quality of care?' *American Journal of Public Health* Vol 91, No. 9 1-5

Harrison S and Pollitt C (1994) *Controlling health professionals*, Open University Press, Buckingham

Harrison S, Hunter DJ and Pollitt C (1990) *The Dynamics of British health policy*, Routledge, London

Hart J Tudor (1971) 'The Inverse Care Law', *The Lancet* 1: 405-12, 27 February

Hart J Tudor (1994) *Feasible Socialism - The National Health Service past present and future*, Socialist Health Association, London

Hart J Tudor J (2003) 'Health care or health trade? A historic moment of choice', June 18, *European Network for the Defence of Public Health*, European Social Forum, Thessaloniki http://www.healthp.org/article.php?sid=203&mode=thread&order=0, accessed 30.06.03

Harvey T (2001) 'Do the performance tables measure up?' *British Journal of Health Care Management* 7 (12): 497-498

Hay C (2001) 'Globalisation, Economic change and the Welfare State: The Vexatious Inquisition of Taxation', in Sykes et al (2001)

Hayward H (2002) *Costing the Casino*, March, War on Want, London

Health GAP (Global Access Project) (2005) *Myths and realities: US pressure on Guatemala regarding data exclusivity, CAFTA and access to medicines*, February 10, Washington www.healthgap.org, accessed 27.03.05

Health Policy Consensus Group (2001) *Why we need market-based health care reform* – in two parts: Part 1 March 1 2001; Part 2 April 1 2001 - Heartland Institute, 9 Jan 2001, www.heartland org

Healy J (2002a) 'Australia', in Dixon & Mossialos (2002)

Healy J (2002b) 'New Zealand', in Dixon & Mossialos (2002)

Heaton A, (2001) *Joint public-private initiatives: meeting children's right to health?* Save the Children Fund UK, May

Hecht R, Overholt C and Homberg H (1995) 'How cost recovery can help rationalise the health care system: lessons from Zimbabwe', in Shaw and Ainsworth (1995)

Heclo, H (1974) *Modern Social Politics in Britain and Sweden: from relief to income maintenance*, New Haven: Yale UP

Heffler S, Levit K, Smith S, Smith C, Cowan C, Lazenby H and Freeland M (2001) 'Health spending growth up in 1999: faster growth expected in the future', *Health Affairs* 20 (2): 193-203

Heffler S, Smith S, Keehan S, Kent Clemens M, Won G and Zezza M (2003) 'Health spending projections for 2002-2012', *Health Affairs* web exclusive www.healthaffairs.org/WebExclusives/Heffler_Web_Excl_020703.htm, accessed 19.06.03

Heffler S, Smith S, Keehan S, Kent Clemens M, Zezza M and Truffer C (2004) 'Health spending projections through to 2013', *Health Affairs* web exclusive, content.healthaffairs.org/cgi/content/abstract/hlthaff.w4.79, February 11, accessed 29.05.04

Hennessy P (1995) 'Social Protection for dependent elderly people: perspectives from a review of OECD countries', *Labour Market and Social Policy Occasional Paper* No. 16, OECD, Paris

Henry-Lee A and Yearwood A (1999) 'Protecting the poor and the medically indigent under health insurance: a case study of Jamaica', *Small Applied Research* No.6 PHR, Abt Associates, Bethesda Ma

Hensher M, Edwards N and Stokes R (1999a) 'International trends in the provision and utilisation of hospital care', *British Medical Journal* 319: 845-8

Hensher M, Fulop N, Coast J and Jefferys E (1999b) 'Better out than in? Alternatives to hospital care', *British Medical Journal* 319: 1127-30

Henwood M (2002) 'No grey areas', *Health Service Journal* Dec 12: 24-27

Herbert S (1996) 'French face standstill as five million go on strike', *Daily Telegraph* October 17

Herbert S (1997) 'Strike taken to minister's doorstep at 4.30am', *Daily Telegraph* April 3

Hesketh T and Zhu WX (1997a) 'Health in China - The healthcare market', *British Medical Journal* 314: 7094; 1616-8

Hesketh T and Zhu WX (1997b) 'Health in China: from Mao to market reform', *British Medical Journal* 314: 1543.

Hewitt Associates (2003) 'HMO rates continue double-digit trend but are lower than last year', *Press release* 23 June, http://was.Hewitt.com/Hewitt/resource/newsroom/pressrel/2003/06-23-0/3.htm, accessed 30.06.03

Hilless M and Healy J (2002) HiT summary: *Australia Health Care Systems in Transition*, European Observatory, WHO, Copenhagen

Himmelstein DU and Woolhandler S (2002a) 'We pay for National Health Insurance but don't get it', *Health Affairs* July, Vol 21 (4) Bethesda

Himmelstein DU and Woolhandler S (2002b) Letter: 'Price adjustments falsify comparison', *British Medical Journal* 324:1332

Himmelstein DU and Woolhandler S (2003) 'National health insurance or incremental reform: aim high, or at our feet?' *American Journal of Public Health* 93(1) 102-105

Himmelstein DU and Woolhandler S et al (30-member writing committee) (1989) *A National Health Program for the United States: a Physicians'*, proposal, www.pnhp.org/publications/archives/000016.php, accessed 10.11.02

Himmelstein DU, Woolhandler S and Wolfe SM (2003) *The cost to the nation, the states and the District of Columbia, with state-specific estimates of potential savings*, www.citizen.org/publications/realease.cfm?ID=7271&secID=1158&catID=126, accessed 15.11.03

Hinkov H, Koulaksuzov S, Semerdjiev I and Healy J (1999) *Bulgaria. Health Care Systems in Transition*, WHO, Copenhagen

Hirst J (2003) 'Patients face a challenge of their choosing', *Public Finance* 11, July25-31

Hirst J (2005) 'Shock and awe', Public Finance (Leader) March 11-17:2

Hlavacka S and Skackova D (2000) *Slovakia. Health Care Systems in Transition*, WHO, Copenhagen

HM Treasury (1997) *An introduction to the private finance initiative*, London, HM Treasury

Hoffman B (2003) 'Health care reform and social movements in the United States', *American Journal of Public Health* 93(1) 75-85, January

Hoffman M (2003) 'Healthcare system needs more than just a Band-Aid', *Sunday Times* 24 June, Johannesburg

Hofrichter R (ed) (2003) *Health and Social Justice: Politics Ideology and Inequity in the distribution of disease*, Jossey-Bass, San Francisco

Hogan MF (1999) 'Public sector mental health care: new challenges', *Health Affairs* Vol 18; 5: 106-111

Hoggett P (1994) 'The politics of the modernisation of the UK welfare state', in Burrows and Loader (1994)

Holland W (2000) 'Extra Money for the United Kingdom National Health Service', *Euro Observer, Newsletter for the European Observatory on Health Care Systems*, Winter /01 Vol 2 No.4 WHO Europe, Copenhagen

Hollander N, Rauch M (1998) Assessment of third party payers in Jordan *Technical Report* No.27 PHR, Abt Associates, Bethesda Ma

Hong E (2000) 'Globalisation and the impact on health: a Third World View', *Prepared for People's Health Assembly, Bangladesh* August, Third World Network, Penang

Hongoro C (1997) 'Hospital Autonomy', *Informing and Reforming* 3 (Jul-Sep): 9-10

Hood C (1991) 'A public Management for all seasons', *Public Administration* 69 (Spring): 3-19

Hope KR and Chikulo BC (2000) 'Decentralization, the new public management, and the changing role of the public sector in Africa', *Public Management* March, 2(1): 25-42

Hornblow A (1997) 'New Zealand's health reforms: a clash of cultures', *British Medical Journal* 314: 1892

Hossain SI (1997) 'Tackling health transition in China', *Policy Research Working Paper*, World Bank August 1997

Howden-Chapman P and Ashton T (2000) 'Public purchasing and private priorities for healthcare in New Zealand', *Health Policy* 54: 27-43

Hryniuk B (2000) 'Report Card on Cancer Care in Canada: why are top Canadian cancer specialists leaving?' September, *Cancer Care in Canada*

Hsiao W (1999) 'International comparison of health systems', *Special Report* No 2 Hong Kong Health Welfare and Food Bureau www.hwfb.gov.hk/hw/English/archive, accessed 10.05.03

Hsiao W (2000) 'Background paper on health care financing', *Flagship course on Health Sector Reform* January 10, World Bank, Washington

Hu S (1997) 'New horizon of health care reform in China', *Informing and Reforming* ICHSRI 1: 5-6 Jan-Mar

Hubbard G and Miller D (eds) (2005) *Arguments against the G8* Pluto Press, London and Ann Arbor

Hughes S (2003) 'The flying carpetbaggers', *Red Pepper* August

Hunter D (1998) 'Public Private mix in health care restructuring', *ILO/PSI workshop on employment and labour practices in health care in Central and Eastern Europe* Part 5, ILO Geneva

Hurst J and Jee-Hughes M (2001) 'Performance measurement and performance management in OECD health systems', *Labour Market and Social Policy Occasional Papers* No. 47, OECD, Paris

Hurst JW (1992) 'The reform of health care - Comparative analyses of seven OECD countries', *OECD* Paris

Hutchinson P and LaFond AK (2004) *Monitoring and evaluation of decentralization reforms in developing country health sectors*, Partners for Health Reformplus, Abt Assiciates Inc, Bethesda

IADB (Inter American Development Bank) (1994) OP-742 *Public Health*, IADB, Washington, www.iadb.org/cont/poli/OP-742E.htm, accessed 01.07.03

ICHRSI (International Clearinghouse of Health System Reform Initiatives) (1997) 'Towards global sharing of experiences', *Informing and Reforming*, No.1, Jan-March, http//:www.insp.mx/ichrsi

ICHRSI (International Clearinghouse of Health System Reform Initiatives) (1998) *Capacity of non-governmental providers in delivery of health care in Kenya*, http://200.15.29.18/ichsri/news/kenya.html accessed 06.10.02

Idelson C (2003) 'The nation's 100 most expensive Operating Rooms New research reveals high mark ups on Operating Room charges', *Press Release* May 15, Califormia Nurses Association www.calnurse.org/can/press/51503.html, accessed 12.07.03

IFC (International Finance Corporation) (2002) *Topical Briefing on health and investing in private healthcare: strategic directions for IFC*, Official use only: restricted circulation February 22, IFC, Washington DC

Ii M (2005) 'Health care financing in Japan, Korea and Taiwan', *Paper for international Symposium on Health Care Systems in Asia*, Hitotsubashi University, Tokyo, www.econ.hit-u.ac.jp/~pppphcs5/paper/Japan_paper.pdf, accessed 24.03.05

ILO/PAHO (1999) 'Overview of the exclusion of social protection in health in Latin America and the Caribbean', *ILO regional tripartite meeting with the collaboration of PAHO*, December, ILO/PAHO, http:/www.oitopsmexico99.org.pe

Imai Y (2002) 'Health Care Reform in Japan', *Economics Department Working Paper* No. 321 February, OECD, Paris

Imai Y, Jacobzone S and Lenain P (2000) 'The changing health system in France', *Economics dept Working Papers* No 269, Nov 2000, OECD, Paris

IMF (1999a) *Zambia: Enhanced Structural Adjustment Facility Policy Framework Paper 1999-2001*, March 10, IMF, Washington

IMF (1999b) 'Africa: Adjusting to the challenges of globalisation', *Proceedings of Seminar held in Paris*, May 4-5 1998, IMF, Washington

Indymedia (2005) *CAFTA passed in Guatemala amid clouds of tear gas*, March 18 http://www.indymedia.org/en/index.shtml, accessed 30.03.05

Ingram M (1995) 'Russia warned of collapse of health system', *British Medical Journal* 311:897

International Confederation of Free Trade Unions, (2000b) 'Achieving poverty reduction, debt relief, social protection and international financial stability', *Joint ICFTU, ITS, TUAC statement to Prague meeting of governors of IMF and World Bank*, Sept, Prague

International Finance Corporation (2002) 'Topical Briefing on health and investing in private healthcare: strategic directions' (For IFC Official use only: restricted circulation) February 22, IFC, Washington DC

International Finance Corporation (2003a) *Health care strategy*, http://ifcln1.ifc.org/ifcext/che.nsf/Content/Strategy, accessed 05.07.03

International Finance Corporation (IFC) (2003b) *Basic facts about IFC*, www.ifc.org/about/basicfacts/basicfacts.html, accessed 14.06.03

International Finance Corporation (IFC) (2003c) *IFC – What we do*, www.ifc.org/about/what/what.html, accessed 14.06.01

Ireland D (2003) 'The bad doctor: Bill Frist's long record of corporate vice', *LA\Weekly* January 10-16 www.laweekly.com/, accessed 12.07.03

Iriart C, Merhy EE and Waitzkin H (2000) 'Managed care in Latin America: transnationalisation of the health sector in a context of reform', *Cad. Saude Publica* 16(1): 95-105, January-March, Rio de Janeiro

Iriart C, Merhy EE and Waitzkin H (2001) 'Managed care in Latin America: the new common sense in health policy reform', *Social Science and Medicine* 52;8: 1243-1253

Iriart C, Waitzkin H and Trotta C (2002) 'Global policies, health care system and social movements in Latin America: a lesson from Argentina', *Global Social Policy* 2(3) 245-248

Ivatts S and Millard P (2002) 'Health care modelling – why should we try?' *British Journal of Health Care Management* 8(6): 218-222

Jacobson C (2003) 'Hospitals cash in on new regulations', *Sunday Times* February 9, Johannesburg

Jacobzone S and Robine JM (1998) 'Long term care services to older people, a perspective on future needs', *Ageing Working Papers* 4.2 OECD, Paris

Jarman B (1993) 'Is London overbedded?' *British Medical Journal* 306: 979-82

Jeong HS and Hurst J (2001) 'An assessment of the performance of the Japanese health care system', *Labour Market and Social Policy Occasional Papers* No.56 December 6, OECD, Paris

Jessop B (2003) 'From Thatcherism to New Labour: neo-liberalism, workfarism and labour market regulation', in Overbeek (2003)

Jing F and Qiongfen X (2001) *Financial Reform and its impact on health service in poor rural China*, September 12, Centre for Business and Government, Harvard, www.ksg.harvard.edu/cbg/Conferences/financal_sector/home.htm, accessed 10.07.03

Johnston T (1998) *The impact of World Bank support to the HNP sector in Zimbabwe*, June 30, Operations Evaluation Department, World Bank, Washington

Johnston T and Stout S (1999) *Investing in Health. Development effectiveness in the Health Nutrition and Population Sector*, Operations Evaluation Department World Bank Washington DC

Jones Fine C (ed) (1999) *Transnational Social Policy*, Oxford: Blackwell

Jones LJ (1994) *The Social Context of Health and Health Work*, Macmillan, Basingstoke

Joy C and Hardstaff P (2003) *Whose development agenda? An analysis of the European Union's GATS requests of developing countries*, April, World Development Movement, London

Kahenya G and S Lake (1994) User Fees and their Impact on *Utilization of Key Health Services*, UNICEF, Lusaka

Kaiser Family Foundation (1999) *Key facts: race, ethnicity and medical care*, October, Kaiser Family Foundation, USA

Kaiser Family Foundation (2003a) *Health Poll report*, Kaiser Family Foundation www.kff.org/healthpollreport, accessed 12.07.03

Kaiser Family Foundation (2003b) *State health facts Online*, Kaiser Family Foundation www.statehealthfacts.kff.org/, accessed 12.07.03

Kamaldien Y (2004) 'Antiretroviral treatment plan way off target', *This Day* Front page, June 8, Johannesburg

Kane-Berman J (2004) 'Minister seems bent on destroying private health care', *News releases* Feb 24, South African Institute of Race Relations www.sairr.org.za, accessed 11.06.04

Kaplan J (2003) 'In need of medical assistance', *Australian Financial Review* November 7

Karcher HL (1997) 'Germany's new health reforms', *British Medical Journal* 314: 845

Karski JB, Koronkiewicz A and Healy J (1999) 'Poland', *Health Care Systems in Transition* WHO, Copenhagen

Kautto M, Fritzell J, Hvinden B, Kvist J and Uusitalo H (eds) (2001) Nordic *Welfare States in the European context*, Routledge, London

Kelsey J (1995) *Economic fundamentalism*, Pluto Press, London

Kemkes J, van der Meer J, Mooren H and de Wildt G (1997) 'Economic adjustment in developing countries is too painful for health care. Time for a signal from the medical profession', *Bulletin medicus mundi* April, www.medicusmundi.cj/bulletin/bulletin641.html, accessed 29.06.02

Kerrison SH and Pollock AM (2001) 'Caring for older people in the private sector in England', *British Medical Journal* 323: 566-9

Khalegian P (2001) 'Immunization financing and sustainability: a review of the literature', GAVI www,gaviftf.info/docs_activities/background_docs.html#planning, accessed 15.11.03

Killick T (1995) *IMF Programmes in developing countries*, Overseas Development Institute (Routledge) London

Kim JY, Shakow A and Bayona J (2000) 'The privatisation of health in Peru', in Bambas et al (2000)

Kimalu PK (2001) 'Debt relief and health care in Kenya', *Kenya Institute for Public Policy Research and Analysis (KIPPRA)*, July 24, Nairobi

Kirby M (chair) (2002) *The Health of Canadians – The Federal Role*, Final Report, Recommendations for action Volume Six Canadian Senate, Ottawa, http://www.parl.gc.ca/37/2/parlbus/commbus/senate/Com-e/SOCI-E/rep-e/repoct02vol6part6-e.htm, accessed 14.11.03

Kirigia J and Emrouznejad A, Sambo LG (2002) 'Measurement of technical efficiency of public hospitals in Kenya: using data envelopment analysis', *Journal of Medical Systems* 26: 1, 39-45

Klein R (2000) *The New Politics of the NHS* (4th edition), Longman, London

Klein R (2004) 'The first wave of NHS foundation trusts', *British Medical Journal* 328:1332 (editorial)

Kleinke JD (2001) *Oxymorons: the myth of a US health care system*, Jossey-Bass, San Francisco

Klugman J and Schieber G (1996) 'A survey of health reform in Central Asia', World Bank *Technical Paper* No. 344, Washington

Kmietowicz Z (2000) 'France heads WHO's league table of health systems', British Medical Journal 320: 1867

Kmietowicz Z (2003) 'Some operating theatres are used only eight hours a week', *British Medical Journal* 326: 1349

Knapp M (2002) 'Mental health: familiar challenges, unprecedented opportunities?' *eurohealth* 8:1 21-24 (Winter 2001-2002)

Knapp M, McDaid D, Mossialos E and Thornicroft G (2003) *Mental health policy and practice across Europe: the future direction of Mental Health Care – Proposal for analytical study*, WHO European Observatory on Health Care Systems www.who.dk/eprise/main/WHO/Progs/OBS/Studies/200211.htm, acessed 23.02.03

Knight R (2004) 'Consumer group attacks "illusion of choice" in public services', *Financial Times* December 1

Knowles JC, Leighton C and Stinson W (1997) 'Measuring results of health sector reform for system performance: a handbook of indicators', *Partnerships for Health Reform*, Bethesda, Sept

Knowles, J (1996) 'Health Sector reform in Cambodia', Feb, *Technical Report* 2, PHR, Harvard

Koivusalo M (2003) 'Health systems solidarity and European Community policies', in Sen (2003)

Koivusalo M and Ollila E (2001) *Making a healthy world: agencies, actors and policies in international health*, Zed Books, London

Kokko S, Hava P, Ortun V and Leppo K (1998) 'The role of the state in health care reform', in Saltman et al (1998)

Konde-Lule JK and Ollello D (1998) 'User fees in government health units in Uganda: implementation, impact and scope', *Small Applied Research* Paper No. 2 June, Partnerships for Health Reform, Bethesda

Kondo J (2005) 'The iron triangle of Japan's health care', *British Medical Journal* 330: 55-6

Korir J (2003) 'Safety nets in Kenya's public health sector', *IPAR policy brief* Vol 9, Issue 7 039/2003 www.ipar.or.ke

Kovac C (2000) 'Norway recruits Hungarian doctors', *British Medical Journal* 321: 136

Kress DH, Fairbank A and Atim C (1998) 'Social Health Insurance Working Group, Meeting in Zimbabwe January 28-30 1998', *PHR Workshop Report No.1* PHR, Abt Associates, Bethesda, Ma

Kroger T (2001) 'Comparative research on social care: the state of the art', February, *European Commission, 5th Framework Programme*, Brussels

Kumar S (2004) 'India's treatment programme for AIDS is premature', *British Medical Journal* 328:70

Kutzin J (2000) 'Towards Universal health care coverage: a goal-oriented framework for policy analysis', *HNP Discussion Paper* July, World Bank, Washington

Kwon S (2003) 'Payment system reform for health care providers in Korea', *Health Policy and Planning* 18(1): 84-92

Kwon S (2004) *Fiscal crisis of the National Health Insurance in Korea: in search of a new paradigm*, Seoul National University, www.econ.hit-u.ac.jp/~appphcs5/paper/korea.pdf, accessed 27.03.05

Kyer K (2002) 'Another bad trade pact: from NAFTA to CAFTA', *Counterpunch* September 12, www.counterpunch.org/kyer0912.html, accessed 02.06.03

Labonte R, Schrecker T and McCoy D (2005) 'Health and HIV/AIDS: fine words and fatal indifference', in Hubbard and Miller (2005)

Labonte R, Schrecker T, Sanders D and Meeus W (2004) *Fatal Indifference – The G8, Africa and Global Health*, University of Cape Town Press, International Development Research Centre

Laghi B (2002a) 'Let health report speak for itself, Romanow warns', Globe and Mail December 4, Toronto

Laghi B (2002b) 'The patchwork of care', *Globe and Mail* December 4, Toronto

Laghi B (2002c) 'Liberals balk at key Romanow principles', *Globe and Mail* December 6, Toronto

Laing & Buisson (2003) *Laing's Healthcare Market Review* (15th Edition) 2002-2003, London

Lamar J (2000) 'Japan's medical insurance system is on verge of bankruptcy', British Medical Journal 321:854

Lampton DM (2003) 'China's health care disaster', *Asia Wall Street Journal* May 6, www.nixoncenter.org/publications/articles, accessed 10.07.03

Landmann Swzarcwald C (2002) 'On the World Health Organisation's measurement of health inequalities', *Journal of Epidemiology and Community Health* 56 (3): 177-82 March

Langer A, Nigenda G and Catino J (2000) 'Health sector reform and reproductive health in Latin America and the Caribbean: strengthening the links', *Bull WHO* 78(5) 667-676

Laporte C (2005) *Overseas nurses: the ethical dilemma*, UNISON, London www.unison.org.uk/features/features/0502nurses.asp, accessed 20.03.05

Laurance J (2004) 'BMA sued for failing to back racism cases', *The Independent* March 30

Laurell AC (1991) 'Crisis, neoliberal health policy and political processes in Mexico', *International Journal of Health Services* Vol 21 No. 3 457-70

Laurell AC and Arellano OL (1996) 'Market commodities and poor relief: the World Bank proposal for health', *International Journal of Health Services* 26 (1) 1-18

Lave JR and Goldman HH (1990) 'Medicare Financing for Mental Health Care', *Health Affairs* Spring 1990

Lavoie J (2003) 'Province set to privatise day surgeries', *CanWest News* Service June 12 http://www.canada.com, accessed 12.06.03

Leason K (2003) 'Carry on doctors?', *Community Care* 24-25, 14-20 August

Leatherman S (2001) 'Measuring up: performance indicators for better healthcare', *OECD Observer* Dec 9, OECD, Paris

Leatherman S and McCarthy D (2002) *Quality of healthcare in the United States: a chartbook*, May 10, www.cmwf.org, accessed 12.07.03

Lee K, Buse K, Fustukian S (eds) (2002) *Health Policy in a Globalising World*, Cambridge University Press

Lee, K and Goodman H (2002) 'Global health networks: the propagation of health care financing reforms since the 1980s', in Lee et al (2002)

Leighton C (1995) '22 Policy questions about health care financing in Africa', *HFS Project* Abt Associates Inc, Bethesda Ma USA

Leighton C and Wouters A (1995) 'Strategies for achieving health financing reform in Africa', *World Development* – Also in HFS Vol 24, no. 9 p 1511-1525, Policy Paper 10, Abt Associates, Bethesda USA

Lenaghan J (1997) *Hard Choices in Health Care*, BMJ Publishing Group, London

Lenin V I (1973) *Imperialism, the Highest Stage of Capitalism*, Foreign Languages Press, Peking

Leon DA, Walt, G and Gilson L (2001) 'International perspectives on health inequalities and policy', *British Medical Journal* 322:591-594

Leppo K (1997) 'Introduction', in Koivusalo and Ollila (2001)

Lethbridge J (2002) 'International Finance Corporate (IFC) health care policy briefing', *Global Social Policy* 2(3) 349-354

Lewis M (2000) *Who is paying for health care in Europe and Central Asia?* World Bank, Washington

Lewis M (2001) 'Who is paying for health care in eastern Europe and central Asia?' *Background material Second ECA Poverty Forum*, World Bank, Washington DC

Leys C (2001) *Market Driven Politics*, Verso, London

Li X, Chen C and Wang L (2001) 'Delivery of basic health care services in China: current status and ongoing reforms', in Molina and del Arco (2001)

Lien L (2003) 'Financial and organisational reforms in the health sector: implications for the financing and management of mental health care services', *Health Policy* Vol 63(1) 73-80, January

Light D (1997) 'The real ethics of rationing', *British Medical Journal* 315: 112-115

Light D (2003) 'Choice bites in Boca Raton', *Health Service Journal* September 25: 18-19

Ling T (2000) 'Unpacking partnership: health care', in Clarke et al (2001)

Lister G (2002) *Hopes and fears for the future of health: scenario for health and care for 2022*, Nuffield Trust, www.ukglobalhealth.org/content/Text/Nuffut.doc, accessed 26.05.03

Lister J (1989a) *Cheap and Cheerless: a response to Kenneth Clarke's proposals for community care*, July, London Health Emergency, London

Lister J (1989b) 'Passing the Buck', *Community Care* 774: 21-22

Lister J (1996a) *Passing the Buck (Cambridge)* April, UNISON Eastern Region, Chelmsford

Lister J (1996b) *Passing the Buck: a survey of health authority policies and eligibility criteria for continuing care in the East Midlands*, August, UNISON East Midlands, Nottingham

Lister J (1996c) *The two-way squeeze: How Cambridge NHS cuts would hit the frail elderly*, October, UNISON Eastern Region, Chelmsford

Lister J (1997a) *Squeezing out the elderly: the impact of NHS eligibility criteria on services for the elderly in Cambridge and Suffolk*, April, UNISON Eastern Region, Chelmsford

Lister J (1997b) *Checking out Community Care: a UNISON campaign kit for health and social services staff*, June, UNISON Eastern Region, Chelmsford

Lister J (1998a) *Taking Liberties, a response to the North Essex Health Authority consultation document Taking the Initiative*, January, UNISON Eastern Region, Chelmsford

Lister J (1998b) *Into the Wilderness: a response of West Hertfordshire Health Authority's document Choosing the right direction*, September, UNISON Eastern Region, www.healthemergency.org.uk, accessed 01.11.03

Lister J (1999) *The Care Gap*, UNISON, London May 27

Lister J (2001) *PFI in the NHS: a dossier*, GMB, London, http://www.gmb.org.uk/docs/pdfs/PFIDossier.pdf, accessed 12.06.04

Lister J (2003a) *SW London Hospitals Under Pressure*, Battersea & Wandsworth TUC, London

Lister J (2003b) *The PFI Experience*, Voices from the frontline, UNISON, London

Lister J (2003c) *Not So Great: voices from the frontline at Swindon's Great Western Hospital*, UNISON, London

Lister J (2004a) *Gambling with our lives: a response to the consultation document from Merton, Sutton and Mid Surrey NHS*, October, UNISON Epsom & St Helier Branch, St Helier Hospital

Lister J (2004b) Beds and jobs axed as Trusts cut back, *Health Emergency* No. 60, December 2004

Lister J (ed) (1988) *Cutting the Lifeline*, Journeyman Press, London

Lister J and Martin G (1988) *Community care: Agenda for disaster*, September, London Health Emergency, London

Liu X and Liu G (1997) 'Regulation of the private medical market in China', *Informing and Reforming* ICHSRI 1: 5-6 Jan-Mar

Liu X, Xu L and Wang S (1996) 'Reforming China's 50,000 township hospitals – effectiveness, challenges and opportunities', *Health Policy* Oct 38(1): 13-29

Liu Y (2000) 'Understanding and setting up the process for health equity', *Bull WHO* 78 (1) 82-83

Liu Y, Rao K and Hu S (2002) *People's Republic of China: Towards establishing a rural health system*, September, Asian Development Bank

Lloyd Sherlock P (2002) 'Ageing and health policy: global perspectives', in Lee et al (2002)

Lobato L and Burlandy L (2000) 'The context and process of health care reform in Brazil', in Fleury et al (2000)

Lockwood DNJ (2002) 'Leprosy elimination – a virtual phenomenon or a reality?' *British Medical Journal* 324: 1516-8

Londono JL and Frenk J (1997) 'Structured pluralism: towards an innovative model for health system reform in Latin America', *Health Policy* 41(1) 1-36

Lonroth K, Thuong LM, Linh PD and Diwan V (1998) 'Risks and benefits of private health care: exploring physicians', views on private health care in Ho Chi Minh City, Vietnam', *Health Policy* Aug 45(2): 81-97

López-Acuña (2000a) 'The Nature of Health Sector Reform in the Americas and its Significance for PAHO's Technical Cooperation', *Background paper for the Annual PAHO's Managers Retreat* September 30, PAHO, Washington

López-Acuña (2000b) *Major trends in health sector reform in Latin America and the Caribbean*, www.reprohealth.org/reprohealthDB/doc/ 02%20Powerpoint%20Presentation%201-%20Lopez_Acuna.pdf, accessed 13.09.03

Lovelace JC (2003) 'Foreword', in Preker and Harding (2003) *Innovations in Health Service Delivery* The Corporatization of Hospitals

Lowery D and Gray V (2000) 'A neopluralist perspective on research on organised interests', April, *paper to Annual Meeting of Midwest Political Science Association*, Chicago

Lund C and Flisher AJ (2001) 'South African mental health process indicators', *Journal of Mental Health Policy and Economics* 4; 1: 9-16

Lyall J (2002) 'Poles apart', *Health Service Journal* 11 July, p14-15

Maceira D (1998) 'Provider payment mechanisms in health care: incentives, outcomes and organisational impact in developing countries', *Major Applied Research 2, Working Paper* 2 PHR, Abt Associates, Bethesda Ma

Macinko JA and Starfield B (2002) 'Annotated Bibliography on Equity in Health, 1980-2001', *International Journal for Equity in Health* 1:1 1-20, May

Mackintosh J (2003) 'Healthcare keeps GM care cheap', *Financial Times* August 20.

Mackintosh J (2005) 'How the wheels fell off at General Motors – and what might fix it', *Financial Times* Monday January 10:17

Mackintosh M (2001) 'Do health care systems contribute to inequalities?' in Leon et al (2001)

Madarasz N (2003) 'A trap for Lula', *News from Brazil* www.brazil-brasil.com/2003/html/news/articles/jul03/p118jul03.htm, accessed 28.07.03

Madlana B (2003) 'African states not buying into NEPAD', The *Mercury Independent online* June 13, www.avmedia.at/nepad/indexgb.html, accessed 09.07.03

Mahler H (1981) 'The meaning of health for all by the year 2000', *World Health Forum* 2 (1) 5-22

Makinen M (1998) 'Demand for care under reforms in Zambia', *Healthwatch* Winter, Abt Associates, Bethesda

Makinen M (1999) 'Health spending inequalities and the government's role in Zambia', *Major Applied Research 3, Working Paper* 4 January, Partnerships for Health Reform, Bethesda

Makinen M and Leighton C (1997) 'Summary of a market analysis for a franchise network of primary health care in Lusaka, Zambia', December PHR, *Technical Report* 15sum, Harvard

Malin N, Wilmot S and Manthorpe J (2002) *Key concepts and debates in health and social policy*, Open University Press, Buckingham

Management Sciences for Health, (2001) *Innovations in Health Care Financing: experiences from Kenya*, Management Sciences for Health, Boston

Manning N (2000) *The new public management and its legacy Administrative and civil service reform*, World Bank http://www1,worldbank.org/publicsector/covilservice/debate.htm, accessed 15.02.03

Manning N and Shaw I (1999) 'The transferability of welfare models: a comparison of the Scandinavian and state socialist models in relation to Finland and Estonia', in Jones Fine (1999)

Marini RA (1999) 'Nonprofit HMOs score higher on quality', *Nurse Week* www.nurseweek.com/news/99-7/39f.html, accessed 04.08.99

Marks A (2003) 'Many doctors call for healthcare system with universal coverage', *Christan Science Monitor* August 13

Marmor T (1994) *Understanding health care reform*, Yale University Press

Marmor T (1999) 'The rage for reform: sense and nonsense in health policy', in Drache and Sullivan (1999)

Marmor T (2002) 'Policy and political fads: the rhetoric and reality of managerialism', *British Journal of Health Care Management* 8(1): 16-23, January

Marmor TR (1998) 'The procompetitive movement in American medical politics', in Ranade (1998)

Marmor TR (2001) 'Comparing Global health systems Lessons and caveats', in Wieners (2001)

Marmot M (2001) 'Future links between socio-economic status and health', *Proceedings of a conference* Health Trends Review, Barbican Centre London

Marree J and Groenewegen PP (1997) *Back to Bismarck: Eastern European health care systems in transition*, Avebury, Ashgate Publishing, Aldershot

Martineau T, Decker K and Bundred P (2002) *Briefing note on international migration of health professionals: levelling the playing field for developing country health systems*, Liverpool School of Tropical Medicine, www.liv.ac.uk/lstm/hsrhome.html, accessed 20.03.05

Martinez E and Garcia A (1997) 'What is "neo-liberalism"? A brief definition for activists', *Corporate Watch* http://www.corpwatch.org/trac/corner/glob/neolib.html, accessed 20.01.01

Marwick C (2002) 'A total of 58 million Americans lack health insurance', *British Medical Journal* 325: 678

Marx K (1852) 'The Eighteenth Brumaire of Louis Bonaparte', in Marx and Engels (1970)

Marx K (1974) *Capital* (Volume 1), Lawrence and Wishart London

Marx K and Engels F (1872) 'Preface', to German edition of *The Communist Manifesto*, in Marx and Engels (1970)

Marx K and Engels F (1970) *The German Ideology*, Lawrence and Wishart London

Maynard A and Bloor K (2000) 'Payment and regulation of providers', *Flagship course on Health Sector Reform*, World Bank Institute, November 2000

Maynard A and Sheldon T (2001) 'Rationing is needed in a national health service', *British Medical Journal* 322: 734

Mayo E and Lea R (2002) *The Mutual Health Service*, November, New Economic Foundation, London

Mays GP, Claxton G and White J (2004) 'Managed care rebound? Recent changes in health plans, cost containment strategies', *Health Affairs* Web Exclusive W4-427, August

Mcauley I (2004) Stress on public hospitals – *why private insurance has made it worse*, Australian Consumers Association, Australian Healthcare Association, http://resources.dmt.canberra.edu.au/imcauley/confs/phpi.pdf, accessed 29.05.04

McCanne D (2003) 'Why incremental reforms will not solve the health care crisis', *Journal of American Board of Family Practice* 16: 257-261

McEuen M (1997) 'Initiatives in health care financing', HHRAA/DDM Southern Africa Regional Workshop Proceedings October 7, *Data for Decision Making Project*, Harvard School of Public Health

McGauran A (2004) 'Moving 15% of procedures to private sector will wreck NHS', *British Medical Journal* 329:1257

McGregor D (2003) 'Democrats commit themselves to healthcare reforms, in all but name', *Financial Times* May 22

McGregor D (2003) 'Senate votes to allow Canada drug purchases', *Financial Times* June 21-22

McIntrye D, Gilson L, Valentine N and Soderlund N (1998) 'Equity of health sector revenue generation and allocation: a South African Case Study', *Major Applied Research 3, Working Paper* 3 August, Partnerships for Health Reform, Bethesda

McIntyre D and Gilson L (2000) 'Redressing Dis-advantage: promoting vertical equity within South Africa', *Health Care Analysis* 8(3): 235-258

McKinlay JB and Arches J (1993) 'Towards the proletarianisation of physicians', *International Journal of Health Services* 15(2) 161-195

McNulty J (2002) 'Concrete examples of failure of for-profit healthcare in Canada', *The Province* November 29, www.Vancouver.indymedia.org/news/2002/11/23151_comment, accessed 26.05.03

McPake B (1993) 'User charges for health services in developing countries: a review of the economic literature', *Social Science and Medicine* 36(11): 1397-405

McPake B (2002) 'The globalisation of health sector reform policies: is "lesson drawing" part of the process?' in Lee et al (2002)

McPake B and Mills A (2000) 'What can we learn from international comparisons of health systems and health system reform?' *Bull WHO* 78 (6) 811-820

Medicover (2002a) *Health care reform in the Czech Republic*, www.medicover.com, accessed 26.05.03

Medicover (2002d) *Health care reform in Estonia*, www.medicover.com, accessed 26.05.03

Medicover (2003) *Health care reform in Poland*, www.medicover.com, accessed 26.05.03

Mehring F (1975) *On historical materialism*, New Park Publications, London

Mekay E (2004) 'Iraq: Debt relief weighed down by IMF burden', *Inter Press service News Agency*, Washington November 23, www.ipsnews.net/interna.asp?idnews=26401, accessed 25.01.05

Merz C (2002) 'The Cuban Paradox', *Harvard Public Health Review* Summer, www.hsph.Harvard.edu/review/677cuba.html, accessed 29.09.03

MGI Report (2000) MGI Report: *why the Japanese economy is not growing*, July, http://www.mckinsey.com/knowledge/mgi/Japan/cases/healthcare.asp

Miller JE (2001) *A perfect storm: The confluence of forces affecting health care coverage*, National Coalition on Health Care, Washington, November 2001

Milliman USA (2003) 'Milliman USA survey foresees average HMO rate increase of 14% for 2004', *Press Release*, July 21, Seattle, www.milliman.com/ press_releases/Survey_Press%20Release_07_21_03.pdf, accessed 29.05.04

Mills A (1998) 'Health care reforms in developing countries', *Informing and Reforming* No.5 2-5 ICHSRI Jan-Mar

Mills A (2002) *Achieving efficient and equitable health care in Africa: What changes are needed?* www.worldbank.org/wbi/attackingpoverty/ programs/seminar_mills.ppt

Mills A, Bennett S and Russell S (2001) *The challenge of health sector reform – What must governments do?* Palgrave, Basingstoke UK

Mills, A, Brugha R, Hanson K and McPake B (2002) 'What can be done about the private health sector in low income countries?' *Bull WHO* 80 (4) 325-330

Mitchell D (2002) 'Managing the new social risks: welfare', in Shiels (2002)

Molina and del Arco (eds) (2001) *Health Services in Latin America and Asia*, Blackwell Publishing, Oxford

Moloney P (1997) *Neo-Liberalism Down-Under: Reflections on the "New Zealand Experiment"*, Victoria University of Wellington, http://www.casi.org.nz/politicaleconomy/moloneynr.html, accessed 23.05.04

Molyneux DH and Nantulya VM (2004) 'Linking disease control programmes in rural Africa: a pro-poor strategy to reach Abuja targets and millennium development goals', *British Medical Journal* 328: 1129-32

Moore M (2000) 'In praise of the future', *WTO News*, speech to *Canterbury Employers Chamber of Commerce* Aug 14 WTO Geneva

Moore W (2000) 'The impossible dream', *Health Service Journal* 8-9, 6

Moran J (2004) 'Medical training Cuban-style', *Irish Times* December 21

Moran M (1999) *Governing the health care state: a comparative study of the United Kingdom, the United States and Germany*, Manchester University Press

Morgan D (2003) 'Senators note health, energy investments', *Washington Post* June 14, www.washintonpost.com, accessed 12.07.03

Morris Z (2000) 'US healthcare really is the business', *Evening Standard* July 25: 10-11, London

Mossialos E and Dixon A, (2002) 'Funding health care in Europe: weighing up the options', in Mossialos et al (2002)

Mossialos E and McKee M (2002) 'Health Care and the European Union', *British Medical Journal* 324: 991-2

Mossialos E and Mrazek M (2002) 'Entrepreneurial behaviour in pharmaceutical markets and the effects of regulation', in Saltman et al (2002)

Mossialos E, Dixon A, Figueras J and Kutzin J (eds) (2002) *Funding health care: options for Europe*, Open University Press, Buckingham

Mpuga P (2004) 'Economic and Welfare Effects of the Abolition of Health User Fees: Evidence from Uganda', *Policy Research Working Paper* 3267, World Bank, April

MSI Healthcare (2000) *MSI healthcare: Germany*, October, MSI, Devon, UK

Mtshali T (2003) 'Physicians who put mercy above money', *Sunday Times* February 23, Johannesburg

Mudyarabikwa O (2000) 'An examination of public sector subsidies to the private health sector: a Zimbabwe case study', *Equinet Policy Series* No. 8 September, Regional Network for Equity in Health in Southern Africa (Equinet), Harare

Mukhopadhyay A (2000) *Public-private partnership in the health sector India*, December, www.adbi.org/PDF/partnership/secondprinting/21muk.pdf, accessed 01.07.03

Munaita P (2003) 'Kenyans to cough up more for health', *The East African on the Web* Monday July 14, accessed 27.03.05

Munishi GK (1995) 'Private sector delivery of health care in Tanzania', *Major Applied Research Paper* No. 14 HFS, Abt Associates, Bethesda MD

Murray Brown J, Timmins N and Wise P (2004) 'Brussels acts to exclude private finance for public works from stability pact rules', *Financial Times* International News February 7

Murray CJL (2001) 'Commentary: comprehensive approaches are needed for full understanding', *British Medical Journal* Response in 323 (7314): 678

Murray CJL and Frenk J (2000) 'A framework for assessing the performance of health systems', *Bull WHO* 78(6): 717-731

Murray CJL and Lopez AD (1996) *The global burden of disease: a comprehensive assessment of mortality and disability*. Harvard School of Public Health, for World Bank, Cambridge, Mass

Murray CJL, Evans DB, Acharya A and Baltussen RMPM *Development of WHO guidelines on generalised cost effectiveness analysis*, www.who.int

Murray CJL, Knaul F, Musgrove P, Xu K and Kawabata K (2001) 'Defining and measuring fairness in financial contribution to the health system', *GPE Discussion paper series*, No.24 WHO, Geneva

Murray CJL, Lopez AD and Wibulpolprasert S (2004) 'Monitoring global health: time for new solutions', *British Medical Journal* 329:1096-1100

Murray V, Walker HW, Mitchell C and Pelosi AJ (1996) 'Needs for care from a demand led community psychiatric service: a study of patients with major mental illness', *British Medical Journal* 312: 1582-1586

Musau SN (1999) 'Community-based health insurance: experiences and lessons learned from East and Southern Africa', *Technical Report* 34 August, Partnerships for Health Reform, Bethesda

Musgrove P (1994) 'Cost effectiveness and health sector reform', *Human Capital development and Operations Policy Working Papers*, World Bank, Washington

Mwabu G, J Mwanzia and Laimbila W (1995) 'User Charges in Government Health Facilities in Kenya', *Health Policy and Planning* 10(2): 164-70

Nandraj S (1997) 'Unhealthy prescriptions: the need for health sector reform in India', *Informing and Reforming* 2: 7-11, Apr-Jun

Nash E (2003) 'The Spanish prototype: efficient, but controversial', *The Independent* May 15: 4 London

National Statistics (2003) 'Experimental total UK health expenditure', 15 may, www.statistics.gov.uk/healthaccounts/experimental.asp, accessed 15.05.03

National Statistics (2003a) 'Experimental total UK health expenditure' www.statistics.gov.uk/healthaccounts/experimental.asp, accessed 31.05.03

National Statistics (2003b) 'A system of health accounts' www.statistics.gov.uk/healthaccounts/system.asp, accessed 31.05.03

Navarro V (1976) *Medicine under capitalism*, Prodist New York

Navarro V (1983) 'Radicalism, Marxism and Medicine', *International Journal of Health Services* 13(2): 179-202

Navarro V (1999) 'Health and equity in the world in the era of "Globalization" ' *International Journal of Health Services* Vol 29 No. 2 215-226

Navarro V (2002) 'The World Health Report 2000: can health care systems be compared using a single measure of performance?' *American Journal of Public Health* 92(1) 31-34

Navarro V (2003) 'Policy without politics: the limits of social engineering', *American Journal of Public Health* 93(1) 64-67

Navarro V (ed) (1992) 'Why the United States does not have a national health program', Baywood Publishing, Amityville NY

Navarro, V. (2000) 'Assessment of the World Health Report 2000', *The Lancet* 356: 1598-601

Naylor DC, Jha P, Woods J and Shariff A (1999) 'A fine balance. Some options for private and public health care in urban India', *Human Development Network* May World Bank Washington

Ncayiyana DJ (2002) 'Africa can solve its own health problems', *British Medical Journal* 324: 688-9

NEHAWU (2001) *Towards a people's hospital: NEHAWU and the reconstruction of Chris Hani Baragwanath*, NEHAWU Johannesburg, www.nehawu.org.za, accessed 07.07.03

NEHAWU (2002) 'Unfilled posts in health department', *Press Release* October 22, NEHAWU Johannseburg, www.nehawu.org.za/documens/pr/2002/pr2210.htm, accessed 07.07.03

NEPAD (2001) *The New Partnership for Africa's Development (NEPAD)*, October, Abuja, www.dfa.gov.za/events/nepad.htm, accessed 09.07.03

New B (1996) 'The rationing agenda in the NHS', *British Medical Journal* 312: 1593-1601

New B (1999) *A Good Enough Service Values, trade-offs and the NHS*, IPPR, London

New B (ed) (1997) *Rationing – Talk and action in health care*, BMJ Publishing Group, King's Fund, London

Newacheck PW, Stoddard JJ, Hughes DC and Pearl M (1998) 'Health insurance and access to primary care for children', *New England Journal of Medicine* 338 (8)

Newbrander W, Collins D, Gilson L (2000) 'Ensuring equal access to health services: User fee systems and the poor', *Management Sciences for Health*, Boston

Newman J (2000) 'Beyond the New Public Management? Modernising public services', in Clarke et al (2001)

News 24 (2003) 'Sama slams health bill', *Wheels* 24 November 19 http://www.news24.com/News24/South_Africa/Politics/0,,2-7-12_1403943,00.html, accessed 12.06.04

Njeru E, Arasa R and Nguli M (2005) 'Social Health Insurance Scheme for all Kenyans: opportunities and sustainability potentia', *IPAR policy brief* Vol 11 Issue 2 060/2004

North N and Peckham S (2001) 'Analysing structural interests in Primary Care Groups', *Social Policy & Administration* 35:4 426-440

Nwuke K and Bekele A (1995) 'Zambia National Conference on Public/Private Sector Partnership for Health', June, *Data for Decision Making*, Harvard

Nyawo MJ (2003) *South African dilemma in the provision of antiretroviral therapy*, (unpublished essay for Coventry University) January 9

Odegbile O (2001) 'Health sector refom and equity: Bolivia and Brazil study cases', *Technical report series* No. 78, November, PAHO, Washington

OECD (Organisation for Economic Co-operation and Development) (1992) 'OECD Health Systems Facts and Trends 1960-1991', *Health Policy Studies* 1(3) OECD, Paris

OECD (Organisation for Economic Co-operation and Development) (1995a) 'New Directions in Health Care Policy', *Health Policy Studies* No. 7, OECD, Paris

OECD (Organisation for Economic Co-operation and Development) (1995b) 'Social protection for dependent elderly people: perspectives from a review of OECD countries', *Labour market and Social Policy occasional paper* No. 16, OECD Paris

OECD (Organisation for Economic Co-operation and Development) (1998b) 'The New Social Policy Agenda A Caring World': OECD, *Press Release* Paris June 24

OECD (Organisation for Economic Co-operation and Development) (1998) *Maintaining Prosperity in an Ageing Society*, OECD Paris

OECD (Organisation for Economic Co-operation and Development) (1999a) *The reform of healthcare*, OECD Paris

OECD (Organisation for Economic Co-operation and Development) (1999b) *A Caring World: The New Social Policy Agenda*, OECD Paris

OECD (Organisation for Economic Co-operation and Development) (2000) *Health Data 2000 (CD)*, OECD Paris

OECD (Organisation for Economic Co-operation and Development) (2001a) *Health at a Glance*, OECD, Paris

OECD (Organisation for Economic Co-operation and Development) (2001b) OECD *Health Project*, OECD Paris, May 2001

OECD (Organisation for Economic Co-operation and Development) (2001c) 'Measuring Up: Improving Health Systems Performance in OECD countries', *Media Information for Ottawa conference* Nov 5-7, OECD, Paris

OECD (Organisation for Economic Co-operation and Development) (2001d) 'What OECD ministers are doing for healthcare', *OECD Observer* Dec 7, OECD, Paris

Office of National Statistics (2004) *Report on Public Sector Productivity*, October London http://www.statistics.gov.uk/pdfdir/healthpr1004.pdf, accessed 19.10.04

Okuonzi SA (2004) 'Learning from failed health reform in Uganda', *British Medical Journal* 329:1173-6

Okwemba A (2004) 'Aids patients quitting treatment', *allAfrica.com* Sept 30, http://allafrica.com/stories/printable/200409300088.html, accessed 03.10.04

Okwii R (1997) 'Uganda. Decentralisation: its impact on the delivery of health services', *Informing and Reforming* 3: 13-14

Ollila E and Koivusalo M (2002) 'The World Health Report 2000: WHO health policy steering off course – changed values, poor evidence and lack of accountability', *International Journal of Health Services* Vol 32 No.3 503-514

Ollila E, Koivusalo M and Baru R (2002) 'Globalisation and national health policies', *Global Social Policy* 2(3) 243-245

Omanga B (2002) 'Ministry reneges on earlier promise', *The Nation* July 23, Nairobi

Omran AR (1971) 'The epidemiologic transition: a theory of the epidemiology of population change', *Milbank Memorial Fund Quarterly* 49: 509-38

Opinion (2005) 'WTO policy a blow to anti-Aids drive', *The Nation* 25 March, http://allafrica.com/stories/printable/200503250620.html, accessed 27.03.05

Opiyo G (2005) 'Crucial bills lined up', *East African Standard* March 19, www.eaststandard.net/news.php?articleid=15838, accessed 27.03.05

Oresaventures.com (2003) 'Analysis of the healthcare sector in central and Eastern Europe', www.oresaventures.com/healthcare.html, accessed 26.05.03

Orlale O (2002) 'MP calls for scrapping of cast sharing', *The Nation (Nairobi)* October 3

Osborn A (2004) 'Half of Russia's doctors face sack in healthcare reforms', *British Medical Journal* 328:1092

Osborne D and Gaebler T (1992) *Reinventing government: how the entrepreneurial spirit is transforming the public sector*, Addison-Wesley, New York

Osborne D and Plastrik P (1997) Banishing bureaucracy: *The five strategies for reinventing government*, Addison-Wesley, Reading Mass, USA

Overbeek H (ed) (2003) *The Political economy of European Unemployment: European Integration and the transnationalisation of the employment question*, Routledge, London

Ovretveit J (1996) 'The Kiwi way: lessons from New Zealand', *British Medical Journal* 312: 645

Owino W and Koris J (1997) *Public health sector efficiency: estimation and policy implications*, December, Institute of Policy Analysis and Research, Nairobi

Owino W, Korir J, Ocholla P and Oloo K (2000) *Decentralisation and health systems development: the question of planning, budgeting and financial structures*, July, Institute of Policy Analysis and Research, Nairobi

Owino W, Odundo P and Oketch T (2001) *Governance of the district health systems: a focus on the health management boards and human resource development teams*, May, Institute of Policy Analysis and Research, Nairobi

Oxfam (2000) *Tax havens: releasing the hidden billions for poverty eradication*, Oxfam, Oxford, UK

Oxfam (2001) 'Pfizer: Formula for fairness. Patient rights before patent rights', *Oxfam Company Briefing Paper* July Oxfam, Oxford

Oxfam Policy Department (1994) A case for reform: *Fifty years of the IMF and World Bank*, Oxfam, Oxford

Oxley H and Jacobzone S (2001) 'Healthcare expenditure: a future in question', *OECD Observer* Dec 9, OECD, Paris

PAHO (Pan American Health Organization) (1998) 'Bolivia', *Health in the Americas*, PAHO, Washington DC

PAHO (Pan American Health Organization) (1998) 'Chile', *Health in the Americas*, PAHO, Washington DC

PAHO (Pan American Health Organization) (1998) 'Colombia', *Health in the Americas*, PAHO, Washington DC

PAHO (Pan American Health Organization) (1998) 'Venezuela', *Health in the Americas*, PAHO, Washington DC

PAHO (Pan American Health Organization) (2000) 'Special Issue on health sector reform', *Pan American Journal of Public Health:* Vol 8, Nos 1-2 PAHO, Washington DC

PAHO (Pan American Health Organization) (2001a) *Evaluating the impact of health reforms on gender equity: a PAHO guide*, 23 April, PAHO, Washington

PAHO (Pan American Health Organization) (2001b) *Regional Consultation on Health Systems Performance Assessment*, May, PAHO, Washington DC

PAHO (Pan American Health Organization) (2001c) *Regional Consultation on Health Systems Performance Assessment (Final Report)*, May, PAHO, Washington DC

PAHO (Pan American Health Organization) (2001d) 'Health Indicators: building blocks for health analysis', *Epidemiological Bulletin* Vol 22 No, 4, December PAHO, Washington DC

PAHO (Pan American Health Organization) (2002) *Health in the Americas 2002 Volume II*, PAHO, Washington, DC

PAHO (Pan American Health Organization) (2002) *Profile of the health services system*, Mexico, April, PAHO, Washington DC

PAHO (Pan American Health Organization) (2003) 'Globalisation and health', *132nd Session of Executive Committee*, April, PAHO, Washington DC

PAHO , WHO and International Development Research Centre (2001) 'Research on health sector reforms in Latin America and the Caribbean: contribution to policymaking', *Paper for pre-summit of the Americas Forum*, March, Montreal, www.idrc.ca/lacro/docs/conferencias/paho_idrc.html, accessed 17.09.03

Palast G (1999) 'Sickness at the heart of private medicine', *The Observer* Business April 25: 10

Palier B and Sykes R (2001) 'Challenges and change: Issues and perspectives in the analysis of globalisation and the European welfare states', in Sykes et al (2001)

Palmer KS (1999) *A brief history: universal health care efforts in the US*, www.pnph.org/print.php, accessed 19.06.03

Palmer N (2000) 'The use of private sector contracts for primary health care: theory, evidence and lessons for low-income and middle-income countries', *Bull WHO* 78(6) 821-829

Palmer S and Torgerson DJ (1999) 'Definitions of efficiency', *British Medical Journal* 318: 1136

PAP News Agency (2000) *Poland health reforms to cost 24,000 jobs*, BBC Monitoring service October 30

Paral R (2004) 'Health worker sortages and the potential of immigration policy', *Immigration Policy IN FOCUS* 3: 1, February Immigration Policy Center, Washington

Park E and Lav IJ (2003) *Proposed expansion of medical savings accounts could drive up insurance costs and increase the number of uninsured*, April 30, Center on Budget and Policy Priorities, Washington

Park M (2004) '58 000 babies saved', *The Star* Front page, June 8, Johanneseburg

Parker G and Clarke H (1995) *The development of long-term care insurance in Britain*, University of Leicester, Nuffield Community Care Studies Unit

Patel D (2004) 'Who's going to heal Ngilu's ailing Ministry of Health?' *East African Standard* Thursday October 7, www.eastandard.net/archives, accessed 27.03.05

Patel K and Rushefsky ME (1999) *Health care politics and policy in America*, ME Sharpe Inc, New York

Patel S and Pretorius L (2002a) 'A summary of the New Partnership for Africa's Development (NEPAD)', *Khanya* 1: August, 22-23, Khanya College, Johannesburg

Patel S and Pretorius L (2002b) 'NEPAD: Integrating Africa into neoliberal globalisation', *Khanya* 1: August, 24-26, Khanya College, Johannesburg

Patel V (2001) 'Poverty, inequality and mental health in developing countries', in Leon et al (2001)

Paterson M (2002) 'Public hospital strengthening', *Insights for Implementers* No. 2, September 2002, PHRplus, Abt Associates, Bethesda Maryland

Paterson R and Walker M (1997) *A very peculiar practice: the case against GP fundholding*, April, UNISON /NHS Support Federation, London

Paton, C (2000) 'New Labour, New Health Policy?' in Hann (2000)

Pauly M (2000) *Foreword to American Health Care*, (ed) Feldman RD, Transaction Publishers New Brunswick (US) and London

Pauly MV (2003) 'Should we be worried about high real medical spending growth in the United States?' *Health Affairs web exclusive* January 8

Payer C (1982) 'The World Bank, a critical analysis', *Monthly Review Press*, New York

Payne D (2001) 'German company offers "package deal ops" to Ireland', *British Medical Journal* 323:471

Pear R (2003) 'New study finds 60 million uninsured during a year', *New York Times* May 13

Pearson M (2000) 'DALYs and essential packages', Briefing Paper DFID HSRC, London June 2000

Peoples Daily (2002a) 'China's health care sector expects enhancement with WTO entry', 29 January http://english.peopledaily.com.cn/, accessed 10.07.03

Peoples Daily (2002b) 'China to give fairer medical service to millions of farmers', 25 January http://english.peopledaily.com.cn/, accessed 10.07.03

Peoples Daily (2002c) 'China's basic medical insurance covers AIDS patients', December 2 http://english.peopledaily.com.cn/, accessed 10.07.03

Peters DH, Elmendorf AE, Kandola K and Chellaraj G (2000) 'Benchmarks for health expenditures, services and outcomes in Africa during the 1990s', *Bull WHO* 78 (6) 761-769

Peters DH, Yazbeck AS, Sharma RR, Ramana G, Pritchett LH and Wagstaff A (2002) *Better health systems for India's poor*, Human Development Network, World Bank, Washington

Petras J and Vieux S (1992) 'Myths and realities: Latin America's free markets', *International Journal of Health Services* Vol 22, No.4 611-617

Petrella R (1996) 'Globalisation and internationalisation: the dynamics of the emerging world order', in Boyer and Drache (1996)

Pfizer (2001) *Annual Report*, Pfizer, New York

PHR (2000) 'Health Insurance models becoming more popular in Africa', *Healthwatch (Abt Associates newsletter)* Fall 2000

PHR (Partnerships for Health Reform) (1998) 'National Health Accounts: Summaries of eight national studies in Latin America and the Caribbean', *Special Initiatives Report* 7, May, Bethesda MD, Abt Associates Inc

Pierson C (1998) *Beyond the Welfare State: the new political economy of welfare*, Polity, Cambridge

Pillay K (2002) 'The National Health Bill: a step in the right direction?' *ESR Review* (3)2 September http://communitylawcentre.org.za/ser/esr2002/2002sept_national.php, accessed 11.06.04

Pillay Y (2004) 'The National Health Bill: Key Issues that Impact on the Public & Private Health Sectors', *Paper delivered at Public Health 2004 Conference*, June 8, Durban www.mrc.ac.za/conference

Pillay Y, Marawa N and Proudlock P (2002) 'Health Legislation', *South African Health Review* 3-12, March, Cape Town

Pillay YG and Bond P (1995) 'Health and social policies in the new South Africa', *International Journal of Health Services* 25(4): 727-43

Pilling D (2003) 'Over-prescription adds $3.5 billion to drugs bill', *Financial Times* May 22

Pink GH and Leatt P (2003) 'The use of "arms length" organisations for health system change in Ontario, Canada: some observations by insiders', *Health Policy* Vol 63(1) 1-15

Plumridge N and Kemp P (2004) 'New dawn for the NHS', *Public Finance* March 12-18: 24-25

PNHP (Physicians for a National Health Program) (2003a) (Unpublished) *Proposal of the Physicians' Working Group for Single-Payer National Health Insurance*, www.pnhp.org accessed 22.06.03 (Password access)

PNHP (Physicians for a National Health Program) (2003b) '31% of health care spending is paperwork', *Press Release* August 20, PNHP, Chicago, www.pnhp.org, accessed 20.08.03

Pollitt C (2000) 'Is the Emperor in his underwear? An analysis of the impacts of public management reform', *Public Management* Vol 2, No.2 pp 181-199

Pollitt C (2003) *The essential public manager*, Open University Press/McGraw Hill, Maidenhead

Pollock AM (2002) 'PFI versus democracy', *Lecture to the Regeneration Institute*, Cardiff University, www.cardiff.ac.uk/news/02-03/021114/lecture.html, accessed 20.10.03

Pollock AM (2003) 'Foundation hospitals will kill the NHS', *The Guardian* May 7

Pollock AM (2004) *NHS plc The privatisation of our health care*, Verso, London

Pollock AM and Dunnigan MG (2000) 'Beds in the NHS: the National Beds Inquiry exposes contradictions in government policy', *British Medical Journal* 320: 461-2

Pollock AM and Price D (2000) *Rewriting the regulations: how the World Trade Organisation could accelerate privatisation in health care systems by undermining the voluntary basis of GATS*, www.unison.org.uk/pfi/rewrite.htm, accessed 30.01.01

Pollock AM and Price D (2003) 'The BetterCare judgment – a challenge to health care', *British Medical Journal* 326: 236-7

Pollock AM and Price D (2003) *In Place of Bevan? Briefing on the Health and Social Care (Community health and standards) Bill 2003*, September, Catalyst, London

Pollock AM, Dunnigan M, Gaffney D, Macfarlane A and Majeed FA (1997) 'What happens when the private sector plans hospital services for the NHS: three case studies under the private finance initiative', *British Medical Journal* 314: 1266

Pollock AM, Price D, Talbot-Smith A and Mohan J (2003) 'NHS and the Health and Social Care Bill: end of Bevan's vision?' *British Medical Journal* 327: 982-5

Preker AS and Harding A (2000) 'The Economics of Public and Private Roles in Health Care: Insights from Institutional Economics and Organizational Theory', *Health Nutrition and Population* June, World Bank, Washington

Preker AS and Harding A (eds) (2003) 'Innovations in health service delivery: the corporatization of public hospitals', *Human development Network Health Nutrition and Population Series*, World Bank, Washington

Press Release JUNE 26 www.usdoj.gov, accessed 4.05.05

Price D and Pollock AM (2002) 'Extending choice in the NHS', *British Medical Journal* 325: 293-4

Price D, Pollock AM and Shaoul J (1999) 'How the World Trade Organisation is shaping domestic policies in health care', *The Lancet* 354: 1889-1891

PSI (Public Services International) (1999) *Health and social services Briefing notes*, Jan PSI, Paris

Publicprivatefinance (2004) *Health FOCUS*, PFP, London

Publicprivatefinance.com (2003) *Edinburgh hospital subject of investigations*, June 9, www.publicprivatefinance.com/pfi/news/, accessed 13.06.03

Purvis G (1997) 'University Teaching Hospital in Zambia: the strategic plan environment', *Technical Report* No. 14 September, PHR, Bethesda

Qadeer I (2003) 'Ethics and medical care in a globalising world: some reflections', in Sen (2003)

RACP (Royal Australasian College of Physicians) (1999) *Health financing: response to the Senate Inquiry into Public Hospital funding*, Health Policy Unit RACP, Sydney

Ranade W (ed) (1998) *Markets and health care a comparative analysis*, Longman, London

Rannan-Eliya R, van Zanten TV and Yazbeck A (1996) 'First year literature review for applied research agenda', *Applied Research Paper 1*, Partnerships for Health Reform Abt Associates, Bethesda MA

RCS (Royal College of Surgeons) (1997) *The provision of emergency surgical services*, June, RCS, London

Reed G (2001) 'Health News from Cuba', *MEDICC review* Vol 11 No. 1 www.medicc.org/Medicc%20Review/III/hiv-aids/news.html, accessed 29.09.03

Reichard S (1996) 'Ideology drives health care reforms in Chile', *Journal of Public Health Policy* 17(1): 80-98

Reilly T (2001) 'Going Dutch on Health', *Public Finance* 21 September

Relman AS (2002) For-profit health care: *Expensive, Inefficient and Inequitable, PNHP*, http://www.pnhp.org//Press/2002/Expensive_Inefficient_Inequitable4.21.02.htm, accessed 22.7.02

Reverte-Cejudo D and Sanchez-Bayle M (1999) 'Devolving health services to Spain's autonomous regions', *British Medical Journal* 318: 1204-5

Reviglio F (2000) 'Health care and its financing in Italy: reform options', *IMF Working Paper*, October, WP/00/166, IMF Washington

Revill J (2003) 'IVF free-for-all may cost £400 million', August 10, *The Observer*

Richardson J, Segal L, Watts J, Carter R, Mortimer D, Peacock S and Robertson I (1999) 'The reform of public hospital funding in Australia', Submission to the Senate Inquiry into Public Hospital funding, *Working Paper 1000* Centre for Health Program Evaluation, Monash University

Rico A (2000) 'Spain', *Health Systems in Transition*, WHO European Observatory, Denmark

Riesberg A and Busse R (2003) 'Cost shifting (and modernisation) in German health care', Euro Observer 5(4):4-5, Winter

Riungu C (2003) 'Payments crisis: HMOs now blame insurers, hospitals', *The East African on the web* Monday December 1, accessed 27.03.05

Rivett G (1998) *From Cradle to Grave*, Kings Fund, London

Roberts D and Alden E (2004) 'Foot to the pedal: US business expects a clear run from a second Bush term', *Financial Times* Friday November 5:17

Robinson R (1998) 'Managed competition: health care reform in the Netherlands', in Ranade (1998)

Robinson R (2002) 'Who's got the master card?' *Health Service Journal* 26 September 22-24

Robinson R and LeGrand J (eds) (1993) *Evaluating the NHS Reforms*, King's Fund Institute, London

Rocco F (2003) 'Bark with a welcome bite', *Financial Times magazine* 11:7, July 5

Romanow RJ (2002a) *Building on values: the future of health care in Canada*, November 2002 Commission on the Future of Health Care in Canada, Ottawa

Romanow RJ (2002b) 'The cost of health care: is it sustainable?' *Notes for a speech to the Weatherhead Center for International Affairs, Harvard University*, October 16, Council of Canadians, www.Canadians.org, accessed 14.11.03

Rondinelli D (1981) 'Government decentralisation in comparative theory and practice in developing countries', *International Review of Administrative Sciences* 47, 133-45

Rondinelli DA and Nellis JR, Cheema GS (1983) 'Decentralization in developing countries: a review of recent experience', *World Bank Staff Working papers* No 581, July, World Bank, Washington

Roper I, Cunningham I and James P (2002) *Assessing the UK government's approach to family friendly policies*, June, www.sase.org/conf2002/papers/c1004.roper_cunningham_james.pdf, accessed 21.12.03

Rowson M (2001) 'Summit fails to agree new deal on world debt', *British Medical Journal* 323: 186

Russell S and Gilson L (1997) 'User fee policies to promote health service access for the poor: a wolf in sheep's clothing?' *International Journal of Health Services* Vol 27 No.2 359-379

Rutten F (2004) 'The impact of healthcare reform in the Netherlands', *PharmacoEconomics* Vol 22, Suppl 2, 65-71

Saadah F and Knowles J (2000) *The World Bank Strategy for Health, Nutrition and Population in the Far East and Pacific Region*, Human Development Network, June, World Bank, Washington

Sachs J (1999) 'Helping the Poorest', *The Economist* 14 August 1999

Sahn D and Bernier R (1995) 'Have structural adjustments led to health sector reform in Africa?' *Health Policy* Apr-Jun 32(1-3): 193-214

Salari N (2003) Are health and care services ready for a surge in Alzheimer's cases? *Community Care* 16-17, 28 August-3Sept

Saltman RB (1991) 'Emerging trends in the Swedish health system', *International Journal of Health Services* Vol 21 No. 4 615-623

Saltman RB (1996) 'The notion of planned markets and fixed budgets', in Schwartz et al (1996)

Saltman RB (1998) 'Health reform in Sweden: the road beyond cost containment', in Ranade (1998)

Saltman RB (2002) 'The Western European experience with health care reform', *European Observatory* 4 April, www.observatory.dk, accessed 23.02.03

Saltman RB and Figueras J (eds) (1997) European Health Care Reform, *Analysis of Current Strategies*, European Observatory on Health Care Systems

Saltman RB and Van Otter C (1992) *Planned markets and public competition Strategic Reform in Northern European Health Systems*, Open University Press, Buckingham

Saltman RB, Busse R and Mossialos E (eds) (2002) *Regulating entrepreneurial behaviour in European health care systems*, Open University Press, Buckingham

Saltman RB, Figueras J and Sakellarides C (eds) (2000) *Critical Challenges for Health Care Reform in Europe*, Open University Press, Buckingham

Samba EM (2004) 'African health care systems: what went wrong?' *Healthcare News* www.news-medical.net/print_article.asp?id=6770, accessed 24.03.05

Sample I (2004) 'Cuban cocktails: The most advanced biotech industry in the developing world exports vaccines around the globe – despite US claims about biological weapons', *The Guardian* March 30, London

Sanchez Bayle M, and Beiras H (2003) 'The trouble with conservative healthcare counter-reforms in Spain', in Sen (2003)

Sandiford P, Gorter A and Salvetto M (2002) 'Vouchers for Health: Using voucher schemes for output-based aid', *Viewpoint* World Bank Private Sector and Infrastructure Network Note No. 243, April 2002

Sanso Soberats FJ (2003) 'Transformation of the Cuban healthcare sector: the past forty years', in Sen (2003)

Sapa-AFP (2004) 'Moms, babies can't leave hospital until they've paid', *Pretoria News* June 4: 4 (news report)

Save the Children (2005) *Whose charity? Africa's aid to the NHS*, London, www.savethechildren.org.uk, accessed 20.3.05

Savedoff WD (2000) 'Is anybody listening? Ignoring evidence in the Latin American health reform debates', *SDS/SOC Health Note* 2 October, IADB, Washington

Sbarabaro J (2000) 'Trade liberalisation in health insurance: Opportunities and challenges. The potential impact of introducing or expanding the availability of private health insurance within Low and Middle-income countries', *CMH Workinf Paper Series* WG4:6, December, Commission on Macroeconomics and Health, WHO Geneva

Scandlen G (2003) *It's up to us*, Feb 1 2003, Heartland Institute, www.heartland org

Schick A (1998) 'Why most developing countries should not try New Zealand reforms', *World Bank Research Observer* Vol 13; 1: 123-31

Schieber G and Maeda A (1997) 'A curmudgeon's guide to financing health care in developing countries', in Schieber (1997)

Schieber GJ (ed) (1997) 'Innovations in Health Care Financing', *World Bank Discussion Paper 365*, March, World Bank, Washington

Schippers E (2002) *Towards a sound system of medical insurance?* www.civitas.org.uk/pdf/dutch pdf, accessed 22.03.05

Schneider P, Diop FP and Bucyana S (2000) 'Development and implementation of prepayment schemes in Rwanda', *Technical Report* No. 45 PHR, Abt Associates, Bethesda Ma

Schreuder B and Kostermans C (2001) 'Global health strategies versus local primary health care priorities – a case study of national immunisation days in Southern Africa', *South African Medical Journal* 91(3): 249-54

Schuftan C (2003) 'Poverty and inequity in the era of globalisation: our need to change and reconceptualise', *International Journal for Equity in Health* 2:4, www.equityhealthj.com/content2/1/4, accessed 30.11.03

Schuftan C and Dahlgren G (1999) *Health Sector Reform measures: are they working? And where do we go from here?* ICHSRI, www.insp.mx/ichsri/news/hanoi.html), accessed 14.09.99

Schuppe M (2002) 'Integrating health across policies', *Issues in European Health Policy*, Issue 6, April, p1,2 and 9

Schwartz FW, Glennerster H and Saltman RB (eds) (1996) *Fixing Health Budgets: Experience from Europe and North America*, John Wiley & Sons, Chichester

Scott C (2001) *Public and private roles in health care systems*, Open University Press, Buckingham

Scott G, McKenzie L and Webster J (2003) 'Maladjustments in the corporatization model: hospital reform in New Zealand', in Preker and Harding (2003)

Seager A (2005) 'Benn to end link between aid and privatisation', *The Guardian* Weds, March 2, London

Sectra Medical Systems (2003) 'Sectra supplies digital technology to Sweden's largest private emergency hospital', *Press Release*, February 21, Sectra, Lingoping, Sweden

Sein T (2001) 'Health Sector Reform – Issues and Opportunities', *Regional Health Forum*, WHO website, http://w3.whosea.org/rh4/4a.htm, accessed 15.02.03

Sen K (ed) (2003) *Restructuring health services*, Zed Books, London

Sexton S (2003) 'Trading healthcare away: the WTO's General Agreement on Trade in Services', in Sen (2003)

Shaw JS (2002) *Public Choice Theory*, Library of economics and Liberty, http://www.econlib.org/library/Enc/PublicChoiceTheory.html, accessed 12.03.04

Shaw RP (2002) 'World Health Report 2000 "Financial fairness indicator": useful compass or crystal ball?' *International Journal of Health Services* 32(1): 195-203

Shaw RP and Ainsworth, M (eds) (1995) 'Financing Health Services through User Fees and Insurance Case Studies from Sub Saharan Africa', *World Bank Discussion Papers* VII, Washington

Shaw RP and Elmendorf AE (1994) *Better Health Care in Africa*, World Bank, Washington

Sheldon T (2004a) 'GP visits excluded from Netherlands', no claims bonus scheme', *British Medical Journal* 329:939

Sheldon T (2004b) 'Manifesto opposes introduction of market forces into Dutch health care', *British Medical Journal* 329:1066

Shelton JD and Johnston B (2001) 'Condom gap in Africa: evidence from donor agencies and key informants', *British Medical Journal* 323: 139

Shepperd S, Harwood D, Gray A, Vessey M, and Morgan P (1998) 'Randomised controlled trial comparing hospital at home care with inpatient hospital care – II: cost minimisation analysis', *British Medical Journal* 316: 1791-1796

Shiels C (ed) (2002) *Globalisation: Australian Impacts*, UNSW Press

Shortt SED (2002) 'Medical Savings Accounts in publicly funded health care systems: enthusiasm versus evidence', *Canadian Medical Association Journal* 167(2): 159-162

Simms C, Rowsan M, and Peattie S (2001) *The bitterest pill of all: the collapse of Africa's health care systems*, Save the Children Fund UK, May

Simon D, Van Spengen W, Dixon C, and Närman A (eds) (1995) *Structurally Adjusted Africa: poverty, debts and basic needs*, Pluto Press, London

Simonian H (2002) 'Berlin ponders radical change in welfare state', *Financial Times* Dec 21-23

Simpson EL and House AO (2002) 'Involving users in the delivery and evaluation of mental health services: a systematic review', *British Medical Journal* 325: 1265

Simpson EL, House AO (2002) 'Involving users in the delivery and evaluation of mental health services: a systematic review', *BMJ* 325: 1265 (November 30)

Skaar CM (1998) 'Extending coverage of priority health care services through collaboration with the private sector: selected experiences of USAID Cooperating Agencies', *Major Applied Research* No 4 *Working Paper 1* PHR, Abt Assiciates, Bethesda, Ma USA

Slack K and Savedoff WD (2001) 'Public purchaser-private contracting for health services', January, IADB, Washington

Smetherham J-A (2004) 'Department, doctors to meet for talks', *Pretoria News* Business Report 12 February

Smith K and Sheaff R (2000) 'Some are more equal than others: differing levels of representation in Primary Care Groups', in Hann (2000)

Smith P (2002) 'Stars in their eyes', *Health Service Journal* 112, No 5816, 10-12

Smith P (2003) 'We might not save flops, judges Dredge', *Health Service Journal* 25 September: 6-7

Smith PC (2002) 'Performance management in British health care: will it deliver?' *Health Affairs* Vol 21, No. 3, 103-115, May/June

Smith PC (ed) (2000) *Reforming Markets in Health Care: an economic perspective*, Open University, Buckingham

Smith PC and Goddard M (2000) 'Reforming health care markets', in Smith PC (ed) *Reforming Markets in Health Care: an economic perspective*

Smith R (1996a) 'Being creative about rationing', *British Medical Journal* 312: 391-392

Smith R (1996b) 'Rationing health care: moving the debate forward', *British Medical Journal* 312: 1553-1554

Smith R (2002) 'A time for global health', *British Medical Journal* 325: 54-5

Smith R (2005) 'NHS at war', *Evening Standard* 18 January, www.thisislondon.co.uk/til/jsp/modules/Article/print.jsp?itemId=15987842, accessed 24.01.05

Social Justice Unit (2002) Urgent action – *El Salvador. Death threats against medical professionals in struggle against privatisation of health services*, October 17, http://www.s-j-c.net/UA1000.htm, accessed 02.06.03

Solomon L (2002) 'Rise of a "zombie" ' *National Post* July 31, Toronto

Spurgeon B (2004) 'French patients will have to go through family doctors to see specialists', *British Medical Journal* 328: 1278

Spurgeon D (2000) 'Canadian government pours money into provincial health budgets', *British Medical Journal* 321:726

Spurgeon D (2002a) 'Canada sees a bigger role for private companies in health care', *British Medical Journal* 324:259

Spurgeon D (2002b) 'Canadians need to spend $C5bn more a year on health care', *British Medical Journal* 325: 1058 9

Staines VS and Lovelace JC (1999) 'The World Bank's Health Sector Strategy for the Europe and Central Asia Region', *Eurohealth* (4) 6 pp 87-93

Standard Team (2004) 'Why Government backed out of Health Bill', *East African Standard* Weds November 7, www.eaststandard.net/news.php?articleid=6097, accessed 18.11.04

Standing H (2000) 'Gender impacts of health reforms: the current state of policy and implementation', July, *Paper for ALAMES meeting* Havana, www.ids.ac.uk/ids/health/alames.pdf, accessed 22.06.03

Statement at conclusion of Forum 8 (2004), Mexico City www.globalforumhealth.org/forum8, accessed 21.03.05

Stenton A (2002) *Comments from Chief Executive of Nairobi Hospital*, (interviewed by John Lister) April, Mombasa

Stewart A (1998) 'Cost effectiveness of SSRIs: a European perspective', *Journal of Mental Health Policy and Economics* 1: 41-49

Stone, D (2001) 'Think tanks, global lesson-drawing and networking social policy ideas', *Global Social Policy* Vol 1 3, Dec, 338-360

Stott R (1999) 'The World Bank: friend or foe to the poor?' *British Medical Journal* 318: 822-823

Sturm R and Gresenz CR (2002) 'Relations of income inequality and family income to chronic medical conditions and mental health disorders: national survey', *British Medical Journal* 324: 1-5, (January 5)

Sussex J (2001) *The economics of the private finance initiative in the NHS*, Office of Health Economics, London

Sutherland R (2002) *Scanning for profit: a critical review of the evidence regarding for-profit MRI and CT clinics*, September, Ontario Health Coalition, Toronto

Suwandono A and Gani A (1997) 'The health sector reform in Indonesia', *Informing and Reforming* No.2, Apr-Jun ICHSRI

Swann C (2005) 'President accused of robbing poor to benefit the rich', *Financial Times* Weds February 9: 8

Sykes R, Palier B and Prior PM (eds) (2001) *Globalization and European Welfare States Challenges and Change*, Palgrave, Basingstoke

Talbot-Smith A, Gnani S, Pollock AM and Pereira Gray D (2004) 'Questioning the claims from Kaiser', *British Journal of General Practice* 54 (503): 415-421

Tamez S and Molina N (2000) 'The context and process of health care reform in Mexico', in Fleury et al (2000)

Tapay N (2001) 'Private insurance, public health', *OECD Observer* Dec 2, OECD, Paris

Taylor M (2003) 'The reformulation of social policy in Chile 1973-2001: Questioning a Neoliberal Model', *Global Social Policy* 3:1; 21-44

Taylor R (2003) 'Singapore's innovative health financing system', *Flagship Online Journal* May, World Bank, www.worldbank.org/wbi/healthandpopulation/oj.html, accessed 22.09.03

Taylor R and Blair S (2002) 'Public Hospitals: options for reform through public-private partnerships', *Viewpoint, World Bank Group Private Sector and Infrastructure Network* January, Note No. 241

Tchernjavski V (1998) 'Russian Federation', *Health Care Systems in Transition* WHO, Copenhagen

Tessa Tan-Torres E (1999) 'North-South research partnerships: the ethics of carrying out research in developing countries', *British Medical Journal* 319: 438-41.

Thakker A (2004) *National Social Health Insurance; framework, flaws and solutions*, July, www.c4idea.com/presentations/NSHIS%20Presentation.ppt, accessed 27.03.05

Therborn G (1996) 'Critical Theory and the legacy of twentieth century Marxism', in Turner (1996)

Timmins N (1995) *The Five Giants, a biography of the welfare state*, Harper Collins, London

Timmins N (2004a) 'Shunned hospitals "may go bust" as patients get choice', *Financial Times* November 23:4

Timmins N (2004b) 'Health service revolution dogged by controversy', *Financial Times* January 13

Timmins N (2005) 'NHS Trusts hit financial trouble despite cash injection', *Financial Times* January 5

Titmuss, R. (1974) Social Policy, Allen & Unwin

Toner R and Pear R (2003) 'States slashing health care for US poor', *New York Times/International Herald Tribune* April 29, www.iht.com, accessed 12.07.03

Tonks A (2002) Letter: 'Summary of responses', *British Medical Journal* 324: 1334

Torrey EF (1997) *Out of the shadows: confronting America's mental illness crisis*, John Wiley, New York

Tragakes E and Lessof S (2003) 'Russian Federation', *Health Care Systems in Transition*, WHO Euro Observatory

Trieman N, Leff J and Glover G (1999) 'Outcome of long stay psychiatric patients resettled in the community: prospective cohort study', *British Medical Journal* 319: 13-16

Trong Hai T and Schuftan C (2001) 'Efficient equity-based health sector reforms in Vietnam', in Molina and del Arco (2001)

Trotsky LD (1936) *Revolution Betrayed*, 1973 edition, New Park Publications, London

Trotsky LD (1977) 'The Transitional Programme', in Breitman and Stanton (1977)

Trumper R and Phillips L (1997) 'Give me discipline and give me death: neoliberalism and health in Chile', *International Journal of Health Services* 27(1): 41-55

Tuffs A (2000) 'Germany expects more hospital privatisation', *British Medical Journal* 320: 1030

Tuffs A (2003a) 'German hospital curtails services because of deficit', *British Medical Journal* 326:11

Tuffs A (2003b) 'German doctors "work to rule" in protest at government plans', *British Medical Journal* 326: 303

Tuffs A (2003c) 'Germany at centre of rationing row as budget in crisis', *British Medical Journal* 327: 414

Tuffs A (2004a) 'German patients rush to doctors before new €10 charge starts', *British Medical Journal* 328:8

Tuffs A (2004b) 'German health reform likely to raise costs for patients', *British Medical Journal* 328:70

Tuffs A (2004c) 'Germany's new charging system has mixed results', *British Medical Journal* 328:366

Tullock G, Brady G and Seldon A (2002) *Government failure: a primer in public choice*, Cato Institute, Washington DC

Turner BS (ed) (1996) *The Blackwell Companion to Social Theory*, Blackwell, Oxford

Turshen M (1999) *Privatising Health Services in Africa*, Rutgers University Press, New Brunswick, New Jersey

Ugwumba C (2000) 'World Bank and IMF: The promotion of "user fees" for health and education', *Bank Information Centre (BIC) Prague 2000 Issue Briefings*, http://www.bicusa.org/ptoc/htm/ugwumba_healthuserfess.htm, accessed 06.10.02

UKCC (United Kingdom Central Council) (1997) *The Continuing Care of Older People*, UKCC, London

UNICEF (United Nations Children's Fund) (1989) *The State of the World's Children*, New York

United Nations (1997) 1997 *Report on the World Social Situation*, UN, New York

United Nations (2002) *Report on the Second World Assembly on Ageing*, United Nations, New York, www.un.org/esa/socdev/ageing/waa/a-conf-197-9b.htm, accessed 08.01.03

UNRISD (United Nations Research Institute for Social Development) (2000) *Visible hands - taking responsibility for social development*, Geneva, UNRISD

US Department of Justice (2003) 'Largest health care fraud case in U.S. history settled. HCA investigation nets record total of $1.7 billion'

USAID (United Nations Research Institute for Social Development) (1999) *Strategic Plan 1998-2003* January, Washington DC

USAID (United Nations Research Institute for Social Development) (2003a) *Security, Democracy, Prosperity Strategic Plan, Fiscal Years 2004 –2009. Aligning Diplomacy and Development Assistance*, USAID, Washington

USAID (United Nations Research Institute for Social Development) (2003b) 'USAID History', www.usaid.gov/about_usaid/usaidhist.html, accessed 31.12.03

USAID (United Nations Research Institute for Social Development) (2003c) 'This is USAID', http://www.usaid.gov/about_usaid/, accessed 31.12.03

Usborne D, Cornwell R and Reeves P (2003) 'Iraq Inc: a joint venture built on broken promises', *The Independent* May 10

Ustun TB (2000) 'Mainstreaming mental health', *Bull WHO* 78; 4: 412

Vaknin S (2002) *Dying breed: health care in Eastern Europe*, May 9, www.aegis.com/news/upi/2002/UP020506.html, accessed 26.05.03

Valentine W (1998) 'WHO spearheads multi-country study of decentralisation and health system change', BRIDGE WHO, http://165.158.1.110/english/hsp/hspbb985.htm, accessed 15.02.03

Valkin V, Bowe C (2003) 'Reputation of US business is tarnished again', *Financial Times* June 13

Vallgarda S, Krasnik A and Vrangbaek K (2001) 'Denmark', *Health Care Systems in Transition*, WHO European Observatory, Denmark

Vallgarda S, Thomson S, Krasnik A and Vrangbaek K (2002) 'Denmark', in Dixon and Mossialos (2002)

Van de Venn WPMM and Schut FT (2000) *The first decade of market oriented health care reforms in the Netherlands*, Institute of Health Care Policy and Management, Erasmus University Rotterdam, www.lse.ac.uk/collections/LSEHealthAndSocialCare/pdf/EHPGFILES/SEP2000/paper3sep2000.pdf, accessed 22.03.05

Van der Gaag J (1996) 'Private and Public Initiatives: working together in health and education', World Bank, www.worldbank.org/html/extdr/hnp/health/ppi/p1option.htm, accessed 08.07.02

Van der Stuyft P and Unger JP (2000) 'Editorial: Improving the performance of health systems: the World Health Report as a go-between for scientific evidence and ideological discourse', *Tropical Medicine and International Health* 5 No. 10: 675-677

Vaughan JP, Modegal S, Kruse S, Lee K, Walt G and de Wilde K (1996) 'Financing the World Health Organisation: global importance of extrabudgetary funds', *Health Policy* 35(3): 229-45

Verdugo JC (2000) 'Moving from a War-time Economy to a Market Economy', in Bambas et al (2000)

Vergara P (1997) 'In pursuit of "growth with equity": the limits of Chile's free market reforms', *International Journal of Health Services* Vol 27 No. 2 207-215

Vienonen M, Jankauskiene D and Vask A. (1999) 'Towards evidence-based health reform', *Bulletin of the WHO* 77(1) 44-47

Vladescu C and Radulescu S (2002) 'Improving primary care – Output based contracting in Romania', in Brook and Smith (2002)

Vladescu C, Radulescu S and Olsavsky V (2000) 'Romania', *Health Care Systems in Transition*, WHO, Copenhagen

Volovitch P (2000a) 'Strikes hit the hospital sector', EIRO online January, European Industrial Relations Observatory, Dublin, www.eiro.eurofound.eu.int//2000/01/features/FR0001136F.htm, accessed 08.06.03

Volovitch P (2000b) 'Universal healthcare insurance introduced', *EIRO online* January, European Industrial Relations Observatory, Dublin, www.eiro.eurofound.eu.int/2000/01/feature/FR0001135F.htm, accessed 08.06.03

Volovitch P (2000c) 'Doctors', organisations opposing current health insurance policy make election gains', *EIRO online* July, European Industrial Relations Observatory, Dublin, www.eiro.eurofound.eu.int/2000/07/feature/FR0007180F.htm, accessed 08.06.03

Volovitch P (2002) 'General practitioners take industrial action', *EIRO online* January, European Industrial Relations Observatory, Dublin, www.eiro.eurofound.eu.int/2002/01/feature/FR0201110F.htm, accessed 06.08.03

Wachino V (2002) *State budgets under stress: how are states planning to reduce the growth in Medicaid costs?* The Kaiser Commission on Medicaid and the Uninsured, July 30

Wagstaff A (2001) 'Poverty and Health', *CMH Working Paper Series*

Wagstaff A (2002) 'Reflections and alternatives to the WHO's fairness of financial contribution index', *Health Economics* Mar 11(2): 103-15

Wagstaff A and van Doorslaer E (2001) *Paying for health care: quantifying fairness, catastrophe and impoverishment, with applications to Vietnam 1993-98*, November, World Bank Development Research Group, Washingon

Wagstaff A (2001) 'Economics Health and Development: some ethical dilemmas facing the World Bank and the International Community', *Journal of Medical Ethics* February www.worldbank.org

Waitzkin, H (1997) 'Challenges of managed care: its role in health system reform in Latin America', *Informing and Reforming* No 4. 2-4 ICHSRI, Oct-Dec

Waitzkin, H, Iriart, C and Estrada A, and Lamadrid S (2001) 'Social medicine then and now: Lessons from Latin America', *American Journal of Public Health* Vol 91, No. 10, 1592-1601

Wakefield Health Authority (1999) *Consultation document: Grasping the Nettle*, Wakefield

Wall A and Owen B (2002) *Health Policy*, Gildredge Social Policy Routledge

Walshe K, Smith J, Dixon J, Edwards N, Hunter DJ, Mays N, Normand C and Robinson R (2004) 'Primary care trusts: premature reorganisation, with mergers, may be harmful', *British Medical Journal* Editorial 329:871-872

Walt G (1994) *Health Policy: an introduction to process and power*, Witwatersrand University Press / Zed Books London

Walt G and Gilson L (1994) 'Reforming the health sector in developing countries: the central role of policy analysis', *Health Policy and Planning* 9(4): 353-70

Wang Y (ed) (2000) Public-Private Partnerships in the Social Sector: Issues and Country Experiences in Asia and the Pacific, ADBI Policy Papers No.1 Asian Development Bank Institute, http://www.adbi.org/PDF/partnerships/secondprinting/04bloom.pdf

Wang',ombe JK (1997a) 'Health sector reform in Kenya', *Informing and Reforming* ICHSRI 1: 5-6 Jan-Mar

Wang',ombe JK (1997b) 'Cost Recovery Strategies in Sub-Saharan Africa', in Schieber (1997)

War on Want (2005) *Profiting from Poverty*, War on Want, London, http://www.waronwant.org/?lid=8740, accessed 25.03.05

Ward A (2002) 'A bitter pill for South Korea's foreign investors', *Financial Times* November 19:13

Ward S (2005) ' "Limit growth" on private care in NHS', *Public Finance* March 11-17:8

Washington Post (1999) *Indonesia Report: Overview*, http://www.washingtonpost.com/wp-srv/inatl/longterm/indonesia/overview.htm, accessed 28.03.05

Wax E (2003) 'In another break with past, Kenyans see hope on AIDS', *Washington Post* May 21, page A01

Ways and Means Committee (2001) *Testimony submitted for the record by the Advanced Medical Technology Association (AvaMed)*, March 7, Washington, www.avamed.org/publicdocs/w&mhearing3-7-01.html, accessed 26.05.03

Weich S and Lewis G (1998) 'Poverty, unemployment and common mental disorders: population based cohort study', *British Medical Journal* 317:115-9 (July 11)

Weiner JP, Lewis R and Gillam S (2001) *US managed care and PCTs. Lessons to a small island from a lost continent*, King's Fund, London

Weiss L (1999) 'Managed openness: beyond neoliberal globalism', *New Left Review* 238: 126-40

Weiss Ratings Inc (2005) *50% of HMOs financially strong as profitability continues*, February 7, www.WeissRatings.com, accessed 09.02.05

Weissman R (2004) *Dying for drugs: How CAFTA will undermine access to essential medicines*, March, Essential Action Washington, www.essentialaction.org, accessed 01.03.05

Wells KP and associates (1998) 'Assessing integrated care as a solution for New Zealand', *Health Care and Informatics Review Online* 2: 11, September 1.www.enigma.co.nz/hcro/website/index.cfm?fuseaction=articledisplay&FeatureID=51, 12.3.04

Went, R (2000) *Globalization: Neoliberal challenge, radical responses*, Pluto Press/IIRE, London

Whitehead M (1992) 'The concepts and principles of equity and health', *International Journal of Health Services 223:* 429-445

Whitehead M (1992) *The Health Divide*, Penguin, London and New York

Whitehead M, Dahlgren G and Evans T (2001) 'Equity and health sector reforms: can low-income counties escape the medical poverty trap?' The Lancet 358: 833-36

Whitfield D (1992) *The Welfare State*, Pluto, London

WHO (World Health Organization) (1992) *Basic documents* (39th edition), Geneva, WHO

WHO (World Health Organization) (1996a) 'The Ljubljana Charter on Reforming Health Care', *Bull WHO* 1999, 77(1) 48-49

WHO (World Health Organization) (1996b) 'Mental Health', *Fact Sheet* No. 130 WHO Geneva August

WHO (World Health Organization) (1996c) 'Mental health and demographic factors', *Fact Sheet* No. 131 WHO Geneva August

WHO (World Health Organization) (1996g) *Psychiatry of the Elderly: a consensus statement*, WHOMNH/MND/96.7 Geneva, February

WHO (1998) *Citation: award of World Health Organisation Health-For-All Gold Medal*, May 15, A51/DIV/7.

WHO (World Health Organization) (1999a) *Health for All Statistical Database*, WHO Copenhagen, www.who.dk

WHO (World Health Organization) (1999b) 'Raising awareness, fighting stigma, improving care', *Press Release* November 12, WHO Geneva

WHO (1999d) 'The "newly defined" burden of mental problems', *Fact Sheet* No 217 WHO Geneva April

WHO (World Health Organization) (2000) *World Health Report*, WHO, Geneva

WHO (World Health Organization) (2001a) *Atlas: country profiles on mental health resources 2001*, WHO, Geneva

WHO (World Health Organization) (2001b) 'Intensifying the response to the conditions associated with poverty', Executive Board May, www.who.int

WHO (World Health Organization) (2001c) *World Health Report*, WHO, Geneva

WHO (2001d) 'Project Atlas: Mapping mental health services around the world', *Fact Sheet*, WHO, Geneva

WHO (World Health Organization) (2001e) Commission on Macroeconomics and Health Paper No. WG1 : 5

Wieners W (ed) (2001) *Global Health Care Markets*, Jossey Bass, San Francisco

Wilensky HL (1975) *The welfare state and equality. Structural and ideological roots of public expenditures*, University of California Press

William AP, Deber R, Baranek P and Gildiner A (2001) 'From Medicare to home care: globalization, state retrenchment, and the profitization of Canada's health-care system', in Armstrong et al (2001)

Williams C and Treloar J (2002) *Trends and Indicators in the changing health marketplace, 2002*, May, Kaiser Family Foundation www.kff.org/content/2002/3161, accessed 12.07.93

Williams F (2003) 'WTO tries to break deadlock on medicines access', *Financial Times* January 28

Williams M (1994) *International Economic Organisations and the Third World*, Harvester Wheatsheaf, London

Williams S (2002) *Alternative Prescriptions* April, Conservative Party, London

Williamson H (2005) 'Medical tourism keeps hospital budgets healthy', *Financial Times* March 1

Williamson J (1990) 'What Washington means by policy reform', in Williamson (2000)

Williamson J (2000) 'What should the World Bank think about the Washington Consensus?' *The World Bank Research Observer* 15; 2: 251-264, August

Woolf ST, Johnson RE, Fryer GE, Rust G and Satcher D (2004) 'The health impact of resolving racial disparities: an analysis of US mortality data', *American Journal of Public Health* 94;12:2078-81

Woolhandler S and Himmelstein DU (2004a) 'The high costs of for-profit care', *Canadian Medical Association Journal* 170(12):1814-1815

Woolhandler S and Himmelstein D (2004b) *Op-ed by Drs David Himmelstein and Steffie Woolhandler on the Kerry Health Plan*, July 23, www.pnhp.org/print.php, accessed 13.03.05

Woolhandler S and Himmelstein DU (2002) 'Paying for National Health Insurance – and not getting it', *Health Affairs* 21; 4: 88-98

Woolhandler S, Campbell T and Himmelstein DU (2003) 'Costs of Health Care Administration in the United States and Canada', *New England Journal of Medicine* 2003; 768-775, Aug 21

World Bank (1987) *Financing Health Services in developing Countries: An Agenda for Reform*, Washington

World Bank (1993) 'Investing in Health', *World Development Report*, Washington

World Bank (1995) *Staff Appraisal Report. Socialist Republic of Viet Nam national health support project*, December, World Bank Human Resources Operations Division, Washingon

World Bank (2000e) 'The role of the World Bank', *Public and Private Initiatives* WB web site, www.worldbank.org/html/extdr/hnp/health/ppi/contents.htm, accessed 08.07.02

World Bank (2001a) *World Bank activities and position on aging*, June, Washington DC www.un.org/esa/socdev/ageing/worldbank200106.htm, accessed 22.02.03

World Bank (2001b) *Mental health at a glance*, www.worldbank.org/hnp, accessed 07.03.03

World Bank (2002) *World Development Indicators*, www.worldbank.org/data, accessed 07.07.02

World Bank (2003a) 'World Bank seeks to ensure CAFTA helps reduce poverty', *Press release* January 9, Web.worldbank.org/WBSITE/EXTERNAL/NEWS/, accessed 02.06.03

World Bank (2003b) *World Development Report 2004*, 21 September, World Bank, Washington

World Bank (2003c) *Argentina Maternal and Child Insurance* SECAL, Initial Project Information Document 26560, July 30

World Bank (2003d) 'Project appraisal document on a proposed loan... to the Russian Federation for a health reform implementation project', February 20, *Report* No: 23260-RU, Human Development Sector Unit, Washington

World Bank Group (1997) *Sector Strategy, Health, Nutrition and Population*, WB, Washington

World Bank Group (2000b) 'Improving Health Care in Uganda is a private matter', *Public and Private Initiatives*, www.worldbank.org/html/extdr/hnp/health/ppi/pubpri2n.htm, accessed 28.10.00

WTO (World Trade Organisation) (2001) *GATS – fact and fiction*, February, WTO, Geneva, www.wto.org

WTO (World Trade Organisation) News (2002a) 'Director-general of WTO and chairman of WTO services negotiations reject misguided claims that public services are under threat', *Press release* Press/299 June 28, WTO, Geneva

WTO (World Trade Organisation) News (2003) 'Decision removes final patent obstacle to cheap drug imports', *Press release* Press/350 30 August WTO Geneva

WTO (World Trade Organisation) Secretariat (1998) *Background Note on Health and Social Services*, 'Restricted', Sep 18, WTO web site, Geneva www.who.dk/eprise/main/WHO/Progs/OBS/Studies/200211.htm, (23.02.03)

Wynne A (2000) 'Banking on the world's poor?' *Public Finance* Sep 22-28, p26-7

Xing L (2002) 'Shifting the burden: commodification of China's health care', *Global Social Policy* 2(3) 248-252

Yang B (2003) 'Korea's recent health financing experience: change in pharmaceutical reimbursement by economic evaluations', *Presentation for Health Care Financing Academic Exchange* December, www.hku.hk/facmed/mhrn/event/16dec2003/6.pdf, accessed 27.03.05

Yip W and Hsiao WC (2001) *Economic transition and urban health care in China: impacts and prospects*, September 12, Centre for Business and Government, Harvard, www.ksg.harvard.edu/cbg/Conferences/financal_sector/home.htm, accessed 10.07.03

Zinn C (2000) 'Australia moves to boost private health cover', *British Medical Journal* 321: 10

Zinn C (2003a) 'Australian public hospitals face only a residual role in surgery', *British Medical Journal* 327: 12

Zinn C (2003b) 'Australia proposes two tier system for paying for GP consultations', *British Medical Journal* 326: 1002

Zúniga MH (2000) 'Nicaragua: The Struggle for Health', in Bambas et al (2000)

Zuvekas SH, Banthin JS and Selden TM (1998) 'Mental health parity: what are the gaps in coverage?' *Journal of Mental Health Policy and Economics* 1: 135-146

Index